The Biology of Oligodendrocytes

Traditionally, oligodendrocytes have been considered to play a supporting role in the central nervous system and their importance has generally been overlooked. For the first time, this book provides a dedicated review of all of the major aspects of oligodendrocyte biology, including development, organization, genetics, and immunobiology. Later chapters emphasize the importance of this often overlooked cell to the mammalian central nervous system by exploring the role of its primary function, myelin synthesis and maintenance, in neural disease and repair. Particular attention is paid to multiple sclerosis, arguably the prime example of an acquired demyelinating disease, with detailed examinations of the current concepts regarding demyelination, oligodendroglial damage, and remyelination in multiple sclerosis lesions.

PATRICIA J. ARMATI is an Associate Professor of Neuroscience and Co-Director of the Nerve Research Foundation, Sydney Medical School at the University of Sydney, Australia. She has a long-standing interest in the cells of the nervous system and their relationship to disease and is editor of *The Biology of Schwann Cells* (Cambridge, 2007).

EMILY K. MATHEY is a postdoctoral scientist at the Brain and Mind Research Institute at the University of Sydney. She has a keen interest in both immunology and neurobiology with particular emphasis on pathogenic antibody responses in demyelinating disease of the peripheral and central nervous systems.

The Biology of Oligodendrocytes

Edited by

PATRICIA J. ARMATI

AND

EMILY K. MATHEY

The University of Sydney,
Australia

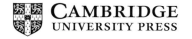

CAMBRIDGE UNIVERSITY PRESS
Cambridge, New York, Melbourne, Madrid, Cape Town, Singapore,
São Paulo, Delhi, Dubai, Tokyo, Mexico City

Cambridge University Press
The Edinburgh Building, Cambridge CB2 8RU, UK

Published in the United States of America by Cambridge University Press,
New York

www.cambridge.org
Information on this title: www.cambridge.org/9780521899659

© Cambridge University Press 2010

First published 2010

Printed in the United Kingdom at the University Press, Cambridge

A catalog record for this publication is available from the British Library

Library of Congress Cataloging-in-Publication Data
The biology of oligodendrocytes / edited by Patricia J. Armati, Emily K. Mathey.
   p. cm.
ISBN 978-0-521-89965-9 (hardback)
1. Neuroglia.   2. Myelination.   I. Armati, Patricia J.   II. Mathey, Emily
K.   III. Title.
QP363.2.B562   2010
611'.0188–dc22

                                2010033562

ISBN 978-0-521-89965-9 Hardback

This book is dedicated to Jonathon Pembroke and Jarrod Glasson.

Contents

The color plate section can be found between pages114 and 115.

Preface

For a long time neurons have blinded neuroscientists with their dazzling array of impulses and synapses. In thrall to these complex neural networks neuroscientists have often concentrated almost exclusively on neurons while the role of the macroglia – the oligodendrocytes and astrocytes – has remained in the shadows. We hope that this book will present a more integrated view of the relationship between oligodendrocytes and neurons and the critical role both cell types play in the central nervous system (CNS).

We aim to set out major aspects of the biology of the oligodendrocyte – a very large, very complex and dynamic cell – highlighting its extraordinarily unique organization and its multiple functions. For example, each oligodendrocyte can produce a plethora of up to 50 elongated paddle-like processes, each of which spirals around an internode of a different CNS axon. This spiraling process forms the compacted myelin lamellae and the associated uncompacted inner mesaxon, lateral paranodal regions and the outer mesaxons so often overlooked. The metabolic requirements and maintenance of such an elaborate organization of membranes depend on the uncompacted and compacted myelin compartments remaining in continuity. This continuity is achieved via the transverse processes and Schmidt–Lanterman incisures and ensures that vital cytoplasmic components have access to the compact myelin membranes. The orchestration of oligodendrocyte interaction with the neurons and other CNS cells is dependent on the precision of developmental processes including cell division, differentiation and migration to exact locations. Damage to this organization or an individual cell type is a major focus of medical research because of the serious consequences of any perturbation of the CNS. We thank Dr. Martin Griffiths, CUP, for his assistance, Professor John Prineas and Dr. Michael Barnett for review of Chapter 9 and all our colleagues who assisted us in the production of this book.

Contributors

Orhan Aktas M. D.
Professor, Heinrich-Heine-Universität, Department of Neurology, Moorenstrasse 5, Dusseldorf, 40225, Germany

Patricia J. Armati Ph.D.
Associate Professor, Brain and Mind Research Institute, The University of Sydney, 94 Mallett Street, Camperdown 2050, NSW Australia

Ariel Arthur Ph.D.
Clinical Neurosciences, Glasgow Biomedical Research Centre, The University of Glasgow, 120 University Place, Glasgow, G12 8TA, Scotland, UK

Udo Bartsch Ph.D.
Klinik und Poliklinik für Augenheilkunde, Universitätsklinikum Hamburg-Eppendorf, Martinistrasse 52, 20246 Hamburg, Germany

Wolfgang Brück M. D.
Department of Neuropathology, University Medical Center, Göttingen, Germany; Institute for Multiple Sclerosis Research, Hertie Foundation and University Medical Center, Göttingen, Germany

Tara M. DeSilva Ph.D.
Instructor of Neurology, Department of Neurology and The F. M. Kirby Neurobiology Center, Children's Hospital and Harvard Medical School, 300 Longwood Avenue, Boston, MA 02115, USA

Janos Groh
Section of Developmental Neurobiology, Neurologische Klinik
der Universität, Josef-Schneider-Str. 11, 97080 Würzburg,
Germany

Hans-Peter Hartung M. D.
Professor and Chair of Neurology, Heinrich-Heine-Universität,
Department of Neurology, Moorenstrasse 5, Dusseldorf, 40225,
Germany

Philip J. Horner Ph.D.
Associate Professor of Neurosurgery, University of Washington,
Institute for Stem Cell and Regenerative Medicine, Box 358056,
Seattle, WA 98195–8056, USA

Lynn D. Hudson Ph.D.
Developmental Genetics Section, Building 49, Room 5A82, 49
Convent Drive, MSC 4479, Bethesda, MD 20892–4479, USA

Grahame Kidd Ph.D.
Department of Neurosciences, Lerner Research Institute – NC30,
Cleveland Clinic, 9500 Euclid Ave, Cleveland, OH 44195, USA

David Kremer M. D.
Heinrich-Heine-Universität, Department of Neurology,
Moorenstrasse 5, Dusseldorf, 40225, Germany

Tanja Kuhlmann M. D.
Universitätsmedizin der Georg-August-Universität, Göttingen,
Abteilung Neuropathologie, Robert-Koch-Strasse 40, 37075
Göttingen, Germany

Patrick Küry Ph.D.
Heinrich-Heine-Universität, Department of Neurology,
Moorenstrasse 5, Dusseldorf, 40225, Germany

Jurate Lasiene
Department of Neurological Surgery, University of Washington,
Seattle, WA, USA

Pierre Lau Ph.D.
Section of Developmental Genetics, National Institute of
Neurological Disorders and Stroke, National Institutes of Health,
Bethesda, MD 20892, USA

Rudolf Martini Ph.D.
Professor and Chairman of the Section of Developmental
Neurobiology, Neurologische Klinik der Universität, Josef-
Schneider-Strasse 11, 97080 Würzburg, Germany

Emily K. Mathey Ph.D.
Brain and Mind Research Institute, The University of Sydney, 94
Mallet St, Camperdown, NSW 2050, Australia

Robert H. Miller Ph.D.
Professor, Department of Neurosciences, School of Medicine,
Case Western Reserve University, Cleveland, OH 44106–4975,
USA

Joseph A. Nielsen Ph.D.
Section of Developmental Genetics, National Institute of
Neurological Disorders and Stroke, National Institutes of Health,
Bethesda, MD 20892, USA

Paul A. Rosenberg M.D. Ph.D.
Senior Associate in Neurology and Associate Professor
of Neurology, Department of Neurology, Children's Hospital
and Harvard Medical School, 300 Longwood
Avenue, Boston, MA 02115, USA

Neil J. Scolding, F.R.C.P. Ph.D.
Burden Professor of Clinical Neurosciences, Institute of Clinical
Neurosciences, University of Bristol, Department of Neurology,
Frenchay Hospital, Bristol BS16 1LE, UK

Bruce D. Trapp Ph.D.
Chairman, Department of Neurosciences, Lerner Research
Institute – NC30, Cleveland Clinic, 9500 Euclid Ave, Cleveland,
OH 44195, USA

EMILY K. MATHEY, ARIEL ARTHUR
AND PATRICIA J. ARMATI

1

CNS oligarchs; the rise of the oligodendrocyte in a neuron-centric culture

If one desired to throw new light on the effect of disease, or injury, and of the process of healing in the brain, the best hope lay in the study of the non-nervous cells.

No Man Alone, Wilder Penfield, 1977 (Gill and Binder, 2007)

NEUROGLIA

For the past 160 or so years the cells of the nervous system have been divided into two main categories: neurons and glia (Kettenmann and Verkhratsky, 2008). Prior to this, ever since the first image of a neuron was published in 1836 by Gabriel Valentin, the nerve cell had been in a class of its own (Lopez-Munoz *et al.*, 2006). Some 20 years later in 1856 the term neuroglia was introduced by the German physician Rudolph Virchow. Virchow, also known as the "Pope of pathology" (Kettenmann and Ransom, 2005; Magner, 2002), described a "connective substance … in which nervous system elements are embedded" and referred to it as "nervenkitt" (or nerve putty). This description led to the use of the term "neuroglia," which derives from archaic Greek, meaning something sticky or clammy. The notion that neuroglia were there merely as neural putty was treated with the reverence usually reserved for a *bona fide* papal encyclical and as such neuroglia remained sidelined for decades to come. Even though Virchow was responsible for the term neuroglia coming into use, at this stage he did not recognize that it was made up of cells rather than an acellular connective tissue. In fact, it would be years until the cellular constituents of the neuroglia were fully defined in a drawn out, confusing and often controversial process (Somjen, 1988). At present glial cells of the central nervous system (CNS) are

The Biology of Oligodendrocytes, eds. Patricia J. Armati and Emily K. Mathey. Published by Cambridge University Press. © Cambridge University Press 2010.

divided into two major categories: macroglia and microglia. The macroglia (also known as neuroglia) are made up of oligodendrocytes, astrocytes, NG2$^+$ cells and ependymal cells. The microglia are derived from myeloid-monocytic cells and are the resident macrophages of the CNS (Tambuyzer *et al.*, 2009).

THE THIRD ELEMENT – DISCOVERY OF THE OLIGODENDROCYTE

The cell that would eventually become known as the oligodendrocyte first appeared in the literature in 1900 when it was identified by the Scottish pathologist W. Ford Robertson. Robertson described a group of small cells with few processes that he believed to be mesodermal in origin and subsequently named them mesoglia. Despite this initial description, the incognito oligodendrocyte went largely unnoticed, or at least ill-defined, for the next two decades. The eminent neuropathologists Ramón y Cajal and del Rio-Hortega spent years debating the cell's very existence and nature. In 1911 Cajal defined a group of cells distinct both from neurons and astrocytes, the only glial cell thus far described. Cajal christened this group of cells with the inscrutable name of "the third element of Cajal." It was not until 1918 that Hortega was able to differentially stain the cell types of the third element of Cajal and introduced the terms microglia and oligodendroglia (Gill and Binder, 2007). However, due to difficulty with staining oligodendrocytes Hortega's mentor Ramón y Cajal could not reproduce the staining of his protégé and denied the existence of oligodendroglia, claiming that the third element was made up solely of microglia (Gill and Binder, 2007). Owing to Cajal's influence as a founding father of neurobiology and Nobel Prize winner, this pronouncement stymied further work on the oligodendrocyte for a number of years. It was not until the neurosurgeon Wilder Penfield visited Hortega's laboratory in Madrid 1924 that the controversy surrounding this enigmatic cell was resolved. In a somewhat avant-garde research proposal for the time, Penfield raised the funds to travel to Madrid where he adapted Hortega's staining methods to confirm the initial classification of glia and resolve the technical problems in specifically staining oligodendrocytes (Penfield, 1924). Hortega reported that these cells were present in large numbers in all regions of the CNS but predominantly in the white matter and that they were frequently located near neurons, blood vessels and in series along nerve fibers. Furthermore he suggested that the membrane

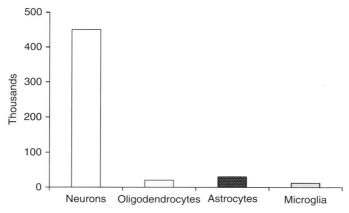

Figure 1.1 Number of publications in Pubmed after searching for each glial cell type.

around central myelinated fibers, identified by Cajal, is actually a derivative of oligodendroglia cells with functions similar to those of Schwann cells of peripheral myelinated fibers. This assertion could not be confirmed until the advent of electron microscopy in the 1960s. Hortega later went on to define perineuronal or interfascicular oligodendrocytes of four classes according to their number of processes and morphology, a classification which remains largely unchanged.

Despite the eventual acceptance of the oligodendrocyte as a distinct cell, the twentieth century was akin to the dark ages for glia. It would be a long time before any of the glia, least of all oligodendrocytes, would be acknowledged as key players in the nervous system in their own right. This can be simply illustrated by a Pubmed search using each cell type as a keyword (Figure 1.1).

MORPHOLOGY OF OLIGODENDROCYTES

Oligodendrocytes far outnumber neurons in the mammalian nervous system (Simons and Trajkovic, 2006) and their organization and structure are integral to a functional nervous system. The name oligodendrocyte, meaning "few branches," was coined at a time when methods for staining the cell were suboptimal and investigators had difficulty visualizing it in its entirety. The name oligodendrocyte is, therefore, something of a misnomer considering the number of its octopus-like processes each of which enwraps a length of axon.

In contrast to Schwann cells, the myelinating cells of the peripheral nervous system (PNS), oligodendrocytes can myelinate axonal lengths or internodes of more than one axon. During development oligodendrocyte progenitor cells (OPCs) migrate from the neural tube into what will become the white matter of the CNS, so called because of its high lipid content and therefore "fatty" or white appearance macroscopically (Simons and Trotter, 2007) (discussed further in Chapter 3). During this migration the OPCs continually extend and retract their processes in an attempt to sense other OPCs in the vicinity so that the cells become uniformly distributed (Kirby et al., 2006). This highly organized distribution of OPCs helps to ensure periodically spaced internodes along the entire length of an axon (Kirby et al., 2006), from where each adjacent internode originates and is myelinated by a different oligodendrocyte (Baumann and Pham-Dinh, 2001). The number of processes that each oligodendrocyte extends out to myelinate individual axonal internodes varies according to the area of the brain and the species of the animal. However, it has been estimated that an individual oligodendrocyte can maintain up to 60 internodal segments (Remahl and Hildebrand, 1990) obliging it to sustain a vast surface area of cell membrane. For example, an average oligodendrocyte with a somal diameter of 12 μm myelinates around 20 axonal segments, each 3 μm in diameter (Siegel et al., 1999). If each of these internodes is 500 μm long with six myelin lamellae the oligodendroglial soma maintains up to 640 times its own surface area in membrane (Siegel et al., 1999). The initiation and maintenance of these vast amounts of plasma membrane during myelination requires the extraordinary coordination of a number of cellular processes and is also discussed further in Chapter 3.

ORGANIZATION OF MYELINATED AXONS

While most references to myelin relate to the compacted, specialized plasma membranes of oligodendrocytes of the CNS or Schwann cells of the PNS, there is now an important understanding of the molecular organization of myelinated axons in regions of the membrane that remain uncompacted. As a result, myelin is now more specifically defined as: (1) compact myelin, those spirals of specialized plasma membrane and (2) non-compact myelin. The use of the term "myelin sheath" throughout the book refers to this complex of compact and non-compact myelin.

Compact myelin

Compact myelin is formed when the oligodendrocyte wraps spirals of plasma membrane around a segment of axon. The cytoplasm is extruded from between the layers so that the lipid-rich oligodendrocyte plasma membranes fuse together. This compaction of the oligodendroglial membrane creates the distinctive, lined, appearance of myelin when viewed by transmission electron microscopy. This lined appearance is the result of the apposing extracellular surfaces of the plasma membrane compacting to form the intraperiod line, while the cytoplasmic surfaces form the major dense line. Myelination of an axon allows the action potential to travel up to 100 times faster than it would along a smaller unmyelinated axon: 430 km/h compared to 3.6 km/h (Karadottir and Attwell, 2007). This specialized compact myelin alone makes the oligodendrocyte indispensible for normal CNS function including all motor, sensory and higher functions of the brain (Nave, 2008). The mechanisms of myelination resulting in the spiraling lamellae of the compact myelin and the signals that regulate this complex process are discussed in greater detail throughout the book.

Non-compact myelin

Although the term myelin is usually used in reference to regions of compact myelin, some of the oligodendrocyte plasma membrane remains uncompacted – the non-compact myelin. This arrangement is better visualized by a conceptual unwrapping of the oligodendrocyte (Figure 1.2). If the myelin were unraveled and stretched out it would be a flat, trapezoid sheet of compacted plasma membrane lined by a tube of cytoplasm. This tube of cytoplasm contains the usual cell organelles and cytoskeletal components and is known as the non-compact myelin. When each trapezoid process is rolled around an axonal length, the non-compact myelin rim forms loops by attaching to the lateral extremities of the myelinated internode. These regions of non-compacted cytoplasm are called the paranodal loops and have a crucial relationship with the axon, forming the axo–glial junction – the largest of all mammalian adhesion complexes (Brophy, 2001). The process of myelination directs the polarization of both the oligodendrocyte and the axon to form distinct domains at the axo–glial junction; the paranode and the adjacent juxtaparanode,

(a)

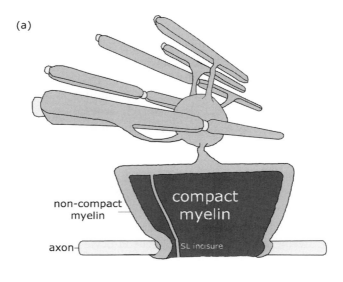

non-compact myelin

compact myelin

axon

SL incisure

(b)

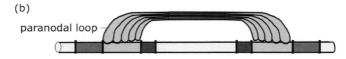

paranodal loop

(c)

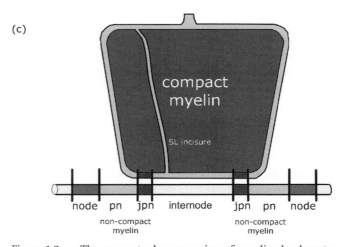

compact myelin

SL incisure

node   pn   jpn   internode   jpn   pn   node

non-compact myelin   non-compact myelin

Figure 1.2a–c The conceptual unwrapping of an oligodendrocyte process reveals the regions of the cell that are made up of compact and non-compact myelin. (a) If the myelin were unraveled and stretched out it would be a flat, trapezoid sheet of plasma membrane with its uncompacted and compacted regions. Occasionally there are also each with different and very specific structural and molecular characteristics. Whether oligodendrocytes also contain channels of uncompacted myelin analogous to the transverse processes and Schmidt–Lanterman incisures of the PNS Schwann cell is somewhat controversial (Ghabriel and Allt, 1981). These regions of non-compact myelin are continuous with the paranodal region and traverse the compacted myelin lamellae – the transverse processes running parallel to the axon and the Schmidt–Lanterman incisures running through the spirals of compact myelin. However, Schmidt–Lanterman incisures, although rare in the CNS, can be frequently seen in large fibers where the axon is at least 2 μm in diameter and whose myelin is at least 0.5 μm thick (Blakemore, 1969). It has been suggested that these regions play a role in the maintenance and metabolism of myelin by allowing the exchange of compounds between the membranous and cytoplasmic compartments of the oligodendrocyte. Further analysis of their function and frequency has been hindered by the lack of specific markers available for their identification in the CNS (Trapp and Kidd, 2004). Nonetheless, domains of non-compact myelin are now recognized as critically important in dissecting disease mechanisms affecting both oligodendrocytes and Schwann cells and are discussed further in Chapter 2. The contributions to saltatory conduction made by compact myelin as an insulator and by non-compact myelin as a diffusion barrier to ion channels vastly increase the speed of nerve conduction such that the acquisition of myelin by vertebrates some 425 million years ago made a significant impact on the course of evolutionary history.

Caption for Figure 1.2 (cont.)
longitudinal channels within the compacted region containing cytoplasm, Schmidt–Lanterman (SL) incisures, that course through the spirally compact myelin. (b) When each trapezoid process is spiraled around an axonal length, the innermost non-compact myelin rim forms the paranode at each end of the myelinated internode and in contact with the axon. (c) These regions of non-compact myelin organize the oligodendrocyte/axon complex into distinct molecular and functional domains vital for saltatory conduction, known as the node of Ranvier, the paranode (pn), juxtaparanode (jpn) and internode and are discussed further in Chapters 2 and 4. Adapted from (Salzer, 2003). See color plate section for color version of this figure.

EVOLUTION OF MYELINATION: MYELIN MAKES
THE WORLD GO AROUND

Animals have developed two different strategies in an attempt to increase the speed of nerve conduction – a distinct evolutionary advantage. The first, and the more primitive, is to send neuronal signals using large or even giant axons (Hartline and Colman, 2007). By increasing the diameter of the axon small invertebrates have been able to acquire an increased conduction velocity. However, this strategy is only effective for relatively small animals ranging from 0.1 to 30 cm in size (Zalc, 2006). The second strategy is to increase conduction velocity by insulating the axons with a myelin or myelin-like covering. Ensheathing neuroglial cells form intimate associations with neurons in all animals except for two phyla, the Ctenophora and the Cnidaria, which include jellyfish, anemone and corals (Schweigreiter et al., 2006). The glial cell–axon pairing is seen in invertebrates ranging from the nematode to the echinoderms (Hartline and Colman, 2007) but only some of these organisms elaborate a myelin-like covering. Indeed, the invertebrates generate an assortment of multilayered glial membranes that act as rudimentary forms of myelin. These structures range from loosely wound to tightly packed membranes ensheathing axons in either a spiral or a concentric arrangement (Schweigreiter et al., 2006). An example of concentric layering of the glial membrane is seen in the copepods, small ocean crustaceans, and is an adaptation that gives these creatures a distinct evolutionary advantage (Davis et al., 1999; Zalc et al., 2008). Myelin allows copepods to move up to 200 body lengths in milliseconds (Davis et al., 1999) providing them with the acceleration needed to escape predators in dangerous ocean environments. This non-compact myelin in invertebrates is sufficient for the needs of small creatures but not for larger vertebrates. In contrast to the diverse myelin organization seen in invertebrates, vertebrate myelin structure is highly conserved from the most ancient myelin present in sharks through to that in humans (Hartline and Colman, 2007). In evolutionary terms, increased conduction velocity bestowed by myelination allows rapid responses, in the sense not only of making a quick getaway in the avoidance of predation but also in attacking prey. The requirement for rapid and more efficient nerve conduction may be related to increasing complexity within the vertebrate CNS. Owing to the restrictions on brain size imposed by the skull, individual oligodendrocytes gained the ability to myelinate multiple axonal lengths, which provided a mechanism by which neuronal numbers could increase without a concomitant increase in oligodendrocyte cell number. This process allowed the brain to increase its complexity with minimal volume increase, enabling a greater capacity for information processing, response to stimuli and more efficient feedback loops (Hartline and Colman, 2007). In this way the acquisition of myelin made vertebrates faster and smarter, setting them on the path to becoming highly evolved. However, hand in hand with this increased complexity comes the potential for dysfunction and the resultant pathological consequences.

OLIGODENDROCYTES MOVE TO THE FORE IN GRAY MATTER DISEASES

Oligodendrocyte involvement in psychiatric disorders

For decades neuroscientists have paid negligible attention to how the study of white matter could contribute to answering the big questions in learning, memory and psychiatric disorders. Instead intense focus was directed towards the inner workings of neurons and their transmission. However, it is apparent that the role of the non-neuronal cells of the CNS in both health and disease has been significantly underrated. As will be discussed throughout this book, study of the "non-nervous" cells of the brain is providing important new leads in the quest for both causes and treatments of neurological diseases. Rapid advances in the understanding of the complexity of the glia/neuron relationship are challenging traditional views. The oligodendrocyte is no longer regarded as an inert axonal comfort blanket but is emerging as a dynamic player in brain function. This paradigm shift is particularly evident with regard to neurodegenerative, psychiatric and mood disorders and pain (Watkins *et al.* 2005) where it once would have been heretical to suggest that oligodendrocytes play an important role. While oligodendrocyte pathology has long been recognized in diseases such as multiple sclerosis where the breakdown of compact myelin is obvious histopathologically, powerful laboratory techniques are now able to define more subtle changes/abnormalities in oligodendrocyte function or specific attack and damage (Antony *et al.*, 2004; Barnett and Prineas, 2004). The use of unbiased genomic and proteomic screening to identify genes or proteins associated with neurodegenerative and psychiatric disorders has revealed unexpected associations with oligodendrocyte and myelin genes. This shift can be exemplified by the spate of reports detailing the dysregulation of myelin-related genes in schizophrenia (Hakak *et al.*, 2001; Karoutzou *et al.*, 2008; Roy *et al.*, 2007; Sugai *et al.*, 2004; Tkachev *et al.*, 2003), bipolar disorder (Adler *et al.*, 2006; Kato *et al.*, 2007) and other psychiatric disorders.

Even mechanisms typically associated with neuronal dysfunction such as deregulation of dopaminergic signaling can be influenced by the oligodendrocyte (Roy *et al.*, 2007). For example, neuregulin-1 (NRG1) and its receptor erb4 are vital for brain development and have previously been genetically linked to schizophrenia (Mei and Xiong, 2008; Stefansson *et al.*, 2002). Although the NRG pathway is important for the development and function of neurons, astrocytes and oligodendrocytes the selective blocking of erb signaling exclusively in oligodendrocytes has significant effects on not only oligodendrocytes but also neuronal functioning (Roy *et al.*, 2007). In transgenic mice, selective blockade of erb signaling in oligodendrocytes resulted in irregularities in oligodendroglial structure such as fewer myelin lamellae ("thinner myelin") as well as changes in neuronal dendritic arborization. Although oligodendrocyte abnormalities could have been predicted, the targeted oligodendroglial disruption of erb signaling also resulted in an unexpected dysregulation of the dopaminergic system. In fact, inactivation of erb4b in oligodendrocytes interfered with dopaminergic neurotransmission to such an extent that behavior was affected in a manner relevant to psychiatric disorders: increased anxiety, enhanced sensitization to amphetamine and hypoactivity (Roy *et al.*, 2007). Such symptoms as these would traditionally have been ascribed to dysfunction of neural transmission; however, in this case they can be directly attributed to oligodendrocyte pathology. This example highlights the often subtle but critical role the oligodendrocyte plays in total brain function.

Perturbation of oligodendrocyte function in transgenic models

Improved technologies have not only been paramount in dissecting the role of oligodendrocytes in disease states but have also exposed previously unknown functions in the normal CNS. Transgenic mouse models for example have become useful in highlighting the importance of oligodendrocyte–axon interaction in the healthy CNS where maintenance of the complex oligodendrocyte myelin architecture – both compact and non-compact – is essential for axonal integrity throughout white matter tracts. Even small perturbations to metabolic processes in oligodendrocytes can have a major impact on both axonal function and survival (Kassmann et al., 2007). This is clearly illustrated by a mouse model in which axons were damaged after the inactivation of oligodendrocyte peroxisomes exclusively (Kassmann et al., 2007). Peroxisomes are membrane-enclosed organelles that are involved in numerous aspects of metabolism including oxidation of fatty acids and detoxification of the resulting hydrogen peroxide (H_2O_2). Although the inactivation of oligodendroglial peroxisomes had no immediate effect on the oligodendrocytes themselves, over the course of some months mice began to exhibit signs of axonal dysfunction such as ataxia and limb weakness. These clinical signs were due to axonal loss and preceded any demyelination – a secondary change. The inactivated peroxisomes had no impact on the survival of the oligodendrocytes themselves (Kassmann et al., 2007). Studies such as these definitively show that oligodendrocytes and their myelin not only facilitate axonal conduction but have an interdependent relationship with the axons they ensheathe. Furthermore, this interdependency can be genetically uncoupled from the process of myelination – previously thought to be the "main function" of the oligodendrocyte (Lappe-Siefke et al., 2003). Transgenic mice deficient in *Cnp1*, a gene coding for the minor myelin protein 2′,3′-cyclic nucleotide phosphodiesterase (Cnp), survive to adulthood and develop normal myelin that is biochemically and morphologically indistinct from wild-type myelin. However, by four months the mice develop drastic and rapidly progressing clinical symptoms including ataxia, hind limb weakness, convulsions and gait abnormalities that result in the death of the majority of the mice within one year (Lappe-Siefke et al., 2003). The reason for this sudden onset of neurological dysfunction is the degeneration of myelinated axons whose myelin remains fully intact and functional throughout the process. This uncoupling of myelination from other less recognized functions of oligodendrocytes now has important implications for neurodegenerative disease. Previously without histological or biochemical defect in the compact myelin the oligodendrocyte was dismissed from any involvement in neurodegeneration. The realization that an abnormality in a minor myelin protein such as Cnp can cause such profound neurodegeneration should now put oligodendrocytes under intense scrutiny.

Myelin model of the human brain

At the other end of the spectrum there are researchers for whom the involvement of oligodendrocytes and their myelin in disease, cognition and behavior is far from unexpected. In the same way that most theories have been neurocentric there are now proponents of a "myelin model" of the human brain (Bartzokis, 2007). According to this model the smooth operation of compact myelin over a human lifetime is the single most important determinant for establishing and sustaining cognition and behavior (Bartzokis, 2007). In fact, two of the distinguishing features of the human brain in comparison with other animals are its high proportion of "white matter" (Fields, 2008c) and continuation of myelination until the age of 50 (Bartzokis, 2005). Although myelination is a developmental process it continues throughout the ordinary lifespan of a human during which myelination of specific brain regions coincides with the acquisition of particular cognitive functions (Nagy *et al.*, 2004) such as reading, speaking (Pujol *et al.*, 2006) and executive decision-making (Fields, 2008b). For example, the frontal lobes, areas of the brain heavily involved in reasoning and judgment, are not completely myelinated until between 25 and 30 years of age (Fields, 2005, 2008c). Conversely, the age-related decline in myelination that begins at around 50 years of age has also been implicated in cognitive decline beginning at this time (Bartzokis *et al.*, 2006).

The myelin model also attributes the learning of complex skills such as piano playing, juggling (Scholz *et al.*, 2009) or perfecting a golf swing to experience-driven myelination of the neuronal circuits involved in performing the activity (Fields, 2008c; Ishibashi *et al.*, 2006; Markham and Greenough, 2004). When the new skill is first practiced, electrical activity in the associated neurons leads to myelination of those neuronal tracts involved with the learning of the skill (Bengtsson *et al.*, 2005). This effect can be seen in concert pianists in whom studies with diffusion tensor imaging show extensive white matter plasticity, particularly if their training began when the fiber tracts involved were still maturing (Bengtsson *et al.*, 2005).

Although this model may seem like a crackpot theory from glial cell fundamentalists it is no more than that claimed on behalf of neurons for over 100 years. Although the interdependent relationship between oligodendrocytes and axons remains far from being completely understood, the idea that it is of critical importance to neurological and psychiatric health, learning and cognition is gaining ever increasing credibility.

NG2⁺ OLIGODENDROCYTE PROGENITOR CELLS
GO WHERE NO GLIAL CELL HAS GONE BEFORE

Classification of NG2⁺ cells

The mantle of housekeeper was assigned to CNS glia based on the dogma that they did not form synapses, were unable to generate action potentials and were thus not involved in information transfer within the nervous system. Although synapses were originally described as "a nexus between neurone and neurone" (Burke, 2007) recent data reveal that a synapse can also be a connection between neurons and glia. One of the most interesting cells able to form synapses with neurons is the NG2⁺ oligodendrocyte progenitor cell (Figure 1.3).

The function and classification of NG2⁺ cells remains somewhat controversial with various proposals that they should be given their

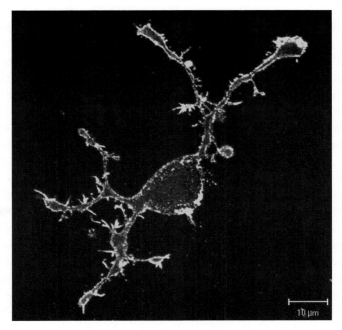

Figure 1.3 Rat OPC stained with rabbit anti-NG2 and Alexafluor 568 nm. See color plate section for color version of this figure.

own categorization. Although NG2$^+$ cells are commonly equated with oligodendrocyte progenitor cells it has been suggested that they are a fourth, distinct, type of glial cell and should be given a separate nomenclature and be christened synantocyte (Butt *et al.*, 2002), polydendrocyte (Nishiyama *et al.*, 2002) or the fifth element (Butt *et al.*, 2005). While some NG2$^+$ glia cells differentiate into myelinating oligodendrocytes during development or after episodes of demyelination, as discussed in Chapters 3, 7, 8 and 9, there is also some controversial evidence that others differentiate into gray matter astrocytes (Zhu *et al.*, 2008) and neurons (Nishiyama *et al.*, 2009). The remaining NG2$^+$ cells survive into adulthood making up 5% of CNS cells (Dawson *et al.*, 2000, 2003; Zhu *et al.*, 2008). Despite differences in nomenclature NG2$^+$ cells have been instrumental in changing the perception of the glial cell since 2000.

NG2$^+$ cells communicate with neurons

Recent data have provided overwhelming evidence that NG2$^+$ cells communicate with surrounding neurons through rapid direct signaling via glial–neuronal synapses (Nishiyama *et al.*, 2009). NG2$^+$ cells extend processes both to synapses and nodes of Ranvier implying that they may monitor or influence neuronal activity. NG2$^+$ cells have also been shown to receive both excitatory and inhibitory input from neurons in gray (Bergles *et al.*, 2000; Lin and Bergles, 2004) and white (Kukley *et al.*, 2007; Ziskin *et al.*, 2007) matter as a normal part of CNS physiology. Not only do NG2$^+$ cells make synapses with neurons but the manner in which they do so is unique and distinct from neurons. NG2$^+$ cells are born with synapses (Kukley *et al.*, 2008); quite remarkably, parent NG2$^+$ cells maintain contact with presynaptic neurons during cell division and pass on this connectivity to their daughter cells (Ge *et al.*, 2009; Kukley *et al.*, 2008). Contrary to the general consensus that cells only differentiate after mitosis, recent work has shown that NG2$^+$ cells can divide while maintaining complex features of differentiation such as morphology, active glutamatergic and GABAergic synaptic responses and the capacity to continue receiving excitatory and inhibitory inputs (Ge *et al.*, 2009). The purpose of this innate interconnectivity is still undefined but it has been suggested that it allows the NG2$^+$ cells to migrate and multiply while still being wired into the surrounding networks (Gallo *et al.*, 2008; Kukley *et al.*, 2008).

NG2$^+$ cells can spike

Having already gained territory on several neuronal functions, NG2$^+$ cells have now laid down their trump card and stolen the last bastion of neuronal exclusivity: neurons are no longer the only cell that can spike (Karadottir *et al.*, 2008). A subclass of the NG2$^+$ OPC, half of those in the rat cerebellum, expresses voltage-gated sodium channels enabling the generation of action potentials (Karadottir *et al.*, 2008). The NG2$^+$ cell action potentials are generated spontaneously or in response to depolarization in the same manner as neuronal action potentials: inward sodium current and voltage-gated outward potassium current. Spiking and non-spiking classes of NG2$^+$ cells have a similar morphology with comparable soma size, number and size of processes, suggesting that they are at equivalent developmental stages (Karadottir *et al.*, 2008). The other important difference between spiking and non-spiking classes of NG2$^+$ cells is their susceptibility to excitotoxicity (Karadottir *et al.*, 2008). Due to the higher level of glutamate- and NMDA-evoked current, spiking NG2$^+$ cells have an increased risk of damage after ischemic injury in the white matter as seen in stroke, spinal cord injury or periventricular leukomalacia (PVL).

Such a revolutionary discovery undoubtedly brings with it considerably more unanswered questions and a flurry of further investigation. The first and perhaps most difficult question to arise from these studies is "What is the function of NG2$^+$ cell signaling?" Although a number of physiological functions have been postulated, none has been confirmed. Direct communication between glia and neurons provides a means for the activity-dependent regulation of a number of cellular processes including glial proliferation and differentiation (Lin and Bergles, 2004; Ziskin *et al.*, 2007). The ability of OPCs to receive electrical signals could enable them to selectively myelinate active axons and in doing so influence development and plasticity in white matter based on activity and experience (Fields, 2008a).

This newly defined ability of OPCs to generate trains of action potentials, previously the defining property of neurons, has blurred the previously inflexible boundaries between neurons and glia. Further research on these synapses will no doubt have clinical implications in a number of developmental and pathological oligodendrocyte disorders. NG2$^+$ OPCs should revolutionize the way scientists think about glial cells and it is hoped that these cells will no longer be pigeon-holed according to traditional paradigms of what it is to be glial or neuronal.

OLIGODENDROCYTES UNDER ATTACK – SITTING
DUCKS OR RAGING BULLS?

Oligodendrocytes have the capacity to defend themselves

Although oligodendrocytes are susceptible to a variety of toxic mediators (See Chapters 7,8,9,10) they are often portrayed as completely vulnerable, sensitive cells that hoist the white flag at the first sign of trouble, surrendering to all comers without the slightest regard for self preservation. However, new data reveal that oligodendrocytes may not be as defenseless as they first appear and may influence their surrounding environment in an attempt at self defense. Microarray and immunohistochemical studies in normal-appearing white matter (NAWM) of multiple sclerosis (MS) patients show that the anti-inflammatory response aimed at protecting the NAWM from damage is mounted predominately by oligodendrocytes (Zeis *et al.*, 2008a). Oligodendrocytes in the NAWM of MS patients upregulate components of the anti-inflammatory STAT6 signaling pathway and express HIF-1α, the master regulator of hypoxia-induced gene regulation. HIF-1α promotes cell survival by regulating the expression of numerous downstream genes after a sublethal injury (Sharp and Bernaudin, 2004). HIF-1α upregulation has also been described predominately in oligodendrocytes in Baló's concentric sclerosis lesions (Stadelmann *et al.*, 2005). Baló's type of lesions are large concentric lesions consisting of alternating layers of normal and damaged compact myelin with the macroscopic appearance of a sliced onion. Intriguingly, HIF-1α is present at the edge of the lesion as well as in the layers of preserved compact myelin suggesting that there is an oligodendrocyte-driven defense mechanism against noxious substances released in adjacent areas of active demyelination (Stadelmann *et al.*, 2005). Complex analyses such as microarray studies are beginning to unearth the finer subtleties of the oligodendrocyte response under a variety of conditions so that the oligodendrocyte's response to injury could be targeted during therapy to augment endogenous protective mechanisms.

Oligodendrocytes secrete soluble mediators

Astrocytes have long been considered the major source of secreted neurotrophic factors that influence neuronal growth and survival.

However, oligodendrocytes have also been shown to secrete a number of neurotrophic growth factors in culture and in vivo (Dai *et al.*, 2003). Neurotrophic factors have a diverse range of actions that affect a variety of neuronal characteristics such as axonal and dendritic growth, synaptic plasticity and long-term potentiation. The suite of growth factors produced by oligodendrocytes includes brain-derived neurotrophic factor (BDNF), nerve growth factor (NGF) (Byravan *et al.*, 1994), glial-derived neurotrophic factor (GDNF) (Wilkins *et al.*, 2003) and insulin-like growth factor 1 (IGF-1) (Wilkins *et al.*, 2001). Neurotrophic growth factors are often upregulated during injury and have the potential not only to provide survival and development signals for surrounding neurons but also to act as autocrine growth factors for oligodendrocytes, and interestingly some cells of the immune system.

There is growing interest in the interplay between CNS and the immune system – the two key adaptive systems in the body. Although immune surveillance does occur normally within the CNS, there is an increase in inflammatory cell infiltration of the CNS during a range of neurological disorders and the secretion of a host of soluble mediators. While most research has focused on the detrimental effects of infiltrating inflammatory cells (see Chapter 7) new data suggest that inflammatory cells may also play a role in neuroprotection and that there is significant cross-talk between inflammatory cells and the cells of the CNS. Bi-directional communication between these seemingly disparate systems is made possible by the overlapping production of cytokines, chemokines and neurotrophins in both the immune system and the nervous system. For example, NGF was discovered as a neurotrophin and described for its role in neuronal development and survival. However, unexpectedly NGF is also produced in the immune system where it acts as a survival factor for memory B cells (Torcia *et al.*, 1996) and can influence cytokine production by T cells (Villoslada *et al.*, 2000). This raises the intriguing possibility that oligodendrocytes can influence not only neurons but also infiltrating immune cells, which could affect the outcome of inflammatory episodes in CNS diseases (see Chapter 7). The realization that nervous system cells and immune system cells can interact in this manner has put researchers in a quandary – as neuroinflammation can be protective as well as destructive and may be a process actively courted by the CNS in some instances. This delicate balance is of critical importance in a number of neurological diseases and further understanding of how it is regulated may give rise to treatments that target the equilibrium between protective and destructive neuroimmune interactions (Kerschensteiner *et al.*, 2009).

WRAP UP

The work described in this book brings to the fore the progress made in recognizing the oligodendrocyte as an important and often overlooked player in both healthy and diseased CNS. However, many pertinent questions remain unanswered. What determines the association between the individual oligodendrocyte and those axonal lengths it enseathes? While the dogma states that neurons are for the most part post-mitotic, what about myelin-forming cells? Are they turned over during a lifetime? Are they subject to programmed cell death? Do the cells undergo apoptosis? As for Schwann cells of the PNS this is not really understood. Far from being sidelined as merely a myelinator the oligodendrocyte is now recognized as an important contributor to the maintenance of a functioning relationship between all cell types in the CNS. It is now well established that contributions of both nerve and glial cells are thoroughly integrated, mutually dependent and essential. It is unlikely that there will be a complete reversal in the ranking of CNS cells where an oligarchy rules supreme; nevertheless, we are now at a stage where oligodendrocytes are no longer only there to fill in the gaps between neurons.

RUDOLF MARTINI, JANOS GROH
AND UDO BARTSCH

2

Comparative biology of Schwann cells and oligodendrocytes

INTRODUCTION

Myelin in the peripheral nervous system (PNS) and central nervous system (CNS) is formed by Schwann cells and oligodendrocytes respectively. The myelin formed by the two glial cell types electrically insulates the axons and restricts the generation of action potentials to the nodes of Ranvier, myelin-free regions separating the myelin segments, allowing for rapid propagation of action potentials along the axons. While there are striking overall similarities in the mechanisms of myelination and the structure and molecular composition of PNS and CNS myelin, there are also important differences between the two glial cell types. For instance, Schwann cells elaborate a single myelin segment around a single axon, while oligodendrocytes may myelinate up to 60 different axons (Figure 2.1). Furthermore, Schwann cells – but not oligodendrocytes – are surrounded by a basal lamina that is continuous with the adjacent internode. In addition, nodes of Ranvier in the PNS are covered by Schwann cell processes, while axons at CNS nodes are bare. A characteristic feature of CNS myelin not present in PNS myelin is the so-called radial component, interlamellar claudin-11-positive strands spanning the myelin. There is also a slight difference in the periodicity of mature compact CNS and PNS myelin, and important differences in the molecular composition of CNS and PNS myelin. For instance, proteolipid protein (PLP) is the major myelin protein in the CNS, while P0 and peripheral myelin protein 22 (PMP22) are exclusively found in PNS myelin. Finally, Schwann cells and oligodendrocytes serve fundamentally different functions in the lesioned nervous system, with Schwann cells fostering and oligodendrocytes limiting long-distance regeneration of injured axons (see Table 2.1 for comparisons).

The Biology of Oligodendrocytes, eds. Patricia J. Armati and Emily K. Mathey. Published by
Cambridge University Press. © Cambridge University Press 2010.

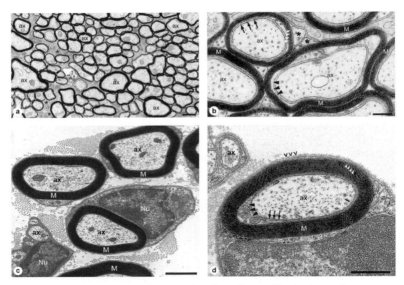

Figure 2.1 Electron micrographs of myelin profiles in the optic nerve
(CNS: a, b) and femoral quadriceps nerve (PNS: c, d) of adult mice. In the
optic nerve, axons are surrounded by oligodendrocytic myelin (a, b),
whereas in the peripheral nerve, larger caliber axons are ensheathed by
Schwann cell myelin (c, d). Note the presence and absence of basal lamina
(empty arrowheads in d) around Schwann cells and oligodendrocytes,
respectively, as one major difference between the two myelinating glial
cell types. Additionally, myelinating Schwann cells always attach to one
single axon (c, d) whereas an oligodendrocyte may myelinate multiple
axons. However, the innermost cytoplasmic aspects of the myelinating
glial cells (black arrowheads in b, d) and the relatively wide periaxonal
space (arrows in b, d) are similarly organized in both glial cell types.
Asterisks in (a), unmyelinated axons; asterisks in (b), external tongue
processes. ax, axon; M, myelin; Nu, Schwann cell nucleus. White
arrowheads in (b) and (d), major dense lines. Bar in (a) and (c): 1 μm; in (b):
0.2 μm; in (d): 0.5μm (a and b reproduced from Bartsch, 2003).

DEVELOPMENT OF OLIGODENDROCYTES

Origin and specification of oligodendrocytes

Oligodendrocyte progenitor cells are highly motile cells that populate all
regions of the CNS where they continue to proliferate in response to
locally expressed mitogens to finally differentiate into mature myelin-
forming oligodendrocytes (Baumann and Pham-Dinh, 2001; Miller,
2002). Although oligodendrocytes are widely distributed throughout

Table 2.1 *Comparison between some features typical for oligodendrocytes and Schwann cells*

	Oligodendrocytes	Myelinating Schwann cells
Morphology	Myelinate mostly multiple axons	Myelinate single axons
	No basal lamina	Basal lamina
	No nodal microvilli (NG2-positive perinodal cells)	Nodal microvilli
	Compact myelin spacing approx. 10–12 nm	Compact myelin spacing approx. 12–15 nm
	Radial claudin-11-positive structures in compact myelin	No radial structures
Origin	Neural tube, multiple domains	Neural crest, neural crest-derived capping cells
Role of neuregulins	React on overexpression of Nrg type I and III with increased myelin thickness	React on overexpression of Nrg type III with increased myelin thickness
	Role during development debated	Nrg type III mediates SCP survival, initiation of myelination and determination of myelin thickness
Contribution to Na^+ channel clustering at nodes	Na^+ channel clustering modulated by (unknown) oligodendrocytic secretion products	Schwann cell microvilli cluster Na^+ channels via gliomedins and nodal CAMs
Myelin molecules	PLP/DM20, MBP, MAG, Nogo, OMgp	P0, PMP22, (PLP/DM20), MBP, MAG
Role during neural damage	Long-time presence of myelin after injury, expression of neurite growth inhibitors Nogo, MAG and OMgp	Rapid destruction of myelin after injury, no expression of neurite growth inhibitors Nogo and OMgp, low expression levels of MAG
	No substantial expression of nerve growth promoting factors	Expression/upregulation of nerve growth promoting factors

CAM, cell adhesion molecule; MAG, myelin-associated glycoprotein; MBP, myelin basic protein; PLP, proteolipid protein; PMP22, peripheral myelin protein 22; SCP, Schwann cell precursors.

the spinal cord and brain, it was generally assumed that spinal cord oligodendrocytes are produced from a singular ventrally located oligodendrocytic domain (for reviews, see Richardson *et al.*, 2006; Rowitch, 2004). However, there was also evidence from in vivo and in culture studies for a dorsal origin (e.g. Cameron-Curry and Le Douarin, 1995; Gregori *et al.*, 2002; Spassky *et al.*, 1998). Recent studies have now provided convincing evidence for multiple ventral as well as dorsal origins of these glial cells in the developing spinal cord and also in more rostral regions of the neural tube, with the ventrally derived cells being produced slightly earlier during development than the dorsally derived cells (Cai *et al.*, 2005; Fogarty *et al.*, 2005; Kessaris *et al.*, 2006; Vallstedt *et al.*, 2005).

The first oligodendrocytes in the spinal cord are generated from the motor neuron progenitor (pMN) domain, a restricted domain of the ventral ventricular zone that sequentially produces first motor neurons and subsequently oligodendrocyte progenitor cells (Lu *et al.*, 2002; Takebayashi *et al.*, 2002; Zhou and Anderson, 2002). Induction of oligodendrocytes in the pMN domain is dependent on sonic hedgehog (Shh) secreted from the notochord and floor plate (e.g. Orentas *et al.*, 1999; Pringle *et al.*, 1996). Shh induces expression of the basic helix-loop-helix transcription factors Olig1 and Olig2, with Olig2 being essential for the specification of both motor neurons and oligodendrocytes in this domain (Lu *et al.*, 2002; Takebayashi *et al.*, 2002; Zhou and Anderson, 2002). Expression of Olig2 in the pMN domain of mutant mice deficient in the homeodomain transcription factors Nkx6.1 and Nkx6.2 is compromised, and the dorsalized cord of Shh null mutants lacks a pMN domain. As a result, production of oligodendrocyte progenitor cells in the ventral cord of both mutant mouse lines is abolished. The absence of ventrally derived oligodendrocyte progenitor cells unmasked a second wave of oligodendrogenesis in the dorsal spinal cord, starting approximately two days later than the ventral oligodendrogenesis in the pMN domain. The dorsally derived oligodendrocyte progenitors, characterized by expression of Olig2, platelet-growth factor receptor α (PDGFRα), SOX10 or NG2, transiently expressed the dorsal progenitor marker Pax7, Mash1 or Gsh1/2, confirming their dorsal identity (Cai *et al.*, 2005; Vallstedt *et al.*, 2005). Cre-lox fate mapping experiments also demonstrated oligodendrogenesis in the dorsal spinal cord and additionally provided evidence that dorsally derived oligodendrocytes develop by direct transformation of radial glia (Fogarty *et al.*, 2005). While generation of ventrally derived oligodendrocytes requires Shh signaling, specification of their dorsally derived counterparts appears to be independent of Shh, demonstrating diversity in the molecular mechanisms that specify oligodendrocytes. Cre-lox fate mapping experiments suggest that oligodendrocytes in the mouse forebrain are also generated in a ventral-to-dorsal sequence, originating first in the medial ganglionic eminence and anterior entopeduncular area, then in the lateral and/or caudal ganglionic eminences and finally within the postnatal cortex (Kessaris *et al.*, 2006). The reasons for the existence of multiple sources of oligodendrocytes and differences in the molecular control of their production in the developing CNS are currently unknown but it is intriguing to speculate that this developmental diversity might correlate with functional differences between the different oligodendrocyte populations (Miller, 2005; Richardson *et al.*, 2006).

Once specified to the oligodendrocyte lineage, the differentiation of oligodendrocyte progenitor cells into myelin-forming oligodendrocytes progresses through various developmental stages that are characterized by the sequential expression of specific developmental markers, typical cellular morphologies, differences in the migratory potential, mitotic activity and the growth factors involved (Miller, 2002; Pfeiffer *et al.*, 1993). Immature oligodendrocyte precursor cells are proliferative and highly migratory cells with a bipolar morphology that express gangliosides recognized by the anti-GD3 and A2B5 antibodies. Based on the capability of these cells to give rise to oligodendrocytes and a subpopulation of cultured astrocytes (type-2 astrocytes), they have been termed oligodendrocyte-type-2 astrocyte (O-2A) progenitor cells (Raff, 1989). O-2A progenitor cells differentiate into still proliferative but less motile and multiprocessed cells, termed pro–oligodendrocytes, that are characterized by the expression of the O4 antigen. Loss of A2B5 positivity and emergence of galactocerebroside recognized by the O1 antibody and of 2′, 3′-cyclic nucleotide 3′-phosphodiesterase (CNP) are indicative for immature oligodendrocytes. Finally, cells terminally differentiate into oligodendrocytes that express myelin proteins such as myelin basic protein (MBP), proteolipid protein (PLP) or myelin-associated glycoprotein (MAG) and elaborate myelin around axons (Pfeiffer *et al.*, 1993).

DEVELOPMENT OF SCHWANN CELLS

Origin and specification of Schwann cells

Recent years have also seen a substantial growth in our knowledge with regard to the origin and differentiation of Schwann cells. It is well established that Schwann cells generally originate from the neural crest (Le Douarin and Smith, 1988). Three basic streams of migratory neural crests cells have been identified in the vertebrate embryo, comprising a lateral-superficial one giving rise to dermal melanocytes, a ventral one giving rise to chromaffin cells, autonomic neurons and their associated glial cells, and a ventrolateral one giving rise to dorsal root ganglion neurons and Schwann cells. The now well established developmental stages of Schwann cells, such as Schwann cell precursors, immature Schwann cells, mature myelinating and mature non-myelinating Schwann cells, have been extensively characterized with regard to their phenotypic profiles and the factors controlling survival and differentiation (Jessen and Mirsky, 2005a, 2005b). A basic prerequisite for neural crest survival is contact with the extracellular matrix (ECM) even in the presence of basic glial survival and differentiation factors, such as neuregulin-1 (NRG1) (Jessen and Mirsky, 2005a; Woodhoo and Sommer, 2008). However, it is not well understood which factors are responsible for neural crest cells adopting a glial phenotype (Jessen and Mirsky, 2005a; Woodhoo and Sommer, 2008). An important prerequisite is the presence of the homeobox gene sox10, as the corresponding knockout mouse embryos lack Schwann cell precursors (Gilmour *et al.*, 2002). The most challenging mechanism contributing to this scenario is that SOX10 might regulate expression of the ErbB3 receptor of the survival factor NRG1 (Woodhoo and Sommer, 2008). Bone morphogenetic proteins, by contrast, appear to inhibit the differentiation pathway leading to glial development (Jessen and Mirsky, 2005a).

Some novel details have been recently described for the origin of Schwann cells populating the dorsal and ventral roots. Although these Schwann cells are morphologically indistinguishable from "regular" Schwann cells of peripheral nerves proper, the root Schwann cells are derived from a unique cell population, namely the so-called boundary caps or boundary capping cells that are found at both the dorsal root entry zones and the exit point of the ventral roots (Jessen and Mirsky, 2005a; Wilkinson *et al.*, 1989). Previous studies identified these cells in ventral root primordia of chicken embryos as putative neural-tube-derived sheath cells using the chicken-neural crest marker HNK-1 (Lunn *et al.*, 1987). Niederlander and Lumsden unequivocally identified these cells as neural crest derivatives using the chick-quail chimera technique (Niederlander and Lumsden, 1996). A reliable marker molecule of the murine capping cells is the transcription factor Egr2/Krox20, which is found in these cells long before its well established expression in myelinating Schwann cells (Wilkinson *et al.*, 1989). By using the transcription factor as a marker, the boundary capping cells could be identified as progenitors of not only the Schwann cells of the spinal roots, but also some nociceptive neurons and satellite cells of the dorsal root ganglia (Aquino *et al.*, 2006; Maro *et al.*, 2004). There is another heterogeneity during early gliogenesis in the PNS: emigrating neural crest cells that express neurogenin develop into Schwann cells of nerve roots, whereas Schwann cells from peripheral nerves proper are derived from neurogenin-negative neural crest cell pools (Woodhoo and Sommer, 2008). The relationship between the neurogenin-positive neural crest cells and the boundary capping cells is, to our knowledge, not yet clarified. Also, and similar to the different origins of oligodendrocytes, it remains an open question whether this diversity of Schwann cell development might reflect functional differences between the peripheral glial cells in roots versus nerves proper.

Stages of Schwann cell development

Function, migration, survival and differentiation of Schwann cell precursors

The molecular markers, some morphological features of Schwann cell precursors (SCPs) and essential factors for their survival have been extensively described elsewhere (Jessen and Mirsky, 2005a; Woodhoo and Sommer, 2008). In brief, SCPs acquire – as opposed to spindle-shaped immature Schwann cells – a flat-shaped appearance in culture. They express cell adhesion molecules, such as L1, N-cadherin and α4 integrin, and the myelin components P0 (myelin protein zero, MPZ), peripheral myelin protein 22 (PMP22) and proteo-lipid protein (PLP), but lack or express very low levels of the glial markers S100β and glial fibrillary acidic protein (GFAP). An exclusive marker for SCPs is cadherin19 (Jessen and Mirsky, 2005a). Most importantly and, as opposed to immature Schwann cells, survival of SCPs is strongly dependent on neuronal contact and this survival function of co-cultured neurons can be substituted by NRG1 (Dong *et al.*, 1995; Jessen and Mirsky, 2005a), most likely mediated through the cognate receptor erbB3. Other survival factors are the platelet-derived growth factor PDGF-B and neurotrophin-3 (NT-3) (Lobsiger *et al.*, 2000) and there are multiple combinations of growth factors, including fibroblast growth factor (FGF), insulin-like growth factor (IGF) and endothelin that promote survival of SCPs in culture (Woodhoo and Sommer, 2008).

In vivo, SCPs are devoid of a basal lamina which is a morphological difference between immature and mature Schwann cells (Jessen and Mirsky, 2005b; Martini, 2005). Electron microscopy revealed that these cells not only intermingle with fasciculating axons but also surround the prospective nerves or nerve fascicles, facing the mesenchyme with their abaxonal surfaces (Bentley and Lee, 2000; Ciutat et al., 1996; Jessen and Mirsky, 2005b; Martini, 1994, 2005). A series of recent sophisticated studies suggests that SCPs are not only transition stages to prospective mature glial cells, but may also fulfill important functions in nerve development (Wanner et al., 2006a, 2006b). During late innervation stages of mouse limbs, these cells form a "mantle" around the fasciculating peripheral axons and cover most of the growth cone surfaces thus separating them from the mesenchymal environment, suggestive of a guidance function for the outgrowing axons as previously speculated (Noakes and Bennett, 1987). Interestingly, the SCPs are strongly N-cadherin-positive during the period of axon outgrowth, but not at later stages of nerve maturation. The view that this cellular microenvironment around growing tips of peripheral nerves is important for nerve guidance and nerve shape formation is in line with observations in various lack-of Schwann cell mutants showing an aberrant and partially maloriented innervation of a predominantly defasciculating phenotype (Gilmour et al., 2002; Morris et al., 1999; Riethmacher et al., 1997). It is, thus, possible that SCPs serve as cellular chaperons (Wanner et al., 2006b) that are instrumental for axon guidance and fasciculation. The latter function may be mediated by the polarized secretion of the repulsive extracellular matrix molecule tenascin-C that has been found previously to surround the abaxonal surfaces of the "mantling" SCPs (Martini and Schachner, 1991; Wehrle-Haller et al., 1991). Additionally, SCPs may serve as sources of trophic support for neurons, since lack-of Schwann cell mouse mutants show a robust loss of neurons projecting into the limbs (Jessen and Mirsky, 2005a). However, this topic needs further attention, since in fish embryos lack of SCPs does not lead to neuronal loss in the lateral line system (Gilmour et al., 2002). It is possible that neuron loss in the glia-deprived mouse mutants results from the failure of misguided axons to innervate their prospective trophic target structures rather than from an interrupted glial-derived trophic support.

Another task for SCPs is their contribution to endoneurial fibro-blasts. Using Cre-recombinase fate mapping, Joseph and colleagues identified neural-crest-derived cells as a possible source for endo-neurial fibroblasts (Joseph *et al.*, 2004). Interestingly, in adult nerves, bone-marrow-derived cells have been found to contribute to peripheral nerve fibroblasts (Maurer *et al.*, 2003), reflecting more complex lineage conditions in the cellular elements of peripheral nerves than previ-ously anticipated.

Immature Schwann cells: autocrine loop for survival as an important prerequisite for axon regrowth after injury

Schwann cell precursors develop into immature Schwann cells under the influence of NRG1; this development is – at least in culture – accelerated by FGF2 (Woodhoo and Sommer, 2008). The most crucial cell biological difference between immature Schwann cells and SCPs is their dependence on survival factors. Whereas SCPs strongly depend on axonal contact/NRG1 in culture and die when deprived of axons or the survival factor, immature Schwann cells are charac-terized by an autocrine survival loop comprising BDNF, IGF-2, PDGF-B, NT-3, leukemia inhibitory factor (LIF) and possibly others (Jessen and Mirsky, 2005a; Meier *et al.*, 1999). This autocrine loop is an important prerequisite for survival of Schwann cells after peri-pheral nerve injury, since mature Schwann cells acquire a differenti-ation state comparable to that of immature Schwann cells when deprived of their axons and can re-acquire the mature state upon re-innervation. Since re-innervation is strictly dependent on the pres-ence of Schwann cells, Schwann cell survival in the injured peri-pheral nerve is one (of several) prerequisites for the regenerative capacity of peripheral nerves (see below). However, denervation for longer than a couple of months eventually results in a substantial loss of Schwann cells with accompanying impaired re-innervation (Hoke, 2006). Although of pivotal clinical relevance, the reasons for Schwann cell wasting under long-term denervation conditions are not known.

Immature Schwann cells: sorting out of myelin-competent axons and switch to the myelination program

Another important function of immature Schwann cells is "radial sorting," achieved by extending cytoplasmic processes in between axon bundles to sort, ensheathe and eventually myelinate them. The larger axons are separated and "forced" to the peripheral margin of the immature axon bundles. Cell surface receptors (β1 integrin; Feltri *et al.*, 2002) and their cognate ligands (laminins; Yu *et al.*, 2005) play a pivotal role in this process, as revealed by the investigation of cell-specific knockout mutants. After having identified these players as essential, particular emphasis was laid on the signal mechanisms downstream of β1 integrin. Two groups independently identified downstream Rho GTPase Rac1 as an important signaling protein for radial sorting (Benninger *et al.*, 2007; Nodari *et al.*, 2007). Additionally, Benninger and colleagues demonstrated that Rho GTPase cdc42 is involved in Schwann cell proliferation. This is an important prerequisite for myelination, since to successfully achieve a 1:1 ratio between myelinating Schwann cells and axons, it is necessary not only that Schwann cell processes protrude in between axon bundles, but also that the appropriate number of Schwann cells is acquired. Another important player in this issue is the focal adhesion kinase FAK. It can be linked to either β1 integrin signaling or ErbB receptor signaling. Conditional deletion of FAK results in normal ErbB phosphorylation reflecting an unimpaired neuregulin signaling pathway in the absence of FAK. However, Schwann cell proliferation was impaired in the absence of FAK whereas process extension was obviously independent of the kinase (Grove *et al.*, 2007). The link between β1 integrin, erbB receptors and FAK regulation is not yet understood.

Having achieved the 1:1 ratio with axons (promyelinating stage), the transition to myelinating profiles is another important step. This stage is transiently mediated by the partially redundant transcription factors Oct-6/SCIP/Brn2 and eventually manifested by Krox-20, ultimately resulting in the induction of the Schwann-cell-related myelin components P0, MBP and Cx32 (Svaren and Meijer, 2008).

MYELINATION

Axonal control of myelination

Oligodendrocytes respond to axonal signals (e.g. Kidd *et al.*, 1990; Scherer *et al.*, 1992), although they can also differentiate in culture and in vivo in the absence of neurons and viable axons, respectively (Dubois-Dalcq *et al.*, 1986; Mirsky *et al.*, 1980; Ueda *et al.*, 1999). In fact, the differentiation of oligodendrocytes follows a default pathway with an intrinsic program controlling the timing of development (Temple and Raff, 1986) and external signals promoting or inhibiting oligodendrocyte differentiation and CNS myelination (Coman *et al.*, 2005; Nave and Trapp, 2008; Simons and Trajkovic, 2006).

Differentiation of oligodendrocytes is influenced by the Notch signaling pathway. In the developing optic nerve, Notch1 is expressed by cells of the oligodendrocyte lineage, and retinal ganglion cells express Jagged1, a ligand of Notch1. Expression of Jagged1 is down-regulated along a time course that parallels that of myelination and Jagged1 strongly inhibits oligodendrocyte differentiation in culture, suggesting that the Jagged-Notch pathway regulates timing of oligo-dendrocyte differentiation and myelination (Wang *et al.*, 1998). The production of prematurely differentiated oligodendrocytes in trans-genic mice with a conditional ablation of Notch1 in oligodendrocyte progenitor cells is in line with this view (Genoud *et al.*, 2002). In con-trast, activation of the Notch/Deltex1 pathway by an alternative axonal ligand, F3/contactin, has been shown to promote oligodendrocyte maturation, possibly implicating MAG (Hu *et al.*, 2003).

Neuronal electrical activity is another factor influencing differ-entiation of myelinating glia and myelination (Demerens *et al.*, 1996; Fields and Burnstock, 2006). While activity-mediated neuronal release of adenosine inhibits oligodendrocyte progenitor prolifera-tion and promotes oligodendrocyte differentiation and myelination through activation of purinergic P1 receptors (Stevens *et al.*, 2002), activity-mediated release of ATP inhibits Schwann cell proliferation, differentiation and myelination through activation of purinergic P2 receptors (Stevens and Fields, 2000). Furthermore, a role for astro-cytes in the activity-mediated control of myelination in the CNS has recently been demonstrated by the observation that ATP released from spiking axons induces astrocytes to secrete the cytokine LIF, which in turn promotes myelination by mature oligodendrocytes (Ishibashi *et al.*, 2006).

Similar to electrical activity, nerve growth factor (NGF) also exerts opposing effects on CNS and PNS myelination. While NGF promotes myelination of TrkA-expressing dorsal root ganglia (DRG) neurons by Schwann cells, it inhibits myelination of these axons by oligodendrocytes (Chan *et al.*, 2004). A recent study has shown that oligodendrocyte- but not Schwann cell-related myelination of DRG neurons is reduced, at least in part, by NGF-induced expression of LINGO-1 (LLR and IG domain-containing Nogo receptor interacting protein), a critical inhibitor of oligodendrocyte differentiation and myelination (Lee *et al.*, 2007; Mi *et al.*, 2005). Blocking LINGO-1 function in cells of the oligodendrocyte lineage or in neurons promoted oligodendrocyte differentiation and myelination, whereas overexpression of LINGO-1 in either cell type inhibited oligodendrocyte differentiation and myelination in culture. Precocious myelination in LINGO-1 knockout mice (Mi *et al.*, 2005) and delayed myelination in transgenic mice overexpressing LINGO-1 in neurons (Lee *et al.*, 2007) confirms a critical role for LINGO-1 in regulating CNS myelination.

The polysialylated form of the neural cell adhesion molecule (PSA-NCAM) is thought to act as another negative regulator of CNS myelination. When PSA-NCAM expression is prematurely decreased by either antibody-mediated internalization or administration of endoneuraminidase N, which specifically hydrolyzes PSA, myelination is increased both in culture and in vivo (Charles *et al.*, 2000). Conversely, permanent expression of PSA-NCAM by oligodendrocytes in transgenic mice results in hypomyelination (Fewou *et al.*, 2007). In line with a proposed function of PSA-NCAM as a negative regulator of CNS myelination, developmental downregulation of this molecule immediately precedes the onset of myelination. Interestingly, PSA-NCAM is re-expressed on demyelinated axons in multiple sclerosis plaques where it may interfere with efficient myelin repair (Charles *et al.*, 2002a).

Neuregulin-1 and ErbB receptor tyrosine signaling plays a critical role at essentially all stages of Schwann cell development (Garratt *et al.*, 2000; Jessen and Mirsky, 2005a; Nave and Salzer, 2006; Nave and Trapp, 2008) (see below). A number of in culture studies and the phenotypic analysis of heterozygous NRG1 type III null mutants or transgenic mice expressing dominant-negative ErbB receptors suggested critical functions of NRG1/Erb signaling also at various stages of oligodendrocyte differentiation, including fate determination, proliferation, survival, differentiation and myelination (Taveggia *et al.*, 2008) (reviewed in Esper *et al.*, 2006; Falls, 2003; Nave and Salzer, 2006; Nave and Trapp, 2008; Simons and Trajkovic, 2006). Unexpectedly, however, a recent study reported apparently normal CNS myelination in heterozygous NRG1 or NRG1 type III null mutants and in various conditional null mutants that completely lacked NRG1 in either the developing CNS or in projection neurons of the forebrain beginning at different developmental stages (Brinkmann *et al.*, 2008). Normal CNS myelination was also observed in young postnatal mice lacking ErbB3 and ErbB4 (and thus neuregulin signaling) in oligodendrocytes. Conversely, a population of CNS axons was hypermyelinated in transgenic mice overexpressing NRG1 type III (in analogy to the PNS) and NRG1 type I (in contrast to the PNS; Brinkmann *et al.*, 2008; Michailov *et al.*, 2004). The combined data suggest that NRG1/ErbB signaling is dispensable for normal myelination in the CNS and further exemplify that distinct mechanisms may regulate myelination in the CNS and PNS.

It is a well established dogma that the axon determines the fate of the Schwann cell with regard to whether it is myelinating or ensheathing. For instance, more than 30 years ago, Spencer and colleagues (Weinberg and Spencer, 1975) and Aguayo and colleagues (Aguayo *et al.*, 1976) independently cross-anastomosed nerves containing myelin-competent axons with nerves containing almost exclusively non-myelinated fibers and found that the axons of the myelinated nerves became myelinated by the Schwann cells from the non-myelinated nerves. Moreover, Voyvodic could show that an originally non-myelinated axon grows in size and induces myelination when supplied with an unusually large neurotrophic target (Voyvodic, 1989). Today, it is well established that the instructive axonal signal that induces ensheathment and myelination in the PNS is NRG1 type III. Using a lentiviral approach Salzer and colleagues (Taveggia *et al.*, 2005) could change the myelin-incompetent fate of NRG-1-deficient neurons into a myelin-competent one. Even more convincingly, lentiviral expression of NRG1 in normally unmyelinated, postganglionic neurons of the sympathetic system of normal mice also induced myelination. Moreover, it was shown that PI 3-kinase is the critical downstream regulator involved (Nave and Salzer, 2006; Taveggia *et al.*, 2005).

By generating and investigating mice expressing various levels of NRG1 in Schwann cells, another important function of the trophic factor could be identified: the determination of myelin thickness (Michailov *et al.*, 2004). Many previous studies have demonstrated that myelin thickness is adjusted to axonal caliber (Friede, 1972; Martini, 2005) and the studies by Michailov and colleagues identified NRG1/III as the "biochemical measure of axon size" (Michailov *et al.*, 2004).

Cell contact in myelination

Previous studies focusing on axon–Schwann cell interactions identified various cell adhesion molecules, such as L1, N-CAM and N-Cadherin, as important mediators of PNS myelination (Bixby *et al.*,

1988; Seilheimer and Schachner, 1988). In line with these finding were immunoelectron microscope investigations showing both axonal and Schwann-cell-borne expression of L1 and N-CAM at early stages of myelination (Martini and Schachner, 1986). Blocking antibodies to L1 and N-CAM impaired neurite–Schwann cell apposition (Seilheimer et al., 1989), ensheathment and eventually myelin formation (Wood et al., 1990). Interestingly, L1 and N-CAM were downregulated at more mature stages of myelin induction, i.e. at time points when MAG and P0 were upregulated (Martini and Schachner, 1986, 1988). These combined observations led to the hypothesis that the respective adhesion molecules are important mediators of axon–Schwann cell interaction during myelination in the PNS (Martini, 1994). Of note, similar observations in the spatiotemporal expression of L1 and N-CAM were made in the CNS, with the substantial difference that oligodendrocytes, in contrast to Schwann cells, did not express L1 (Bartsch et al., 1989).

The roles of the above-mentioned adhesion molecules have been further investigated by scoring the respective knockout mutants. Unexpectedly, both L1- and N-CAM-deficient mice lacked myelin abnormalities in both the PNS and CNS, probably reflecting redundant functional roles during the myelinating process (Carenini et al., 1997; Cohen et al., 1998; Dahme et al., 1997; Haney et al., 1999). While MAG-deficient mice showed a delay in myelination in the CNS, myelination in the PNS was initially normal but was then followed by axon and myelin degeneration (Bartsch, 2003; Bartsch et al., 1997; Carenini et al., 1997; Fruttiger et al., 1995; Li, C. et al., 1994; Montag et al., 1994). These studies strongly argued for the involvement of other, non-redundant, molecules in the initiation of myelination in both the PNS and CNS. By screening cDNA libraries of Schwann cells and DRG neurons, Peles and colleagues as well as Salzer et al. identified several members of the nectin-like (Necl) family of adhesion molecules. These molecules all contain three extracellular Ig-like domains, a transmembrane domain and an intracellular domain containing FERM- and PBZ-binding sites (Maurel et al., 2007; Spiegel et al., 2007). Interestingly, Necl4 is localized to the internodal, juxtaparanodal and paranodal, but not to the nodal, regions of myelinating Schwann cells, whereas one of its cognate ligands/receptors, Necl1, is expressed on the axon membrane. Using myelinating co-culture systems, both groups identified Necl4 as Schwann cell- and Necl1 as axon-related molecules that heterophilically interact with each other and mediate Schwann cell myelination (Maurel *et al.*, 2007; Spiegel *et al.*, 2007). Of note, preliminary observations with Necl1-Fc, Necl3-Fc and Necl4-Fc binding fragments suggest that a similar molecular arrangement may appear during CNS myelination (Spiegel *et al.*, 2007). Indeed, by an independent approach Necl3 has been identified on myelinated CNS axons (Pellissier *et al.*, 2007) where it might interact with oligodendrocytes (Spiegel *et al.*, 2007).

Myelin-specific components of oligodendrocytes and Schwann cells

In addition to the above-mentioned molecules involved in myelination there are some components left that deserve attention with regard to their presence in either CNS or PNS myelin or both. For instance, the major oligodendrocytic tetraspan component PLP/DM20 has previously been supposed to be predominantly expressed in CNS myelin while Schwann cells do not incorporate substantial amounts of the protein into the myelin (Puckett *et al.*, 1987). However, a functional role of PLP in PNS myelin is demonstrated by the observation that patients with a PLP null mutation (but not with other PLP mutations) develop features indicative of demyelination in peripheral nerves (Garbern *et al.*, 1997). In contrast, however, mice deficient in PLP show normal peripheral myelin, with impaired axonal transport and axonal survival being restricted to the CNS (Edgar *et al.*, 2004; Klugmann *et al.*, 1997). Nevertheless, under certain conditions, Schwann cells are able to incorporate substantial levels of PLP into compact myelin: Colman and colleagues demonstrated the presence of PLP in compact Schwann cell myelin of bony fish and amphibians (Yoshida and Colman, 1996). Furthermore, inactivation of the P0 gene in mice leads to an upregulation of PLP in myelin-related structures (Giese *et al.*, 1992). Nevertheless there is a common view that PLP is a major component of mammalian CNS myelin, and that mutations in the plp gene are implicated in a variety of human CNS disorders, such as Pelizaeus–Merzbacher disease, spastic paraplegia type 2 and possibly multiple sclerosis (Gorman *et al.*, 2007; Hudson *et al.*, 2004; Nave and Griffiths, 2004; Warshawsky *et al.*, 2005).

Another protein prominently expressed in CNS myelin is myelin basic protein (MBP). In contrast to PLP, it is not an integral membrane protein but associated with the cytoplasmic aspect of the myelin membrane. Due to its positive charges, it is thought to mediate the formation (compaction) of the major dense lines (MDL) by electrostatically interacting with apposed phospholipid residues of the cell membrane (Inouye *et al.*, 1985) in both CNS and PNS myelin. However, the absence of MBP from the shiverer mutant leads to myelin decompaction at the MDL only in the CNS, but not in the PNS (Kirschner and Ganser, 1980; Privat *et al.*, 1979; Rosenbluth, 1980a, 1980b). The only defect observed in the PNS of shiverer mice is an elevated number of Schwann-cell-related Schmidt–Lanterman incisures (Gould *et al.*, 1995). The lack of Schwann cell myelin decompaction in the absence of MBP can be best explained by compensatory functions of the positive charges of the intracellular portion of the P0 protein (Martini *et al.*, 1995). The latter protein is – at least in mammals – exclusively expressed in Schwann cell myelin (Lemke, 1986; Nave *et al.*, 2007; Niemann *et al.*, 2006) (in addition to low levels in SCPs, see above). Interestingly, oligodendrocytes of lower vertebrates incorporate P0 into their compact myelin (Schweitzer *et al.*, 2006; Yoshida and Colman, 1996). In addition to its adhesive function, the protein has been proposed to be involved in signal transduction (Xu *et al.*, 2001). Similar to P0, PMP22 is another component of compact myelin that is exclusively found in PNS myelin (and in some other neural and non-neural cell types; Baechner *et al.*, 1995; Parmantier *et al.*, 1995). Whereas the role of P0 as an adhesive molecule involved in myelin compaction is well established, the role of PMP22 is still not clearly understood, although it is the major culprit gene for inherited demyelinating neuropathies of Charcot–Marie–Tooth type 1A (Berger *et al.*, 2006; Nave *et al.*, 2007; Niemann *et al.*, 2006; Scherer and Wrabetz, 2008). Other myelin components of either CNS (Nogo, OMgp) or both CNS and PNS myelin (MAG) are discussed later in the context of axonal regrowth after neural injury. More extensive overviews of the biology of myelin components and their relationship to myelin disorders are given elsewhere (Berger *et al.*, 2006; Nave *et al.*, 2007; Niemann *et al.*, 2006; Scherer and Wrabetz, 2008).

The contribution of myelinating glial cells to the formation of nodal compartments

A typical component of myelinated fibers is the node of Ranvier and its associated regions, the paranodes and juxtaparanodes. While the node of Ranvier is at first glance an exposed axonal domain with a high concentration of voltage-gated ion channels, it has become clear that myelinating glial cells strongly contribute to the formation of this functionally important structure (Bhat *et al.*, 2001; Poliak and Peles, 2003; Salzer, 2003; Salzer *et al.*, 2008; Schafer and Rasband, 2006). The mechanisms through which this structure is formed and maintained are best understood in the PNS.

The node of Ranvier proper

In the PNS, the nodal compartment consists not only of the exposed axolemma, but also the ECM-related nodal gap substance that contains tenascin-C among other ECM constituents such as syndecan-3, collagen V and versican V1 (Martini *et al.*, 1990; Melendez-Vasquez *et al.*, 2005). Additionally, multiple slender Schwann cell protrusions abutting the axolemma are typical. Due to the presence of the microvillus-related proteins ezrin, radixin and moesin, these structures have been termed Schwann cell or nodal microvilli (Melendez-Vasquez *et al.*, 2001).

In the CNS, nodes of Ranvier are also associated with distinct ECM components, which, however, differ in their composition, in that syndecan-3 is lacking and tenascin-R may replace tenascin-C at the PNS node (Bartsch *et al.*, 1993; Melendez-Vasquez *et al.*, 2005). Another difference to PNS nodes is the absence of nodal microvilli. Instead, cellular processes of cells expressing the proteoglycan NG2 protrude into the nodal gap of myelinated CNS fibers (Butt *et al.*, 1999). These cells are thought to be derived from the oligodendrocytic lineage and form a perinodal cellular ring around the nodal area that is decorated with the neurite-outgrowth inhibitory molecule OMgp (Huang *et al.*, 2005).

A characteristic molecular and functionally relevant feature of the node of Ranvier is the clustering of voltage-gated Na^+ channels (Poliak and Peles, 2003; Salzer, 2003; Salzer *et al.*, 2008; Schafer and Rasband, 2006). Considerable knowledge has been gained about the molecular mechanisms leading to the formation of channel clusters at the node, particularly in the PNS. Importantly, correct clustering is dependent on intact Schwann cells, as indicated by the abnormal ion channel clustering demonstrated in Schwann cell mouse mutants (Devaux and Scherer, 2005; Ulzheimer *et al.*, 2004). During the process of Na^+ channel clustering, important players are distinct cell adhesion molecules, such as NF186 and Nr-CAM (Koticha *et al.*, 2006), but also cytoskeletal elements, such as ankyrin G, which itself binds to the cytoplasmic (axoplasmic) domain of the voltage-gated Na^+ channels and its "anchor" protein βIV-spectrin (Dzhashiashvili et al., 2007; Salzer, 2003; Yang et al., 2007). Further pivotal players are the gliomedins, Schwann cell microvilli-related and secreted molecules that interact with the extracellular domains of Nr-CAM and NF186 and, in this way, appear to direct and fix a molecular complex consisting of the two CAMs and the nodal cytoskeletal and Na^+ channel components (Eshed et al., 2005, 2007). A proof of principle demonstrating the pivotal role of neurofascins was provided by investigating corresponding knockout mice that show defective Na^+ channel clustering at nodes (Sherman et al., 2005). Other Schwann cell-derived molecules involved in correct ion channel clustering include laminin 2 and its receptor component dystroglycan (Occhi et al., 2005). The combined findings unequivocally demonstrate the important roles that Schwann cells play during the clustering of voltage-gated Na^+ channels.

The mechanisms underlying Na^+ channel clustering in the CNS are not as well understood. Based on the aforementioned structural differences between nodes in the PNS and CNS, it is not surprising that the mechanisms of channel clustering are not identical in the different nervous tissues. For example, it appears that direct contact between oligodendrocytes and axolemma is not required for Na^+ channel clustering on retinal ganglion cell axons (Kaplan et al., 1997, 2001). This finding goes along with the observations that gliomedin is not expressed by oligodendrocytes (Eshed et al., 2005, 2007) and that one of its potential ligands, Nr-CAM, is lacking in CNS nodes. An oligodendrocytic contribution may be the secretion of an as yet unknown factor that initiates cluster formation on the axolemma of cultured retinal ganglion cell axons (Kaplan et al., 1997; Simons and Trajkovic, 2006). One candidate may be tenascin-R: the interaction of this ECM component with $\beta 2$-subunits of Na^+ channels suggests a significant role in proper cluster organization and, more indirectly, tenascin-R-deficient mice show decreased axonal conduction in the CNS (Weber et al., 1999). Other node-related glial components are possibly provided by the processes of the $NG2^+$ perinodal cells (Butt et al., 1999). In conclusion, more work is necessary to further characterize the molecular mechanisms that induce and stabilize the clustering of ion channels at CNS nodes.

Paranodes

The nodes of Ranvier proper are flanked by the paranodal loops, i.e. cytoplasmic pockets of the respective myelinating glial cells.

In both PNS and CNS, the paranodal loops are linked to the associated axolemma by specialized septate junctions that are thought to form diffusion barriers for membrane components and soluble molecules of larger size. Laterally, Schwann cell paranodes are connected by adherens junctions (Fannon *et al.*, 1995). In the PNS, the organization of the paranodal loops is strongly dependent on axon diameter: while the loops of smaller caliber axons are regularly organized along the longitudinal extension of the axon, they appear less regular in larger fibers where not all loops are in contact with the axolemma (Martini, 2005). Such differences have – to our knowledge – not yet been described for oligodendrocytic paranodes.

Molecularly, there are similarities, but also clear differences between PNS and CNS paranodes. Common molecular features include the presence of NF-155, the putative ligand of the axonal components contactin and Caspr, contributing to the organization of the septate-like junctions (Salzer *et al.*, 2008; Schafer and Rasband, 2006; Scherer and Arroyo, 2002; Spiegel and Peles, 2002). Interestingly, mice lacking one of these molecular components fail to form paranodal junctions both in the PNS and CNS (Bhat *et al.*, 2001; Sherman *et al.*, 2005).

In the CNS, paranodal interactions are detected before nodal protein clustering, in striking contrast to the PNS (Schafer and Rasband, 2006). CNS and PNS paranodes also differ with respect to the gap-junction component Cx32. While this molecule forms reflexive junctions in paranodal loops and Schmidt–Lanterman incisures of Schwann cells, where it may allow rapid radial connection between the axonal and abaxonal Schwann cell cytoplasm (Balice-Gordon *et al.*, 1998; Scherer *et al.*, 1995), the channel component is lacking in paranodal regions of oligodendrocytes (Scherer *et al.*, 1995). Interestingly, mutations in Cx32 lead to the X-linked dominant form of inherited peripheral neuropathies (Scherer and Wrabetz, 2008).

Juxtaparanodes

Compared to the paranodal regions, juxtaparanodal aspects are morphologically less conspicuous domains of the myelinated fibers that are molecularly defined by the presence of TAG-1 on both the glial and axonal sites and by Caspr2 and voltage-gated K^+ channels on the axonal site (Poliak and Peles, 2003; Salzer *et al.*, 2008; Scherer and Arroyo, 2002; Traka *et al.*, 2003). Caspr2 may associate with K^+ channels via an unidentified PDZ-domain protein (Rasband *et al.*, 2002) and with the cytoskeleton through 4.1B (Denisenko-Nehrbass *et al.*, 2003).

In contrast to the CNS, juxtaparanodal regions are morphologically defined in the PNS, particularly in large caliber fibers (Martini, 2005). A typical feature as revealed by electron microscopy is the juxtaparanodal network between axonal and glial membranes (Gatzinsky *et al.*, 1997). Interestingly, this compartment appears particularly vulnerable to molecular changes in Schwann cells, such as reduced expression of P0 (Martini *et al.*, 1995) or lack of β4 integrin and dystroglycan (Nodari *et al.*, 2008), that lead to macrophage-related myelin destruction. The disorganization of the juxtaparanodal structures in myelin-related mutants, and also in aging wild-type rodents, might be a pathological consequence of a labile, molecularly specialized structure that comprises not only the K$^+$ channel compartment and Caspr2 molecules but also the juxtaparanodal network between axonal and glial membranes. It might be important to focus future research on the characteristics that define the juxtaparanodal compartment as the "Achilles' heel" of the peripheral nerve fiber and the possible link to degenerating features implicating macrophage activation and further damage (Wang Ip *et al.*, 2006).

ROLE OF MYELINATING GLIAL CELLS
AFTER NEURAL INJURY

Impact of oligodendrocytes

In contrast to the PNS or the embryonic CNS, neurons in the adult mammalian CNS usually fail to regenerate their axons after injury. The limited regenerative potential of adult CNS neurons might be partly attributed to a decrease in their intrinsic capability to regrow damaged axons as they mature. However, adult neurons are able to regrow severed axons over long distances through a growth-permissive environment, such as a peripheral nerve graft (David and Aguayo, 1981; Richardson *et al.*, 1980). Similarly, dorsal root ganglion neurons can regenerate their peripheral but not their central processes, and cultured neurons extend neurites into sciatic nerve explants but not into optic nerve explants (Schwab and Thoenen, 1985). These and other observations indicate that the adult CNS comprises a non-permissive or inhibitory environment that prevents long-distance axonal regeneration. Indeed, a variety of growth inhibitory factors have been identified including chondroitin sulfate proteoglycans (CSPGs) associated with glial scarring (Laabs *et al.*, 2005; Silver and Miller, 2004) and myelin-associated inhibitors of neurite growth expressed by oligodendrocytes (Chaudhry and Filbin, 2007; Filbin, 2003; Liu *et al.*, 2006a; Schwab, 2004; Schwab and Bartholdi, 1996; Yiu and He, 2006).

The myelin-associated inhibitors Nogo, MAG and OMgp
and their impact on axon regeneration

Central nervous system myelin and mature oligodendrocytes induce growth cone collapse and inhibit neurite elongation from neurons in culture (Bandtlow *et al.*, 1990; Carbonetto *et al.*, 1987; Schwab and Caroni, 1988; Schwab and Thoenen, 1985). Furthermore, axonal regeneration occurs in CNS fiber tracts in which myelination has been delayed experimentally (Keirstead *et al.*, 1992; Savio and Schwab, 1990). These and other observations clearly suggest the presence of oligodendrocyte-derived and myelin-associated inhibitors that prevent successful axonal regeneration in the adult CNS. Part of the inhibitory activity of CNS myelin has been shown to be associated with two protein fractions of 35 and 250 kDa (NI-35 and NI-250). An antibody raised against NI-250, termed IN-1, partly neu-tralized the inhibitory activity of CNS myelin and oligodendrocytes in culture and promoted axonal regeneration and functional recov-ery after a partial spinal cord injury in vivo (Bregman *et al.*, 1995; Caroni and Schwab, 1988a, 1988b; Schnell and Schwab, 1990). Following the publication of the partial protein sequence of the bovine homolog of rat NI-250 (Spillmann *et al.*, 1998), three groups independently identified the nogo gene (Chen *et al.*, 2000; GrandPre *et al.*, 2000; Prinjha *et al.*, 2000). Nogo is a member of the reticulon family and exists in three isoforms, Nogo-A (NI-250), Nogo-B and Nogo-C. Nogo-A is particularly enriched in oligodendrocytes and myelin but is also expressed in neurons (Huber *et al.*, 2002). Nogo-A contains two neurite growth-inhibitory domains: a 66-amino-acid loop (Nogo-66), which is located in the C-terminal part of the protein and is common to all Nogo isoforms, and a second domain in the N-terminal part of the protein (amino-Nogo), which is not shared by Nogo-B or Nogo-C (Chen *et al.*, 2000; Fournier *et al.*, 2001; GrandPre *et al.*, 2000; Oertle *et al.*, 2003).

In addition to Nogo, two other myelin proteins – myelin-associated glycoprotein (MAG) and oligodendrocyte-myelin glycopro-tein (OMgp) – also induce growth cone collapse and inhibit neurite outgrowth in culture (Filbin, 2003; Yiu and He, 2006). MAG, a mem-ber of the immunoglobulin superfamily, is expressed by both

oligodendrocytes and Schwann cells and has been shown to participate in the formation and maintenance of myelin (Bartsch, 2003;
Schachner and Bartsch, 2000). Interestingly, the inhibitory effect of
MAG on neurite growth is restricted to adult neurons, whereas
neurite outgrowth from embryonic neurons is promoted by MAG
(Cai et al., 2001; Johnson et al., 1989; Mukhopadhyay et al., 1994).
OMgp is a glycosylphosphatidylinositol- (GPI-) anchored protein that
is expressed by oligodendrocytes and neurons (Vourc'h and Andres,
2004). OMgp induces growth cone collapse and potently inhibits
neurite outgrowth from cultured nerve cells (Kottis et al., 2002;
Wang et al., 2002b). Furthermore, OMgp has recently been implicated
in the stabilization of nodes of Ranvier and in preventing collateral
axon sprouting from nodes of Ranvier in the normal CNS (Huang
et al., 2005).

While the putative neuronal receptor for amino-Nogo is not
yet known, Nogo-66 binds to a GPI-anchored neuronal leucine-rich
repeat (LRR) protein termed Nogo-66 receptor (NgR1) (Barton et al.,
2003; Fournier et al., 2001; He et al., 2003). Remarkably, MAG and
OMgp also bind to NgR1 (Domeniconi et al., 2002; Liu et al., 2002;
Wang et al., 2002b). MAG can also mediate inhibition through the
structurally related receptor NgR2 (Venkatesh et al., 2005). NgR1 lacks
an intracellular signaling domain, and requires the low-affinity neurotrophin receptor p75 (p75NTR) and LINGO-1 as co-receptors to
transmit inhibitory signals to the axon (Mi et al., 2004; Wang et al.,
2002a; Wong et al., 2002). TROY (also known as TAJ) has been identified as an alternative co-receptor that can substitute for p75NTR
within the NgR1 receptor complex (Park et al., 2005; Shao et al.,
2005). Binding of ligands to the NgR1 receptor complex leads to
activation of the GTPase RhoA, which in turn activates its downstream effector Rho-associated kinase (ROCK), ultimately resulting
in neurite growth inhibition (Fournier et al., 2003; Niederost et al.,
2002).

Administration of the IN-1 antibody or newly developed anti-
Nogo antibodies resulted in axon regeneration, anatomical plasticity
and functional recovery in a variety of lesion paradigms in vivo (see
e.g. Bregman et al., 1995; Brosamle et al., 2000; Liebscher et al., 2005;
Merkler et al., 2001; Schnell and Schwab, 1990; Wiessner et al., 2003).
The use of other neutralizing agents also suggested a critical role for
Nogo in restricting axon regeneration in the adult CNS. For example,
administration of NEP1–40 – a Nogo-66 fragment that competes with
Nogo for binding to NgR1 – to the hemisected spinal cord of rats at

the time of lesioning or to the lesioned spinal cord of mice a few days after the lesion also resulted in improved regeneration and locomotor recovery (GrandPre *et al.*, 2002; Li and Strittmatter, 2003). In comparison, assessment of the regenerative phenotype of four different Nogo knockout mouse lines provided less consistent results (Kim *et al.*, 2003; Simonen *et al.*, 2003; Zheng *et al.*, 2003). While myelin from the various Nogo-deficient mouse lines was less inhibitory towards neurite growth than myelin from control mice in assays in culture, there were marked differences between the different knockout lines with regard to the regenerative growth of corticospinal tract (CST) axons following a dorsal hemisection. One group analyzed a gene trap mutant deficient in Nogo-A and Nogo-B and reported robust regeneration of CST axons in young adult Nogo-A/B knockout mice (Kim *et al.*, 2003). Another group studied a Nogo-A-deficient mouse line (with a markedly increased expression of Nogo-B predominantly in oligodendrocytes), and found only moderately improved regeneration of CST axons (Simonen *et al.*, 2003). Remarkably, however, significantly enhanced regeneration of CST axons was observed in the same mutant mouse line after it had been backcrossed into a pure genetic background (Dimou *et al.*, 2006). The third group analyzed mice lacking either Nogo-A and Nogo-B or all three Nogo isoforms and found no evidence for enhanced regeneration of the CST in either mutant line (Zheng *et al.*, 2003). The genetic background of mutant mice, the age of experimental animals at the time of lesioning, differences in experimental procedures, compensatory mechanisms and/or the nature of the mutant allele are among the factors that may account for the discrepant findings in the different Nogo knockout mouse lines.

Evidence for a role of MAG in limiting axonal regeneration in vivo comes from experiments demonstrating enhanced regeneration of peripheral nerves in MAG null mutants that had been crossed with C57BL/Wlds mice to delay the rapid lesion-induced degeneration of PNS myelin (Schafer *et al.*, 1996). In the CNS of MAG-deficient mice, in comparison, one study reported only moderate improvement of CST regeneration (Li, M. *et al.*, 1996), while another study did not find enhanced regeneration of either CST axons in the hemisected spinal cord or retinal ganglion cell (RGC) axons in the intraorbitally crushed optic nerve (Bartsch *et al.*, 1995a). Finally, a recent study has reported that OMgp-deficient mice on a mixed 129/Sv-C57BL/6, but not on a pure C57BL/6, background show enhanced regeneration of serotonergic fibers (but not CST fibers) and improved functional recovery following complete spinal cord transection or dorsal hemi-section (Ji *et al.*, 2008).

Because Nogo, MAG and OMgp all bind to NgR1, targeting this receptor was expected to neutralize a significant fraction of the inhibitory activity of oligodendrocytes and myelin and to result in robust axonal regeneration. Administration of the soluble function-blocking NgR1 ectodomain NgR(310)ecto that competes with endogenous NgR1 for the binding of MAG, Nogo and OMgp indeed promoted regeneration of raphespinal and corticospinal axons and improved locomotor recovery in rats (Li, S. *et al.*, 2004) and mice (Li, S. *et al.*, 2005). Similarly, transgenic expression of a dominant-negative form of NgR1 also robustly promoted regeneration of RGC axons, but only when combined with lens injury to revert RGCs to an active growth state (Fischer *et al.*, 2004). Assessment of the regenerative phenotype of NgR1-deficient mice, in comparison, revealed enhanced regeneration of rubrospinal and raphespinal fibers but not of corticospinal axons (Kim *et al.*, 2004b; Zheng *et al.*, 2005). Compensatory upregulation of other inhibitory pathways in knockout mice and/or additional regenerative effects of neutralizing agents in acute perturbation experiments might account for these discrepant findings (Kim *et al.*, 2004b; Simonen *et al.*, 2003; Teng and Tang, 2005; Zheng *et al.*, 2005). In addition, recent in-culture work has provided evidence that while NgR1 is required for myelin-inhibitor-induced growth cone collapse, chronic neurite growth inhibition might be mediated by an NgR1-independent mechanism, at least for certain types of neurons (Chivatakarn *et al.*, 2007; Kim *et al.*, 2004b; Zheng *et al.*, 2005). Mutant mice lacking multiple inhibitory molecules at the ligand and/or receptor level will eventually help to define more clearly the contribution of myelin-associated inhibitors to the regenerative failure in the mature CNS.

Axon guidance molecules as oligodendrocyte-derived inhibitors of neurite growth

In addition to Nogo, MAG and OMgp, several axon guidance molecules may contribute to the inhibition of axonal regeneration by oligodendrocytes and myelin. For instance, ephrin-B3 is expressed by myelinating oligodendrocytes and accounts for a significant fraction of the inhibitory activity of CNS myelin as shown by culture studies (Benson *et al.*, 2005). Netrin-1 might also function as a myelin-associated inhibitor as netrin-1 is expressed by oligodendrocytes and its repulsive UNC5 receptors are localized to axons in the lesioned adult spinal cord (Manitt et al., 2006). Indeed, blocking of netrin-1 enhances neurite outgrowth from UNC5-positive spinal motor neurons on adult rat spinal cord myelin in culture, and netrin-1-expressing fibroblast grafts inhibit axon regrowth in the lesioned spinal cord in vivo (Low et al., 2008). Furthermore, Sema4D, which repels neurites from cerebellar granule cells and DRG when offered as a substrate in a stripe assay, is transiently upregulated in oligodendrocytes in the injured adult spinal cord near the lesion site (Moreau-Fauvarque et al., 2003). Another semaphorin, Sema5A, is expressed by oligodendrocytes and their precursor cells, but not in CNS myelin. Sema5A induces growth cone collapse and inhibits neurite growth from embryonic and postnatal RGCs, and neutralizing antibodies to Sema5A significantly enhance RGC axon growth on postnatal and adult optic nerve explants (Goldberg et al., 2004). Repulsive guidance molecule A (RGMa) is yet another axon guidance molecule expressed by myelinating oligodendrocytes. Expression of RGMa in the lesioned spinal cord is upregulated around the lesion site, and intrathecal administration of neutralizing RGMa antibodies results in improved regeneration of the corticospinal tract and enhanced locomotor recovery (Hata et al., 2006). The extracellular matrix glycoprotein tenascin-R is also expressed by oligodendrocytes and additionally by some neuronal cell types. Tenascin-R is expressed in the lesioned optic nerve, and strongly inhibits neurite outgrowth of adult RGCs in culture (Becker et al., 2000).

The functional role of myelin-associated inhibitors under physiological conditions is unknown, but it has been hypothesized that they might serve to stabilize the neural circuitry of the adult CNS. Observations that are in line with this view include the sprouting of Purkinje cell axons in normal adult cerebella treated with the IN-1 antibody (Buffo et al., 2000), collateral axon sprouting in OMgp-deficient mice (Huang et al., 2005), or the persistence of ocular dominance plasticity in Nogo-A/B and NgR knockout mice well beyond the critical period (McGee et al., 2005).

Impact of Schwann cells

It is well known that the PNS has a much higher capacity to regenerate lesioned axons than the CNS. There are several glial-related differences that explain the distinct regenerative capacity of the PNS versus the CNS. First, denervated Schwann cells survive axonal transection due to the above-mentioned autocrine survival cues. Second, in the course of the so-called Wallerian degeneration of the distal part of the transected nerve, denervated Schwann cells proliferate, form cellular chains called Bands of Büngner, and de-differentiate, resulting in dramatic changes of the Schwann cells' molecular phenotype, including downregulation of myelin molecules and upregulation of molecules that are normally expressed by immature Schwann cells. Third, alongside these processes, some obstructive structures are relatively quickly removed, such as the myelin, whereas others – preferentially ECM structures such as the Schwann cell basal laminae – are maintained as scaffolds that guide regrowing axons. These features are in marked contrast to the situation in the CNS, where oligodendrocytes that have been deprived of axonal contact degenerate by apoptosis or atrophy (Vargas and Barres, 2007). However, the oligodendrocytic myelin with its associated nerve growth inhibitors remains preserved for extended time periods after axonal injury (Stoll *et al.*, 1989; Vargas and Barres, 2007) which is one of the most significant obstacles for axon regrowth. It is worthwhile mentioning in this context that injury-related myelin removal in the PNS is predominantly mediated by nerve- and blood-derived macrophages (Mueller *et al.*, 2003; Stoll and Muller, 1999), which are activated by a sophisticated communication with the Schwann cells, implicating distinct cytokines, chemokines and other signals (Martini *et al.*, 2008). Such a communication might be missing in the CNS, due to the atrophy and poor survival of denervated oligodendrocytes. In addition, oligodendrocyte-related cues inhibiting the macrophage-activating complement system might prohibit myelin clearance by microglial cells and macrophages (Vargas and Barres, 2007). Additionally, the tumor necrosis factor TNF-α2 from astrocytes might also inhibit macrophage-like cells from phagocytosing myelin (Stoll *et al.*, 2004). Furthermore, oligodendrocytes by themselves appear unable to clear myelin (Stoll *et al.*, 1989; Vaughn and Pease, 1970), whereas Schwann cells are capable of phagocytosing myelin (Fernandez-Valle *et al.*, 1995; Hall, 2005; Stoll *et al.*, 1989).

Expression of Schwann-cell-related nerve growth-promoting molecules and lack of persistent nerve growth inhibitors foster axonal regrowth in the PNS

Schwann cells do have to de-differentiate to allow axon regrowth, as reflected by cross anastomosis experiments showing that mature

Schwann cells in intact nerves are non-permissive for axonal regeneration (Hall, 2005). Early axonal changes after injury are mediated by Ca^{2+}-dependent and Ca^{2+}-independent deterioration of the axolemma and granular disintegration of the axonal cytoskeleton (Coleman and Perry, 2002; George et al., 1995; Vargas and Barres, 2007). Early Schwann cell responses implicate transient activation of ErbB2 receptors on the nodal Schwann cell microvilli and the corresponding downstream signaling via mitogen-activated protein kinase (Guertin et al., 2005). Another molecular cue underlying the switch from mature to immature Schwann cells has recently been identified. Parkinson and colleagues have shown that, in transected nerves, c-Jun mediates the de-differentiation of myelinating Schwann cells into immature ones, probably by inhibiting the myelin-related transcription factor Krox20 (Parkinson et al., 2008). However, the complete mechanism leading from axon damage to the multiple molecular changes observed in axon-deprived Schwann cells remain incompletely understood (Vargas and Barres, 2007). The molecular mechanisms triggering Schwann cell proliferation are also poorly defined, but involvement of erbB2 and the cognate neuregulin ligands has been suggested (Carroll et al., 1997; Vargas and Barres, 2007). Since some experiments suggest that myelin debris might be mitogenic for Schwann cells (Yoshino et al., 1987), it is probable that multiple factors induce Schwann cells to proliferate (Hall, 2005). However, the functional relevance of Schwann cell proliferation is not entirely clear. Blockade of Schwann cell proliferation by mitomycin C leads to impaired nerve regeneration and remyelination (Hall and Gregson, 1974). However, in a genetic approach, absence of cyclin D1 abolished detectable Schwann cell proliferation after injury, but the functional recovery and myelination of regrown axons was similar in mutant mice and control mice (Yang et al., 2008). Paradoxically, the typical shortening of internodal length that is indicative of a numerical Schwann cell increase was not altered in cyclin D1-deficient mice (Yang et al., 2008).

During and after Wallerian degeneration, the injured axons regrow in a particular microcompartment, namely the interface between the Schwann cell surface and the inner aspect of the Schwann cell basal lamina (Ide et al., 1983; Martini, 1994; Martini and Schachner, 1988; Scherer and Easter, 1984). This at least partially reflects the presence of the nerve growth-promoting components in the peripheral nerve, comprising Schwann cell-related molecules and distinct ECM components. Among such components, the cell adhesion molecules L1 and ninjurin have been identified as possible Schwann-cell-related mediators of axon regrowth (Araki and Milbrandt, 1996; Martini, 1994). Of note, these components are not expressed/upregulated in axon-deprived oligodendrocytes. Furthermore, the basal lamina component laminin is an important mediator of axon regrowth (Cornbrooks et al., 1983). Among the ECM components, tenascin-C, which is strongly upregulated after injury, may also contribute to the nerve growth-promoting features of the injured peripheral nerve (Martini, 1994), but it is also possible that it "retains" the axons within the scaffold of the basal lamina. Remarkably, there are multiple trophic factors and cytokines that are upregulated by Schwann cells of injured nerves that may also foster regeneration. Among those, NGF, BDNF, GDNF and IGF might be the most relevant outgrowth-related neurotrophic factors in the injured peripheral nerve (Chen et al., 2007b; Heumann et al., 1987; Stoll and Muller, 1999; Sulaiman et al., 2005; Vargas and Barres, 2007), while cytokines and chemokines, such as IL-6, LIF, TNFα, IL-1 and MCP-1, are also relevant, partially for fostering axon growth and partially for macrophage recruitment (Martini et al., 2008; Stoll and Muller, 1999; Sulaiman et al., 2005; Tofaris et al., 2002). Thus, the upregulation of secreted and membrane-bound nerve growth-promoting components by Schwann cells may create a highly regeneration-promoting environment for damaged axons. Because of these nerve growth-promoting properties of denervated Schwann cells, the peripheral glia cells are considered as a suitable and promising cell type for autologous grafts to foster axonal regrowth after CNS damage (Bunge and Pearse, 2003; Pearse et al., 2004), or to remyelinate axons in demyelinating disorders of the CNS (Kocsis and Waxman, 2007; Lavdas et al., 2008; Papastefanaki et al., 2007; Woodhoo et al., 2007).

Another important issue is the absence of growth-inhibitory myelin constituents in the distal stump of injured peripheral nerves where axons are "ready to go." While Nogo-A is not detectable on Schwann cell surfaces, it is a potent inhibitor of axon regeneration in the PNS when experimentally and constitutively expressed on Schwann cells (Pot et al., 2002). Among the inhibitory molecular cues in the PNS, Schwann cell basal lamina-related chondroitin sulfate proteoglycans (CSPGs) might be a relevant component of axon growth inhibition (Hall, 2005). However, along with the reactive changes during Wallerian degeneration, Schwann cells upregulate matrix metalloproteinases that digest CSPGs and thus abolish or attenuate these inhibitory components (Hall, 2005; Zuo et al., 1998).

MAG is a constituent of the axon-related aspect of the Schwann cell myelin and of the abaxonal compartment that is theoretically on the "route" of the regrowing axons (Hall, 2005; Martini and Schachner, 1986). However, the inhibitory role of MAG is not very relevant to axon regrowth in the PNS due mainly to two reasons: (1) Schwann cells express only 10% of the amount of MAG found in oligodendrocytes and downregulate myelin molecules after injury (Schachner and Bartsch, 2000), and, more importantly, (2) Schwann-cell-related MAG molecules are rapidly removed after nerve injury in the course of Wallerian degeneration and are, thus, usually not "seen" by the regrowing axons (Vargas and Barres, 2007). Additionally, culture experiments suggest that neurite-outgrowth-promoting ECM components might override the inhibitory function of MAG (David *et al.*, 1995). That MAG theoretically could be a significant inhibitor of axonal regeneration in the PNS has been demonstrated in MAG-deficient/Wlds mice which, as mentioned above, are characterized by a delayed clearance of myelin and thus exposed to MAG for a prolonged time in the lesioned peripheral nerve (Schafer *et al.*, 1996). Thus, although MAG has no obvious nerve growth-inhibitory relevance in lesioned nerves of normal animals, it has another interesting function in the lesioned PNS that is related to phagocytosing macrophages. After Wallerian degeneration and removal of myelin debris by macrophages, repulsive MAG molecules on the surface of the new myelin are instrumental in "cleaning" the endoneurial tubes of NgR-positive macrophages thus terminating the inflammatory conditions in the repaired endoneurial tube (Fry *et al.*, 2007).

Schwann-cell-related limitations in peripheral nerve regeneration: long-term denervation and pathway cues

One of the major problems in peripheral nerve regeneration is the regeneration distance, particularly in proximal nerve lesions of larger individuals (e.g. humans). Based on an axonal regrowth rate of approximately 0.5–1 mm/day, the consequence of long regeneration distances is that distal aspects of lesioned nerves become reinnervated relatively late after the insult. Long-term denervation of Schwann cells leads to Schwann cell atrophy and possibly to loss of nerve-growth-promoting Schwann cell basal laminae, resulting in the halt of regeneration and the failure of functional reconstitution (Hoke, 2006).

Another limiting aspect of peripheral nerve regeneration concerns pathway specificity, particularly in injured mixed nerves with completely disrupted endoneurial tubes. However, there is clear evidence for Schwann-cell-related pathway specificity in peripheral nerves. In a series of elegant experiments combining sophisticated nerve surgery and retrograde labeling techniques, Brushart developed the concept of "preferential motor reinnervation" by motoneurons after pruning of erroneously grown motor axons into sensory nerves (Brushart, 1993, 1990). This concept is in line with the observation that the HNK-1-carbohydrate epitope fosters neurite outgrowth of cultured motor neurons and that motor-axon-associated Schwann cells express the epitope in mouse peripheral nerves and roots (Martini *et al.*, 1992; Martini and Schachner, 1988). Interestingly, cross-anastomosis experiments revealed that – with regard to post-lesion HNK-1 expression – Schwann cells appear to maintain a "memory" of their previous association with motor axons (Martini *et al.*, 1994). Moreover, short-term electrical stimulation of lesioned and surgically repaired femoral nerves leads to a BDNF/TrkB-dependent motor-nerve-specific enhancement of HNK-1 expression and to an acceleration of muscle reinnervation (Eberhardt *et al.*, 2006). In addition, Schwann cells in motor nerves and ventral roots express higher levels of GDNF and pleiotrophin than sensory nerves and dorsal roots, which express more BDNF and NGF (Hoke *et al.*, 2006). These combined observations suggest that Schwann cells express distinct motor- versus sensory-related phenotypes that may be relevant to appropriate pathway selection of regrowing axons.

ROBERT H. MILLER

3
_____

Control of oligodendrocyte development and myelination in the vertebrate CNS

INTRODUCTION

The oligodendrocyte lineage is among the best studied and most well understood of all the lineages in the vertebrate central nervous system (CNS). Oligodendrocytes are the cells responsible for the formation of CNS myelin. Structurally compact as distinct from non-compact myelin appears as concentric wraps of modified plasma membrane that ensheathe individual lengths, i.e. internodes, of neuronal processes or axons, that connect neurons with their targets. This compact internodal myelin is discontinuous as each of the up to 50 oligodendrocyte processes forms only one internode. The myelination by the oligodendrocyte processes results in accelerated conduction of signals along the axons and lowering of the threshold for propagating such signals. In the adult CNS, myelination is critical for the normal functioning of the CNS such that diseases and injury that result in the loss of myelin lead to functional deficits. The ability to isolate and grow cells in culture that will generate oligodendrocytes has allowed researchers to understand some of the fundamental steps that lead from a neural stem cell to a myelinating oligodendrocyte in the adult CNS. The identification of oligodendrocyte-lineage-specific cell surface molecules, growth factor receptors and transcription factors has facilitated the labeling and manipulation of the lineage both in vivo and in culture. These studies have revealed extensive plasticity in the development of oligodendrocytes and provided critical insights into the behavior of oligodendrocytes and their oligodendrocyte precursor cells during development in a variety of different regions of the CNS as well as under a number of pathological conditions. This chapter will review the major recent advances

The Biology of Oligodendrocytes, eds. Patricia J. Armati and Emily K. Mathey. Published by Cambridge University Press. © Cambridge University Press 2010.

in the understanding of oligodendrocyte development in the context of classical knowledge.

INDUCTION OF THE FOUNDER CELLS
OF THE OLIGODENDROCYTE LINEAGE

Oligodendrocyte precursors and stem cells

During early vertebrate embryonic development a defined region of the dorsal epithelium becomes specified to generate the neural tube, which ultimately gives rise to the vast majority of cells in the central and peripheral nervous systems. The specification of this region is a consequence of patterning that occurs at the time of gastrulation and establishes the major axis of the developing organism. Within the CNS classical studies defined three major classes of cells: *neurons*, electrically excitable cells that form the interconnecting networks that underlie all CNS function; and two classes of macroglial cells, namely *astrocytes*, star-shaped cells that provide trophic support and structural organization in the CNS, and *oligodendrocytes*, the myelinating cells of the CNS. All three cell types are derived from the original cells of the neural tube as a result of periods of coordinated cell induction, proliferation and differentiation. Early studies suggested that the first wave of cells to emerge from the neural tube were neurons, followed by astrocytes and then oligodendrocytes (Jacobson, 1978). While generally correct, studies over the last two decades have indicated that, perhaps not surprisingly, CNS development is more dynamic and complex than previously thought. One of the most surprising insights from studies on the cellular and molecular control of neural development is that many of the cells of the early neural tube possess characteristics of stem cells (Gage, 2000; Reynolds and Weiss, 1992). For example, they appear to be self-renewing and multipotent as well as capable of generating all major classes of neural cells (Gage, 2000). Even more remarkable is that some neural cells retain these stem-cell-like properties into adulthood (Reynolds *et al.*, 1992).

The realization that the developing CNS contained cells with the self-renewing, multipotent characteristics of stem cells led to an intense search for instructive cues that guide the fate choices of neural stem cells. The most common approach to address these issues is to generate neurospheres (Reynolds and Weiss, 1992). When neural tissue is dissociated into single cells and these cells are grown in a medium supplemented with epidermal growth factor (EGF) and basic fibroblast growth factor (bFGF) under conditions where adherence to the substrate is minimal the vast majority of cells die. However, a small proportion of the cells survive and go on to proliferate and generate a floating sphere of cells. Plating the neurospheres on an adherent substrate allows for the differentiation of sphere-derived cells into the three major classes of neural cells. Such spheres can be passaged repeatedly without losing their potential to generate neurons, astrocytes and oligodendrocytes. The best interpretation of these studies is that the founding cell(s) of the neurosphere is a neural stem cell that can be repeatedly subcloned. Among the cell types that develop from such neurospheres are oligodendrocyte progenitor cells (OPCs) that will differentiate into oligodendrocytes, the myelinating cells of the CNS. Surprisingly, since myelin is largely localized to white matter regions of the CNS, the vast majority of neurospheres derived from virtually every region of the neural tube have the capacity to generate oligodendrocytes in culture (Hall and Miller, 2004). These studies suggest that the potential to give rise to cells of the oligodendrocyte lineage is ubiquitously distributed throughout the developing CNS.

Localized origins of oligodendrocyte precursors

The ability to identify the founder cells of the oligodendrocyte lineage in embryos of multiple species has allowed a detailed description of the timing and localization of their appearance (Ono *et al.*, 1995, 1997; Orentas and Miller, 1996; Pringle and Richardson, 1993). Given that neurospheres from most regions of the CNS can generate oligoden-drocytes in culture it was somewhat unexpected to find that during normal development in vivo the appearance of the earliest detectable OPCs was restricted to specific regions of the neural tube (Orentas and Miller, 1996; Pringle and Richardson, 1993). In the developing spinal cord for example, the founder cells of the oligodendrocyte lineage arise in a distinct location at the ventral midline directly dorsal to the floor plate (Figure 3.1). Much later in development a second smaller source of OPCs arises from a discrete location in the dorsal spinal cord (Cai *et al.*, 2005). Other regions of the germinal zone do not appear to give rise to oligodendrocytes although they generate both neurons and astrocytes. In more rostral regions of the CNS similar discrete sources of OPCs have been defined (Spassky *et al.*, 1998). These include the floor of the third ventricle, which generates a subset of cells that migrate down the optic nerve (Gao and Miller,

BMP

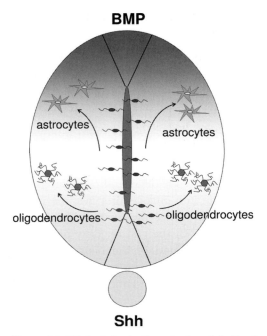

Shh

Figure 3.1 Glial origins in the spinal cord. In the developing vertebrate spinal cord the earliest OPCs arise in a distinct region of the ventral ventricular zone and subsequently migrate throughout the tissue. Other more dorsal regions of the germinal zone generate the majority of astrocytes. Distinct subtypes of neurons arise from distinct domains of the germinal zone with motor neurons sharing a common source with oligodendrocytes. BMP, bone morphogenetic protein; Shh, sonic hedgehog. See color plate section for color version of this figure.

2006), and the medial ganglion eminence (Perez Villages *et al.*, 1999; Spassky *et al.*, 1998; Timsit *et al.*, 1995), which contributes oligodendrocytes to particular domains of the CNS. More recent studies indicate that distinct populations of oligodendrocytes arise in different regions of the mouse forebrain at distinct times (Kessaris *et al.*, 2006) and that their progeny subsequently intermingle.

In the developing vertebrate spinal cord the earliest oligodendrocyte precursors arise in a distinct region of the ventral ventricular zone and subsequently migrate throughout the tissue. Other more dorsal regions of the germinal zone generate the majority of astrocytes. Distinct subtypes of neurons arise from distinct domains of the germinal zone with motor neurons sharing a common source with oligodendrocytes.

Extracellular cues controlling the initial appearance of OPCs

The localized appearance of the earliest OPCs is a reflection of local signals that control stem cell fate. In the spinal cord some of the molecular signaling controlling the initial appearance of OPCs has been defined. Positive cues that promote the appearance of OPCs include the morphogen sonic hedgehog (Shh) (Orentas *et al.*, 1999; Orentas and Miller, 1996; Pringle *et al.*, 1996). During early development Shh is expressed in the notochord, a transient mesodermal structure located ventrally to the developing neural tube (Jessell, 2000). The high concentrations of Shh released by the notochord influence adjacent cells in this ventral neural tube to develop into motor neurons and subsequently OPCs (Jessell, 2000; Rowitch, 2004). It is thought that the graded signaling of Shh from the notochord and overlying floor plate establishes a series of ventral to dorsal domains in the ventricular zone in which precursor cells become specified for distinct cell fates such as motor neurons and different classes of interneurons (Jessell, 2000). In dorsal regions of the caudal neural tube similar domains are established from the roof plate ventrally that give rise largely to sensory interneurons. The dorsal domains do not generate oligodendrocytes until much later in development and then only in small numbers (Cai *et al.*, 2005). One mechanism that appears to inhibit the dorsal development of OPCs is the localized expression of bone morphogenetic proteins (BMPs), specifically BMP4 (Gomes *et al.*, 2003; Miller *et al.*, 2004). The BMPs are members of the transforming growth factor beta superfamily and signal through the Smad pathways. Initial culture studies implicated BMPs in inhibiting oligodendrocyte development, and they appear to antagonize the inductive signaling of Shh (Gomes *et al.*, 2003; Miller *et al.*, 2004). It seems likely however that several pathways facilitate the appearance of OPCs. For example, neurosphere studies have demonstrated that in hedgehog-null preparations, OPCs can be induced and that this appears to depend on bFGF signaling. Likewise there are likely to be several mechanisms that antagonize OPC induction including signaling through the Wnt pathways.

One common theme that emerges from the in-vivo studies is that the initial appearance of OPCs is highly localized. This localization is not only the consequence of gradients of signaling molecules such as Shh but also reflects interactions between the inducible precursor cells and neighboring (inducer?) cells. Several lines of evidence are consistent with this hypothesis. At the cellular level, oligodendrocyte precursors that ultimately generate at least a subpopulation of oligodendrocytes in the optic nerve are derived from a distinct rostral/caudal portion of the floor of the third ventricle (Gao and Miller, 2006). These cells or their progeny then migrate along the nerve toward the retina (Gao and Miller, 2006; Prestoz et al., 2004). During their migration the cells proliferate, differentiate and ultimately myelinate the retinal ganglion cell axons. The appearance of the founder cells in the floor of the third ventricle has been proposed to be dependent on the ingrowth of retinal ganglion cell axons. In vivo there is a spatial and temporal correlation between the appearance of OPCs in the floor of the third ventricle and axonal growth to the region (Gao and Miller, 2006) and removal of retinal axons results in reduced numbers of OPCs generated in this region. More direct evidence for axonal induction of OPCs comes from culture studies where, in compartmental culture systems, retinal ganglion cell axons in the absence of any soluble signals from the cell body were able to induce oligodendrocytes in tissues such as dorsal spinal cord (Figure 3.2) (Gao and Miller, 2006). This induction required signaling by Shh and possibly another axonal expressed protein neuregulin 1 (Vartanian et al., 1999) as well as additional ill-defined factors. The notion that axons are competent to induce OPCs from naïve tissue is an attractive idea since they represent the ultimate target for the progeny of OPCs. Whether all axons have the capacity to induce OPCs or whether this is a characteristic of only those neurons that express Shh remains to be determined.

Relationships between oligodendrocytes, astrocytes and neurons

An unusual characteristic of OPCs is that at least in culture they have the capacity to generate a specific population of astrocytes in addition to myelinating oligodendrocytes (Raff et al., 1983). Purification of OPCs from the rat optic nerve showed that when grown in the presence of serum additives these cells rapidly developed into astrocytes positive for glial fibrillary acidic protein (GFAP$^+$ astrocytes) and lost the capacity to generate oligodendrocytes (Raff et al., 1983). For this reason these cells were termed oligodendrocyte-type-2 astrocyte progenitors (O-2A cells) (Raff et al., 1983). While it is clear that OPCs can give rise to astrocytes in culture the capacity of O-2A cells to generate astrocytes in the developing brain has proven controversial

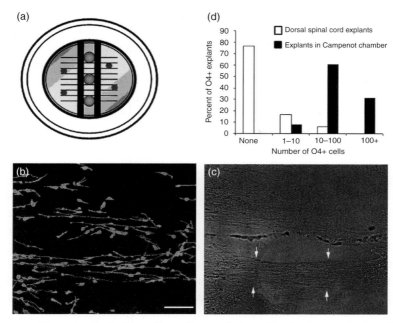

Figure 3.2 Retinal ganglion cell axons induce oligodendrocytes in dorsal spinal cord. (a) A representation of the culture conditions. The green circles represent retinal explants placed in the central chamber whose axons grow through a barrier into the lateral chambers where the blue circles represent dorsal spinal cord explants grown on the axons. (b) OPCs (green) develop in large numbers (c) adjacent to the axons. (d) Quantitation of the results. See color plate section for color version of this figure.

(Miller, 2002). Recent studies using cell lineage reporters have, however, provided good evidence that both during normal development (Goldman *et al.*, 1986) and in response to some neural injuries OPCs generate a subset of astrocytes that might contribute to CNS responses to injury.

Transcriptional control of OPC induction

The localized origin of oligodendrocytes allowed for the identification of distinct transcription factors that are associated with different stages of oligodendrogenesis (Rowitch, 2004). Perhaps the most well studied of the transcription factors involved in the early development of OPCs are the olig genes: olig1 and olig2 (Lu *et al.*, 2000, 2002). These genes encode basic helix proteins and, as the name implies, they are essential for the development of the oligodendrocyte lineage. Detailed analysis of the role of the olig genes suggests that they also contribute to the development of particular populations of neurons. In the spinal cord for example, the domain that generates motor neurons also generates OPCs and both appear to be dependent upon the expression of olig2. Olig1 and olig2 have similar but non-overlapping roles during CNS development. In the absence of olig2, oligodendrocytes are completely absent from the spinal cord but are present in hindbrain and forebrain. The development of these cells is dependent upon olig1. See Rowitch (2004) for an excellent review of these issues.

Precisely how the olig genes regulate cell fate during development is not entirely clear. In the spinal cord the domain that gives rise to oligodendrocytes also gives rise to motor neurons and it seems likely that these two cell types are derived from a common precursor. One attractive hypothesis to explain the function of the olig genes is that the olig proteins act as transcriptional repressors that shut off proteins that antagonize the development of motor neurons and oligodendrocytes and that this inhibition of repressors allows for the emergence of the targeted cell types (Rowitch, 2004). Whether this repression model is correct and operates throughout the neural tube is currently unclear. Other transcription factors that have been implicated in the development of OPCs include Nkx2.2 (Kitada and Rowitch, 2006) and Sox10 (Kitada and Rowitch, 2006). The timing at which these transcription factors operate appears to be complex. For example, expression of olig2 and Nkx2.2 promotes an ectopic expression of oligodendrocytes in the chick spinal cord. The interaction between olig2 and Nkx2.2 appears to be predominantly active at later stages in the oligodendrocyte lineage, where it likely controls differentiation, namely the transition of OPCs to oligodendrocytes. In the absence of Nkx2.2 oligodendrocytes fail to develop, presumably because this factor is part of the regulatory mechanism that controls oligodendrocyte differentiation. Thus, Nkx2.2 is a complex transcription factor in the oligodendrocyte lineage where early on it contributes with olig2 to promote the induction of OPCs and later regulates the differentiation of those OPCs to oligodendrocytes. Similarly, Sox10 appears to be important for the maturation of OPCs but, in contrast to Nkx2.2 and olig2, Sox10 is not required for the initiation of OPCs. A complete understanding of the transcriptional control of oligodendrocyte is lacking and it seems likely there are other major regulatory pathways that have yet to be defined.

Are all oligodendrocyte precursors equivalent?

Several lines of evidence suggest that oligodendrocytes are not a homogenous population of cells. Morphological studies demonstrate that in white matter regions such as the optic nerve an individual oligodendrocyte may myelinate up to 60 different internodes of individual axons in the spinal cord, while in the ventral spinal cord some oligodendrocytes myelinate only a single axon. Likewise, it remains unclear whether the OPCs derived from the dorsal spinal cord (Cai et al., 2005) are destined to myelinate a specific population of axons. In the forebrain, it appears that the origin of OPCs does not simply dictate where their progeny will ultimately reside. During development three distinct waves of OPCs are generated in a ventral to dorsal temporal gradient (Kessaris et al., 2006). The earliest born cells migrate dorsally where they intersperse with later arising dorsally derived cells (Kessaris et al., 2006). Somewhat surprisingly those cells that develop earliest appear to be eliminated during later development. These findings have led to the proposal that there is competition between different pools of oligodendrocytes for a limited number of target axons (Richardson et al., 2006). This notion of competition for limiting target-derived signals may be similar in concept to the mechanisms by which distinct pools of neurons are matched to their targets.

REGULATION OF OLIGODENDROCYTE PRECURSOR PROLIFERATION AND MATURATION

The ability to isolate OPCs from the developing CNS permitted the identification of a series of reproducible stages through which OPCs mature during their progression from an immature OPC to a myelinating oligodendrocyte. In the rodent, the earliest clearly identifiable OPCs are bipolar, highly motile cells that express antigens on their surface recognized by the monoclonal antibody A2B5 (Figure 3.3a). These cells also express NG2 antigens although the precise correlation between NG2$^+$ and A2B5$^+$ cells remains unresolved (Baracskay et al., 2007). With further maturation, OPCs become what are known as prooligodendrocytes (Bansal and Pfeiffer, 1992) and develop immune reactivity to a series of antigens recognized by the mAb O4 termed POA. The O4$^+$ (Figure 3.3b) cells rapidly become multiprocessed and non-motile. Differentiation into oligodendrocytes is marked by expression of galactocerebroside (O1) (Raff et al., 1978), cessation of proliferation and the expansion of an arborization of processes (Figure 3.3c).

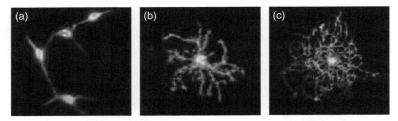

Figure 3.3 Biochemical and morphological characteristics reveal
distinct stages in OPC development. (a) Immature OPCs are bipolar
and express cell surface antigens recognized by the mAb A2B5.
(b) Pro-oligodendrocytes are multiprocessed and express antigens
recognized by the mAb O4. (c) Differentiated oligodendrocytes are
non-proliferative, have a small cell body with many processes and
express galactocerebroside, a major myelin lipid, on their surface.
See color plate section for color version of this figure.

While originally defined in tissue cultures, labeling of tissue sections
of developing rodent CNS suggests that similar stages of maturation
occur in the CNS and the oligodendrocytes then myelinate following
upregulation of expression of the major myelin proteins such as
myelin basic protein (MBP) and proteolipid protein (PLP).

Major mitogens for oligodendrocyte precursors

A remarkable array of growth factors has been shown to influence the
biology of OPCs both in culture and in vivo. Perhaps the best characterized of OPC mitogens is platelet-derived growth factor A (PDGF-A)
that stimulates OPC proliferation through binding to PDGF receptor
α (PDGFRα) (Richardson et al., 1988). The expression of PDGFRα is
often used as a defining characteristic of OPCs and it is clearly
expressed on the majority of OPCs at least at some stage in their
development (Pringle et al., 1992).

A second class of growth factors important for oligodendrocyte
development is formed by the FGFs. The initial indication that FGFs
might play a role in oligodendrocyte development came from culture
studies in which a combination of PDGF and bFGF was shown to
promote the continuous proliferation of OPCs and to inhibit their
differentiation (Bogler et al., 1990). This approach has been used in
the intervening time as a mechanism for generating large numbers
of OPCs. The precise nature of the cells generated following exposure
to PDGF and bFGF in culture may not be identical to that of cells

arising during normal development (Bansal and Pfeiffer, 1997). Indeed, treatment of more mature oligodendrocytes with bFGF has been proposed to cause reversion to a more immature phenotype (Bansal and Pfeiffer, 1997; Grinspan et al., 1993). More recent studies suggest multiple roles for different members of the FGF family and their receptors in the development of oligodendrocytes, including regulating survival and proliferation at specific stages in the lineage (Fortin et al., 2005). Several other growth factors have been implicated in the development of oligodendrocytes including insulin-like growth factor (IGF) (McMorris and Dubois-Dalcq, 1988; Zeger et al., 2007) and thyroid hormone (Franco et al., 2008; Harsan et al., 2008). How these different signals integrate together to regulate OPC development and whether a hierarchy or temporal requirement for mitogenic stimulation exists remain to be determined.

MIGRATION OF OLIGODENDROCYTE PRECURSORS DURING DEVELOPMENT

The finding that OPCs initially arise in specific domains of the ventricular zone of the CNS and yet their progeny are widely disseminated throughout the adult brain and spinal cord indicates the critical requirement for dispersal of the progenitor cells. Unlike migrating neurons or their growth cones, the targeting of OPC migration is less critical since they simply have to populate regions rich in axons. The ability to specifically identify OPCs in culture and in vivo has allowed their dispersal and migration to be studied in culture and in fixed and living tissue (Tsai et al., 2002, 2003, 2006). Multiple factors have been implicated in regulating the migration of OPCs. In some cases these factors simply promote extensive motility, while in other cases they act as chemoattractants or chemorepellents to guide the directive migration of precursor cells throughout the CNS. For example, Eph and ephrins have been proposed to regulate the migration of OPCs down the optic nerve (Prestoz et al., 2004). Perhaps the best characterized regulator of OPC migration is PDGF. Culture studies demonstrate that PDGF is a strong chemoattractant for OPCs from multiple regions of the CNS and is strongly implicated in facilitating the widespread dispersal of these cells. It seems likely, however, that PDGF is not directing OPCs to particular locations. It is relatively ubiquitously distributed throughout the CNS and consequently appears to act as a general dispersal cue or simply to promote motility (Frost et al., 2009). In the spinal cord, several studies have implicated Netrin-1 as a chemorepellant for OPCs (Tsai *et al.*, 2003, 2006). In the absence of netrin-1, OPCs are generated but fail to disperse throughout the CNS and remain concentrated at their source of origin around the central neural canal.

The signaling pathways that regulate OPC migration are less well understood. In the case of PDGF it is clear that ligand binding to the alpha receptor promotes migration of progenitor cells and recent studies indicate that transient stimulation of the PDGF receptor is sufficient to promote a long-lasting migratory response. This response appears to be mediated through the MAP kinase pathways (Frost *et al.*, 2009). The specific mitogen activated protein (MAP) kinase signaling cascade that regulates precursor migration has yet to be defined and recent studies have implicated p38 MAP kinase in the regulation of OPC migration (Haines *et al.*, 2008). Not all migratory events are dependent upon similar signaling pathways. Indeed, signaling through GABA(B) receptors on OPCs has been implicated in promoting the migration of those cells (Luyt *et al.*, 2007) while activation of the sphingosine 1-phosphate receptor (sip5) has been implicated in inhibiting OPC migration (Novgorodov *et al.*, 2007). In the case of netrin-1 regulation, a critical role for DCC (i.e. the netrin-1 receptor called deleted in colorectal cancer) in mediating the chemorepulsive cue has been identified and it seems likely that an additional, and as yet unidentified, receptor is required to fulfill that event (Tsai *et al.*, 2003). The involvement of additional non-receptor tyrosine kinases such as Fyn has been proposed to modulate OPC migration, particularly in response to the phosphorylation of WAVE2 (Miyamoto *et al.*, 2008). The role of WAVE proteins in both migration and myelination of OPCs is an area of emerging interest. Overall, the broad spectrum of regulators of OPC migration suggests that multiple environmental cues mediate the ability of these cells to disperse throughout the CNS. It seems likely that the control of migration of OPCs is going to be closely linked to their ability to proliferate and undergo cell division. Emerging studies have demonstrated a critical association between effective migration and localized proliferation of OPCs in the developing spinal cord (Tsai *et al.*, 2009).

The final localization of OPC to presumptive white matter reflects the arrest of OPC migration that is mediated by stop signals. One such signal appears to be the local expression of the chemokine CXCL1 by a subset of astrocytes (Tsai *et al.*, 2002). In the absence of CXCR2, the receptor for CXCL1, OPCs continue to migrate and fail to effectively populate spinal cord white matter resulting in long-term functional deficits (Padovani-Claudio *et al.*, 2006).

Intrinsic timers of oligodendrocyte differentiation

Studies on OPCs from the optic nerve suggest that the switch from a proliferative precursor cell to a non-proliferative differentiated oligodendrocyte can be regulated in large part by intrinsic timing mechanisms (Temple and Raff, 1986). Classical studies using clonal analysis revealed that OPCs separated early in their proliferative phase and, grown separately, generated clones of similar sizes that differentiated synchronously (Temple and Raff, 1986). These studies raise the possibility that the induction of differentiation is established by cell intrinsic timers. Subsequent studies in the optic nerve have provided molecular substrates for such inductive timers. These include regulators of the cell cycle, such as p21 and p57. How an intrinsic mechanism modulates cell differentiation is not entirely clear. However, it has been proposed that mitogenic signaling cascades may be diminished with each cycle such that, ultimately, the progenitor cell ceases division and differentiates constitutively. Support for this hypothesis comes from studies in which removal of growth factors drives precocious differentiation of OPCs and the continued proliferation in the presence of PDGF and FGF (Bogler *et al.*, 1990).

Recent studies suggest that in the intact nervous system regulation of OPC differentiation is a reflection of both intrinsic and extrinsic cues. One emerging area of interest is the role of epigenetic factors in controlling oligodendrocyte differentiation. Culture studies have suggested that HDAC1 is a critical modulator of genes that regulate oligodendrocyte differentiation. Manipulation of HDAC1 results in altered timing of oligodendrocyte appearance both in culture and in vivo.

The signaling cascades that regulate this phenomenon have yet to be resolved. It is clear, however, that multiple external cues influence the differentiation of OPCs. In high-density cultures and in vivo, clonally derived OPCs do not differentiate synchronously. While some cells retain characteristics associated with early oligodendrocytes, others undergo extensive myelination. Whether such cells express similar proliferative histories is not clear. Thus it may be that local

exposure to growth factors drives a proliferative response and precocious myelination in some cells while sister-derived OPCs have yet to
achieve the capacity to differentiate.

While clearly an understanding of oligodendrocyte differentiation awaits further study it seems likely that early OPCs are intrinsically refractory to signals that promote differentiation. With further
maturation these cells become susceptible to differentiative cues.
Should such cells be present, they would then be capable of undergoing
terminal differentiation. It seems likely that the genesis of adult
OPCs reflects the interplay between the intrinsic cues and extrinsic
signals that regulate oligodendrocyte differentiation.

CONTROL AND MECHANISMS OF MYELINATION IN THE CNS

The control of the onset of myelination

Several factors are likely to control the onset of CNS myelination.
Traditionally it was believed that the trigger to myelinate an axon
was when the axon reached a specific diameter. This simple notion is
probably incorrect since axons with a wide range of diameters are
myelinated. Furthermore, myelination itself alters axonal diameter,
thus myelinated axons are larger because they are myelinated. It
seems likely that the trigger to form myelin has at least three components. The axon has to have achieved a level of maturation at which
myelination can be initiated, the oligodendrocyte has to be competent
to engage the myelination machinery and there has to be a release
of inhibitory cues that block myelination. While specific signals
such as neuregulin-1 have been identified that modulate the levels
of myelination, at least in the periphery (Vartanian et al., 1997),
the axonal competence cues in the CNS are unknown. Likewise the
instructive signal that activates the myelination program in mature
oligodendrocytes remains to be defined. One area in which there
has been recent progress is the definition of signals that inhibit or
block myelination. Several candidates have emerged including the
notch-Delta pathway, the expression of the polysialylated form of
the neural cell adhesion molecule (PSA-NCAM) and the transmembrane
glycoprotein LINGO-1 (Mi et al., 2005, 2007). Reducing expression of
LINGO-1 drives precocious myelination in culture and in vivo and
inhibiting LINGO-1 binding promotes remyelination in models of
demyelination (Mi et al., 2005, 2007). It seems likely that controlling

the timing of myelination is important since myelin is inhibitory for axonal growth and precocious myelination might severely impair subsequent connectivity by later born neurons.

The mechanisms of myelination

The cellular mechanisms that result in the formation of compact myelin in the CNS remain obscure. The rapid generation of myelin requires the coordinated synthesis and assembly of a range of proteins and lipids, and how this is regulated at the level of individual oligodendrocytes is not well understood. The formation of myelin requires cellular motility and this may reflect the formation of a leading process that enwraps an axon and then a compaction phase in which residual cytoplasm is eliminated and the inner and outer membrane leaflet fuse. Currently this model is speculative as there is no effective model of CNS myelination in culture that allows for careful analysis of the active process.

CONSEQUENCES FOR MYELIN REPAIR

One emerging focus for the studies on oligodendrocyte development is the potential to influence the progression of demyelinating diseases such as multiple sclerosis (MS). In MS, areas of the brain and spinal cord are subject to attack from specific cells of the immune system and a major consequence is that myelin is lost, resulting in a lack of axonal conduction. Studies in development have begun to reveal some of the critical pathways that regulate the initial formation of myelin and it seems likely that myelin repair will have similar regulatory steps. The ability to influence CNS myelination in both positive and negative directions will lead to the development of new therapeutic strategies for myelin repair in the future.

GRAHAME KIDD AND BRUCE D. TRAPP

4

Molecular organization of the oligodendrocyte and myelin

INTRODUCTION

Oligodendrocytes are remarkable cells. In vertebrate evolution, the advent of oligodendrocytes and myelination transformed the CNS by allowing fast and energy efficient communication between neurons, ultimately fostering the evolution of animals with complex, highly integrated motor, sensory and cognitive functions. In humans, myelination underlies most of the early developmental neurological milestones, and new myelination continues to be important into the third and fourth decades. Human diseases involving oligodendrocyte dysfunction are devastating, and those such as multiple sclerosis (MS) account for a significant proportion of neurological disease. Since the first studies of myelin protein biochemistry in the late nineteenth century, myelin proteins and lipids have received intense experimental investigation. Extensive reviews of the biochemistry, genetics, immunogenicity and localizations of the major myelin proteins and lipids have been published. Recent genomic and proteomic studies have begun to provide a complete list of myelin and oligodendrocyte-enriched molecules. The goal of this chapter is to consider the contributions of different myelin proteins and lipids to (1) the structure of central nervous system (CNS) myelin, (2) the cell biology of myelin formation and (3) their roles in vital interactions between oligodendrocyte and axons. The emerging picture of oligodendrocyte myelination is a process that is extremely fault tolerant and inextricably intertwined with axonal function.

OLIGODENDROCYTES HAVE A HIGHLY POLARIZED SHAPE

Few cells have as extreme a shape as myelinating oligodendrocytes. Before discussing their molecular organization, it is therefore important

The Biology of Oligodendrocytes, eds. Patricia J. Armati and Emily K. Mathey. Published by Cambridge University Press. © Cambridge University Press 2010.

to have a clear picture of oligodendrocytes and their myelin membranes. Mature oligodendrocytes have modestly sized cell bodies (Figure 4.1) with cell processes that extend radially from the cell body. Although evident in the preparations of del Rio Hortega and Penfield (Penfield, 1924), confocal microscopy of mouse oligodendrocytes expressing green fluorescent protein permits the tracing of fine oligodendrocyte processes in three dimensions (Figure 4.1). The processes branch frequently to contact lengths of a number of axons – up to 50 – with each process spiraling around its region of axon to form the complex "internode." The major biosynthetic organelles of the secretory pathway such as the rough endoplasmic reticulum (RER) and Golgi apparatus are concentrated in the cell body and proximal processes. The number of processes and their orientation depend upon the axons being myelinated. Oligodendrocytes myelinating small axons in the cortex have numerous fine processes (Figure 4.1a), while those myelinating fewer, larger axons in striatum have a small number of well-defined processes (Figure 4.1c). An oligodendrocyte producing a single myelin internode on a large spinal motor axon may have only a few processes that all wrap helically around the outer margin of the myelin internode (Figure 4.1b), superficially resembling the uncompacted paranodal loops of myelinating Schwann cells (see also Chapter 1).

Myelin internodes are an extension of the oligodendrocyte plasma membrane that is partitioned into a systematic patchwork of biochemically and functionally diverse membrane domains. Compact myelin comprises the majority of the myelin internode and, as the

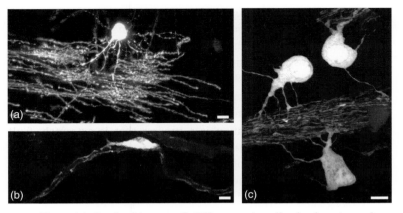

Figure 4.1 Confocal images of eGFP-expressing oligodendrocytes and their processes from (a) cortex, (b) spinal cord, and (c) striatum. eGFP, enhanced green fluorescent protein. Scale bar 10 μm.

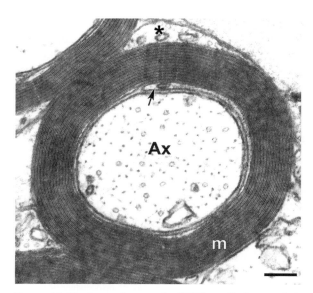

Figure 4.2 Electron micrograph of CNS myelin internode in transverse section. Ax, axon; m, compact myelin; arrow, inner oligodendrocyte tongue process; *, outer oligodendrocyte tongue process. Scale bar 0.1 μm. Reproduced from Tabira *et al.* (1978) with permission.

term "compact" suggests, contains little cytoplasm (Figure 4.2). Non-compact myelin membranes encompass several different membrane domains, including Schmidt–Lanterman incisures, the paranodal loops (Figure 4.3, asterisks), the adaxonal membrane and inner mesaxon (Figure 4.2, arrow indicates inner tongue process), and the abaxonal membrane and outer mesaxon of the outer tongue process (Figure 4.2, asterisk). Non-compact regions retain cytoplasm that is continuous with that in the cell body. These cytoplasmic regions serve as conduits for vesicular transport and sites of protein synthesis by free ribosomes. The complex interrelationships between myelin internodal regions and the oligodendrocyte cell body can be easily visualized as an "unrolled" membrane expansion (Figure 4.4), although this configuration does not occur in vivo. Each internode is effectively a large, flat, sheet-like expansion of the oligodendrocyte plasma membrane. A central, cytoplasm-free region of compacted plasma membrane forms the compact myelin. Around the margins of compact myelin, cytoplasm-filled channels are retained and these form inner and outer tongue processes and paranodal loops. Paranodal loops are so named because, although they are a continuous rim of cytoplasm-containing oligodendrocyte (Figure 4.4), when rolled around the axon cylinder and

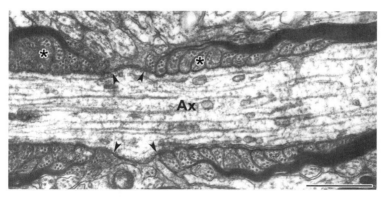

Figure 4.3 Electron micrograph of CNS node in longitudinal orientation. Ax, axon; *, paranodal loops. Arrowheads define nodal region. Scale bar 1 μm. Reproduced from Peters *et al.* (1991) with permission.

examined by electron microscopy (EM) in longitudinal section, they appear as loops (Figure 4.3 asterisk). Midway along each internode, the outer tongue process connects to a somatic branch from the oligodendrocyte cell body. In this way, newly synthesized molecules and biosynthetic organelles such as mitochondria can be transported to different areas of the myelin internode using the cytoplasmic channels as conduits. These cytoplasmic channels may also participate in ion and metabolite redistribution. Plasma membrane subdivision into different domains is not unique to oligodendrocytes, but while most cells have a few distinct types of surfaces (e.g. apical and basolateral in epithelial cells), oligodendrocytes, like myelinating Schwann cells, are unusual in having at least five.

From Figure 4.4, it should also be apparent that oligodendrocytes are extremely large cells with substantial surface areas. The ultimate size and area of each oligodendrocyte depends on the internodal size and number of internodes produced. Morphological data indicate that oligodendrocytes myelinating small axons (1.5 μm) produce internodes of ~200 μm length with about 20 lamellae. Typically, these oligodendrocytes myelinate 30–50 axons and have a total myelin surface area of ~1.5 mm² (Blakemore, 1981; Hildebrand *et al.*, 1993). Figure 4.4 depicts such an oligodendrocyte drawn to scale. Oligodendrocytes ensheathing large (10 μm) axons produce only a single internode that may be 1250 μm long and have more than 120 wraps, with a total surface area of ~14 mm². By comparison, absorptive epithelial cells have surface areas around 0.002 mm². The number of internodes formed by each oligodendrocyte is regulated by the

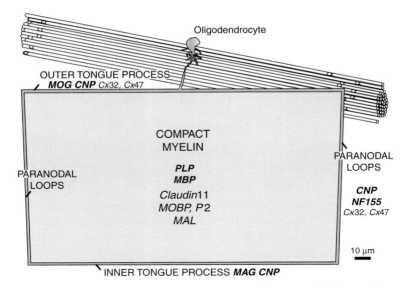

Figure 4.4 Summary diagram of an oligodendrocyte and its internodes, including an "unrolled" internode with localization of major myelin proteins indicated. CNP, 2′,3′-cyclic nucleotide 3′-phosphodiesterase; MAG, myelin-associated glycoprotein; MAL, myelin and lymphocyte protein; MBP, myelin basic protein; MOBP, myelin oligodendrocyte basic protein; MOG, myelin oligodendrocyte protein; PLP, proteolipid protein. Drawn to scale. Scale bar 10 μm.

axons it surrounds (Blakemore, 1981; Hildebrand *et al.*, 1993) in addition to their myelin length and thickness, i.e. number of lamellae (discussed below in "Molecular mechanisms of myelin membrane formation"). Formation of multiple myelin internodes is a major difference between oligodendrocytes and Schwann cells, which produce only a single internode (see Chapter 2), and is a characteristic that greatly reduces the number of cells required for myelination of the CNS compared with the peripheral nervous system (PNS), minimizing the space occupied by their nuclei and cell bodies.

Schwann cell internodes also have prominent and regularly spaced Schmidt–Lanterman incisures, which are cytoplasmic channels through areas of compact myelin. Incisure-like structures that resemble PNS incisures have been identified in some larger CNS myelin internodes (Blakemore, 1969), but are rare among smaller CNS internodes and little is known about their molecular composition.

MOLECULAR COMPOSITION OF MYELIN
AND OLIGODENDROCYTE MEMBRANES

In common with all plasma membranes, myelin is composed of a lipid bilayer augmented by intrinsic and extrinsic proteins. Nevertheless, CNS myelin membranes are biochemically unique. Purified myelin (mainly compact myelin) has 50% and 75% less total protein than plasma membranes from erythrocytes and liver cells, respectively (Guidotti, 1972) and products of two genes make up 80% of dry weight protein. As compact myelin serves primarily as insulation, a lipid-rich membrane with a few small proteins and no bulky ion pumps, metabolite transporters, or cytoskeletal-anchoring proteins is appropriate. Localization of the major and several minor myelin proteins is illustrated in Figure 4.4.

Myelin lipid composition is also unusual. Much richer in cholesterol than most biological membranes [up to 50%, (Norton and Cammer, 1984)], myelin is also characteristically enriched with galactose-containing glycolipids. Galactosylceramide (GalC; cerebroside) and sulfatide make up 20–30% of myelin membrane (Norton and Cammer, 1984). Oligodendrocytes switch to expression of UDP-galactose:ceramide galactosyltransferase (CGT) during development as progenitors in vivo. Myelin lipids also contain saturated very long chain fatty acids, which reduce membrane fluidity and may balance the fluidizing effect of cholesterol and other unsaturated lipids. As Schwann cells also express galactosyl lipids, these lipids were thought to be selectively important for myelin assembly or maintenance. Mice null for CGT or for cerebroside sulfotransferase (CST) (Bosio et al., 1998; Dupree et al., 1998), which catalyzes conversion of GalC to sulfatide, produced ample compact myelin, although abnormalities occurred at the region of the paranode and mice suffered neurological deficits (Bosio et al., 1998; Dupree et al., 1998; Honke et al., 2002; Marcus et al., 2000). The other major myelin lipid is cholesterol, which provides fluidity to compact myelin membranes. Mice whose oligodendrocytes were deficient in squalene synthetase, a key enzyme in cholesterol biosynthesis, showed greatly reduced numbers of myelinated axons and fewer myelin lamellae (Saher et al., 2005). With increasing age, the extent of myelination increased as exogenous cholesterol was recruited to the compact myelin. The normal stoichiometry of cholesterol to other lipids was preserved in squalene-synthetase-null myelin. These results suggest that, in contrast to galactolipids, cholesterol is essential for myelination and cholesterol levels are rate-limiting. Detailed distributions for myelin proteins have been constructed from immunostaining, but lipids distributions are less amenable to staining in vivo. For this reason, few details are available regarding lipid distributions in specific membrane domains.

Compact myelin and roles of the major myelin proteins

Most of the myelin internode consists of compact myelin. By EM, compact myelin is characterized by a lamellar structure of alternating dark and light lines that spiral around the axon (Figures 4.2, 4.5). In the compacted spiral, apposing extracellular leaflets called intraperiod or intermediate lines (IPL) are separated by 2.0 nm in the CNS (Figure 4.5). The intracellular leaflets appear fused and form the major dense lines (MDL). The spiral membranes of compact myelin have a periodicity (distance from dense line to dense line) of approximately 13–14 nm when fixed with aldehydes, which is slightly less than in PNS myelin. Extracellular spacing in compact myelin is unusually narrow for cell–cell contact, which is normally of the order of 20 nm or more. Partly this may reflect the absence of large carbohydrate-containing proteins on the compact myelin membrane surface. The extreme regularity of the lamellar spacing suggests adhesion between proteins in extracellular leaflets. In peripheral nerves and in the CNS of lower vertebrates, homotypic adhesion of immunoglobulin gene (Ig) superfamily adhesion molecule P0 in both *cis* and *trans* binds apposing membrane leaflets together at both

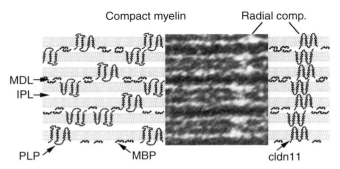

Figure 4.5 Major CNS myelin proteins showing organization in the membrane lipid bilayer. cldn11, claudin-11; IPL intraperiod line; MBP, myelin basic protein; MDL, major dense line; PLP, proteolipid protein.

extracellular and intracellular faces. In oligodendrocyte myelin, a combination of proteins maintains myelin structure, utilizing largely electrostatic forces rather than adhesive binding.

The most abundant CNS myelin protein is the *proteolipid protein (PLP)*. At ~30 kDa, PLP is a comparatively small protein. PLP is a hydrophilic protein with four membrane-spanning domains and both the amino and carboxy termini reside in the cytoplasm (Figure 4.5) (reviewed by Griffiths *et al.*, 1998a; Lees, 1998). The PLP gene has alternative transcription start sites and an abundant alternative splice form called DM20. DM20 predominates early during initial myelin wrapping but is much less abundant than PLP in mature compact myelin. DM20 lacks a 35-amino-acid segment of the internal peptide loop (Macklin *et al.*, 1987a; Nave *et al.*, 1987). Both PLP and DM20 are rendered additionally hydrophobic by acylation (Agrawal *et al.*, 1982; Bizzozero *et al.*, 1986) through palmitoylation or addition of oleate or stearate fatty acids. PLP has six acylation sites (Weimbs and Stoffel, 1992), two of which are present in the extra amino acids not found in DM20. Fatty acylation may serve in targeting proteins to compact myelin (discussed in the next section) and may impose order on surrounding membrane lipids. The prominence of PLP in CNS myelin suggested adhesive functions for PLP, but in-culture adhesion studies and protein structure comparisons indicate that PLP/DM20 is not likely to be a major adhesion protein (Timsit *et al.*, 1992). Furthermore, rodents expressing PLP mutations that reduce or eliminate PLP in compact myelin (Duncan *et al.*, 1988; Griffiths *et al.*, 1998b; Klugmann *et al.*, 1997) produce compact myelin that is not radically disrupted (Figure 4.6a), except for either fusion of the extracellular leaflets (Klugmann *et al.*, 1997) (Figure 4.6d) or separation by >2 nm. PLP-null myelin is prone to IPL splitting due to osmotic challenge (Rosenbluth *et al.*, 2009). The primary structural role of PLP in compact myelin therefore appears to be to maintain a constant close spacing between extracellular leaflets, which may involve weak electrostatic interactions with itself or myelin lipids. Human patients and rodents that lack PLP ultimately develop pronounced neurological deficits that result from axonal defects and degeneration (Edgar *et al.*, 2004; Garbern *et al.*, 2002; Griffiths *et al.*, 1998b; Klugmann *et al.*, 1997; Yin *et al.*, 2006). The roles of and significance for PLP in axonal maintenance are discussed in the later section entitled "Reciprocal interactions between oligodendrocytes and axons regulate myelination and promote axonal survival".

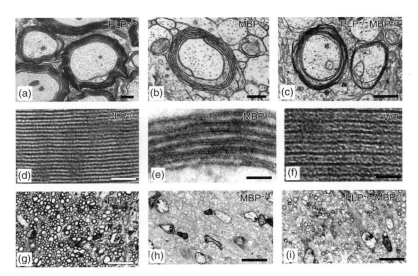

Figure 4.6 Consequences of myelin protein loss on myelin ultrastructure (a–f) and extent of myelination (g–i) for oligodendrocytes lacking PLP (a,d,g), MBP (b,e,h), both MBP and PLP (c,i) and WT (f). Scale bars a–c = 0.5 µm, d–f = 25 nm, g–i = 10 µm. Reproduced from (Uschkureit *et al.*, 2000) (a, g), (Kwiecien *et al.*, 1998) (b); (Stoffel *et al.*, 1997) (c,e,h,i) and (Duncan *et al.*, 1988) (d,f) with permission.

Myelin basic proteins are the other major compact myelin protein component. A family of small proteins varying from 14 to 21.5 kDa (Barbarese *et al.*, 1978; Zeller *et al.*, 1984), MBPs are generated from a single gene by alternative splicing. MBP transcripts come from a larger gene structure, called GOLLI (gene of the oligodendrocyte lineage), which generates transcripts unrelated to MBP mRNAs and may serve regulatory roles in other cells, but does not appear to be expressed in oligodendrocytes (Campagnoni *et al.*, 1993). MBPs are extrinsic membrane proteins of compact myelin and are localized at the intracellular surface of compact CNS and PNS myelin (Figure 4.5) (Omlin *et al.*, 1982). In MBP-deficient *shiverer* myelin, the intracellular leaflets of compact CNS myelin are not fused (Figure 4.6b,e) (Privat *et al.*, 1979). MBPs therefore maintain the major dense line of CNS myelin. Regardless of splicing, MBPs have a high percentage of charged amino acids, with a net excess of basic amino acids. The inner leaflets of many membranes are negatively charged and MBPs may interact with the membrane through this means. In addition, MBPs also have hydrophobic stretches, which may partly insert into the myelin membrane. MBPs are heavily phosphorylated along most of their length (Carnegie *et al.*, 1974; Miyamoto *et al.*, 1974) and arginylation, citrullination and methylation have all been described (see review by Boggs, 2006). The charges and phosphorylation sites on MBPs allow them to interact not only with myelin membranes but also potentially with a large number of positively charged proteins, and roles in the nucleus and the cytoskeleton have also been suggested (see review by Boggs, 2006).

Of all the myelin proteins identified so far, MBPs appear to be the most critical to sustained spiral growth. In *shiverer* mutant mice and Long Evans *shaker* rats, genetic defects that prevent MBP synthesis result in axonal ensheathment with minimal spiral growth (Figure 4.6b) and fewer myelinated axons than PLP-null tissue (Figure 4.6g and h) (Kwiecien *et al.*, 1998; Privat *et al.*, 1979; Readhead *et al.*, 1987). A single MBP cDNA transgene rescues the mouse *shiverer* phenotype (Kimura *et al.*, 1989) establishing that classic MBPs, rather than GOLLI transcripts, are required and that the effect is not dependent on multiple splice forms or intronic sequences. Alone, these observations seem to suggest a direct structural requirement for MBP in spiral growth. However, when the *shiverer* defect was bred into PLP-null (Figure 4.6c,f,i) or PLP-null/MAG-null mice (Stoffel *et al.*, 1997; Uschkureit *et al.*, 2000) substantial spiral membranes were produced in the absence of both MBP and PLP. This suggests that a regulatory mechanism for coordinating PLP and MBP production exists, in which spiral growth is inhibited when PLP is present but MBP is absent.

Several other less abundant compact myelin proteins have also been identified, and many are either four-pass transmembrane proteins like PLP or small basic proteins with similarities to MBPs. *Myelin-oligodendrocyte basic proteins (MOBPs)* are a family of small (7–14 kDa) proteins produced by a single gene (Holz *et al.*, 1996; Yamamoto *et al.*, 1994). As their name suggests, they are positively charged and are found at the MDL like MBPs. They are abundant but they cannot compensate for loss of MBPs, and their functions remain unknown (see review by Montague *et al.*, 2006). P_2 *protein* is another extrinsic protein that is enriched at the MDL in PNS myelin and is also detected in CNS myelin of rabbits, humans, cattle and horses (Trapp *et al.*, 1983), though not in the CNS of mice or rats. P_2 belongs to a family of proteins that function in fatty acid transport. In the CNS of those species that contain P_2 protein it is abundant in spinal cord and brainstem myelin but not in cerebral cortex myelin. Reasons for this heterogeneous distribution and indeed the functions of P_2 in myelin remain a mystery. *Myelin and lymphocyte (MAL, VIP17/MVP17) protein* is a tetraspan protein enriched in compact myelin (Frank, 2000;

Schaeren-Wiemers *et al.*, 1995) and in other cells. In epithelial cells MAL associates with glycolipid-rich membranes and contributes to protein targeting (Cheong *et al.*, 1999). Its role in compact myelin is unclear. *Tetraspanin family member CD9* is expressed by oligodendrocytes and enriched in myelin membranes (Kagawa *et al.*, 1997; Terada *et al.*, 2002a) and may associate with other tetraspanins, Tspan 2 and Tspan 81. Mice lacking CD9 have no CNS myelin-related phenotype, although PNS paranodal effects were observed (Ishibashi *et al.*, 2004).

Radial component of compact CNS myelin

The radial component is often overlooked ultrastructurally because it is not contrasted by conventional EM preparations, but when ideally prepared it appears in transverse sections as registered lines of intralamellar junctional complexes that extend partially or totally across the thickness of the myelin sheath (Figure 4.7a). Radial components resemble tight junctions in that extracellular leaflets appear fused (Figure 4.5). Visualized in longitudinal orientation, radial components are also in register and extend from paranode to paranode. The major dense line shows little variation in the radial component (Figure 4.5). In the mature myelin internode, radial components are common beneath the outer tongue process and often extend to the inner tongue process, which frequently lies in the same quadrant (Figure 4.7a,b). Where adjacent myelin internodes make contact, the

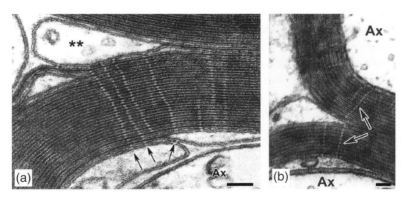

Figure 4.7 Radial component of compact myelin (arrows) traverses compact myelin from inner mesaxon to outer mesaxon (a). Radial components in adjacent internodes are aligned (b, arrows). Ax, axon; **, outer tongue process. Scale bars 0.1 μm. Reproduced from (Tabira *et al.*, 1978) with permission.

radial components often align with each other between internodes (Figure 4.7b). In certain pathological conditions such as hexachlorophene (HCP) or triethyl tin intoxication, white matter edema develops and large intramyelinic vacuoles appear from the splitting of the extracellular leaflets of compact CNS myelin (Tabira *et al.*, 1978). These myelin vacuoles remain tethered to the axons in the area of the inner tongue process where a tight-junction-like radial component is present (Tabira *et al.*, 1978). Thus the molecules that make up the radial component provide focal points of lamellar adhesion that extend longitudinally along the compact myelin.

Assembly of the radial component depends on *Claudin-11* (also called oligodendrocyte-specific protein, OSP), a 22-kDa protein that constitutes ~7% of CNS myelin protein (Gow *et al.*, 1999; Morita *et al.*, 1999) (Figure 4.5). Like PLP, the claudins are integral membrane proteins with four transmembrane domains and cytoplasmically oriented amino- and carboxy-termini. Unlike PLP, the claudins adhere with one another between adjacent plasma membranes and are capable of binding both homotypically and heterotypically in *cis* and *trans* (Krause *et al.*, 2008). They are common components of tight junctions, and claudin-11 is also found in tight junctions between oligodendrocyte cell bodies, between paranodal loops (below) and in other cells, including epithelial cells of the ependyma and testis (Gow *et al.*, 1999). Superficially the radial component resembles a tight junction, but neither an ultrastructural cytoplasmic plaque nor the tight junction complex proteins such as ZO-1 are detectable elements of the radial component. The close registration of radial components between myelin lamellae of even different internodes suggests that the protein interacts both extracellularly and intracellularly. Claudin-11-null mice exhibit few phenotype or myelin defects (Gow *et al.*, 1999), but mice that lack both claudin-11 and PLP/DM20 have a severe phenotype (Chow *et al.*, 2005) that features prominent IPL separation, suggesting that one or the other is required to stabilize compact myelin during spiral growth.

Non-compact myelin domains and axonal organization at the node

Non-compact myelin membrane domains include the paranodal loops, periaxonal membrane and the abaxonal membrane, and they are fundamental to saltatory conduction. Non-compact membranes are key sites of interaction with the axonal surface (Figure 4.8).

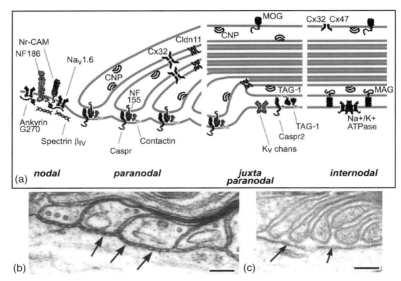

Figure 4.8 Localization of proteins in CNS non-compact myelin membranes and their axonal binding partners (a). EM of wild-type node (b) illustrates septate paranodal junctions (arrows) and their loss in contactin-null mice (c). Cldn11, claudin-11; CNP, 2′,3′-cyclic nucleotide 3′-phosphodiesterase; Cx, connexin; MAG, myelin-associated glycoprotein; MOG, myelin oligodendrocyte protein; TAG-1, transient axonal glycoprotein-1. Scale bar = 0.1 μm. Reproduced from (Bosio *et al.*, 1998) (b) and (Boyle *et al.*, 2001)(c) with permission.

Although contiguous with compact myelin, non-compact membranes differ ultrastructurally and have distinct mutually exclusive protein compositions (Figure 4.8a). While compact myelin features small four-pass proteins with modestly sized extracellular domains, non-compact myelin domains are often characterized by the presence of large adhesion molecules with substantial extracellular projections. Mixing of proteins between compact and non-compact domains does not normally occur. Some non-compact myelin proteins serve more generalized functions and are enriched in multiple non-compact membranes, while others perform specialized functions at one particular site.

One protein common to all non-compact myelin regions is *2′,3′-cyclic nucleotide 3′-phosphodiesterase (CNP)*, an extrinsic membrane protein (Figures 4.4, 4.8a) (Braun *et al.*, 1988; Trapp *et al.*, 1988). CNP consists of two highly basic proteins of 46 kDa (CNP1) and 48 kDa (CNP2) produced as multiple transcripts and alternative splicing from a single gene. They are modified by carboxy-terminal isoprenylation and also by fatty acylation, and these post-translational modifications mediate interaction with the inner leaflet of the non-compact membranes. As its name implies, CNP is capable of catalyzing the hydrolysis of 2',3' nucleotides into their corresponding 2' nucleotides; however a CNS substrate for this enzymatic activity has not been identified. CNP may interact with cytoskeletal components, and CNP promotes process outgrowth when transfected into COS-7 cells (Lee et al., 2005). Absence of CNP expression does not inhibit initial CNS myelination, and myelin internodes exhibit a largely normal ultrastructure of compact and non-compact membranes (Lappe-Siefke et al., 2003). Delayed paranodal disruption does occur (Rasband et al., 2005), however, and is followed by widespread and progressive axonal swelling (Lappe-Siefke et al., 2003). When overexpressed in oligodendrocytes in mice, CNP is mislocalized to compact CNS myelin membranes and compaction is prevented (Yin et al., 1997). These membranes are deficient in MBP and do not form major dense lines. CNP therefore may help target MBP to compacting myelin membranes and serve to prevent compaction of an MDL in regions where cytoplasm is required.

Non-compact CNS myelin membranes also commonly contain connexins, which are channel-forming proteins found in gap junctions. Products of several different genes, connexins are four-pass transmembrane proteins which, like PLP, have carboxy- and amino-termini in the cytoplasm. Connexins homo- and heterodimerize into connexons, which are hemi-junctional complexes of six connexins that are capable of binding connexons in apposing membranes to form gap junctions between cells (Orthmann-Murphy et al., 2008). Oligodendrocytes express at least three connexins: Cx32, Cx47 and Cx29 (Dermietzel et al., 1989; Li, J. et al., 1997; Micevych and Abelson, 1991; Nagy et al., 2003; Rash et al., 2001; Scherer et al., 1995). Different connexins have different distributions in oligodendrocytes. Cx32 is the best characterized and is found on the membranes of the oligodendrocyte cell body, at the paranodes and some abaxonal membranes (Kamasawa et al., 2005; Kleopa et al., 2004). Cx47 localizes to cell bodies, processes and the outer tongue process. Cx32 and Cx47 are present in ultrastructurally defined gap junctions between oligodendrocytes and astrocytes and in reflexive junctions between apposing paranodal loops (Figure 4.8a). Mutations in Cx32 cause X-linked Charcot–Marie–Tooth disease (Bergoffen et al., 1993; Bruzzone et al., 1994), a heritable dysmyelination of the human PNS, but central myelination continues in the absence of either Cx32 or Cx47 in knockout mice (Menichella *et al.*, 2003; Scherer *et al.*, 1998), although some compact myelin vacuolation was reported in Cx47 knockout mice (Odermatt *et al.*, 2003). Animals lacking both Cx32 and Cx47 die as neonates with thin or absent CNS myelin sheaths (Menichella *et al.*, 2003). Mutations affecting Cx47 cause human Pelizaeus–Merzbacher-like disease (Orthmann-Murphy *et al.*, 2008; Uhlenberg *et al.*, 2004). Connexin-based gap junctions mediate exchange of ions and small molecules between oligodendrocytes and astrocytes. This is likely to be very important for oligodendrocytes, as there is little extracellular space around individual internodes in white matter tracts, which presumably impedes metabolite and ion exchange via extracellular pathways. Reflexive gap junctions between oligodendrocyte compartments may also facilitate ion exchange (described below).

The nodal region

Unlike Schwann cells, oligodendrocytes do not extend their cellular processes into the nodal gap, but in other ways oligodendrocytes are integral to node formation. As illustrated in Figure 4.8a, the nodal axolemma contains voltage-gated Na^+ channels and is especially enriched for the $Na_v1.6$ isoform (Black *et al.*, 1990). Na^+ entry through these channels in response to an action potential generates the sudden voltage drop that results in channel opening at the next node, thereby propagating the signal along the axon. Nodal membrane contains other proteins as well, including the adhesion protein neurofascin186 (NF186) (Davis *et al.*, 1996; Tait *et al.*, 2000) and Nr-CAM (Grumet *et al.*, 1991; Moscoso and Sanes, 1995). Nodal axolemma is characterized electron microscopically by the dense, 20-nm-thick layer beneath the axolemma (Figure 4.3), which represents a specialized submembranous cytoskeleton. This submembranous cytoskeleton contains two alternately spliced isoforms of the ankyrin$_G$ (270 and 480 kDa) (Kordeli *et al.*, 1990, 1995), spectrin βIV (Berghs *et al.*, 2000; Lacas-Gervais *et al.*, 2004) and f-actin (Kordeli *et al.*, 1990). Ankyrin$_G$ associates with Na^+ channels in the neuronal cell body and assists in targeting Na^+ channels to the node (Bennett and Lambert, 1999; Kordeli *et al.*, 1995). Oligodendrocyte contact is essential to node formation and maintenance. Without oligodendrocytes, the nodal channels diffuse laterally into the internodal plasma membrane (Black *et al.*, 1990; Craner *et al.*, 2003, 2004) and $Na_v1.6$ is replaced by $Na_v1.2$, an isoform associated with continuous rather than saltatory conduction. It is unknown precisely how oligodendrocytes promote node formation, but it is presumed to involve interactions between paranodal membranes triggering signaling kinase cascades within the axoplasm that promote dynamic cytoskeletal assembly/reorganization subadjacent to the nodal axolemma.

Paranodal loops

As compact myelin approaches the node, the major dense line "opens up" to accommodate cytoplasm (Figure 4.3, 4.8a,b). A characteristic lateral spacing of 12–14 nm is maintained between paranodal loop extracellular leaflets, but the molecular basis for this is unclear; unlike PNS paranodal membranes, there is no myelin-associated glycoprotein (MAG, see below) or E-cadherins in the paranodal loops. CNP is present but is not essential for paranodal loop formation (Lappe-Siefke et al., 2003); it may, however, contribute to paranodal maintenance (Rasband et al., 2005). GalC and/or sulfatide are important for paranodal loop formation, as major paranodal abnormalities are detected in CGT- and CST-null mice (Dupree et al., 1998, 1999), which are unable to make one or both glycolipids. Paranodal defects include reversed paranodal loops, nodal widening and heminode formation (Dupree et al., 1998, 1999) and absence of paranodal junctions with the axonal surface. Glycolipids have been suggested to act as ligands for axonal receptors, as mediators of protein targeting (below), or as structural lipids, but their precise functions are unclear at this time. Autotypic reflexive junctions are present between adjacent paranodal loops. Claudin-11-containing tight junctions tether the lateral paranodal loop membranes to each other (Gow et al., 1999; Morita et al., 1999; Schnapp and Mugnaini, 1976) (Figure 4.8a). Tight junctions are assumed to prevent extracellular entry of ions into compact myelin and they may structurally support the paranodal loops. Gap junction component Cx32 is also present and forms Cx32/Cx32 channels (Kamasawa et al., 2005; Kleopa et al., 2004) between adjacent paranodal loops (Figure 4.8a). The significance of these gap junctions has been debated, but evidence suggests that they facilitate passage of small ions, particularly K^+, between adjacent loops, creating a "short-cut" between the juxtaparanodal and nodal compartments (Kamasawa et al., 2005; Kleopa et al., 2004).

   Where the paranodal loops appose the axolemma adjacent to the node, evenly spaced densities connect the two membranes

(Figure 4.8b). Originally called transverse bands, these densities represent a septate-like junctional complex and are a major adhesive apparatus between the abaxonal membrane of the oligodendrocyte process and the axolemma (Einheber *et al.*, 1997; Peters *et al.*, 1991). The septate axoglial junction between the paranodal loops and axolemma serves at least two purposes. It creates a diffusion barrier that impedes passage of nodal ions to the internodal periaxonal space and it also compartmentalizes the molecules in the axonal surface. The major oligodendrocyte component of the axoglial septate junctions is *Neurofascin 155* (NF155), which is also found at Schwann cell paranodal loop membranes (Charles *et al.*, 2002b; Tait *et al.*, 2000) with a different isoform NF186– on the axolemma (see also Chapter 3). A 155-kDa member of the Ig superfamily of adhesion molecules, NF155 has homology with the neural adhesion molecule L1 and structurally resembles primitive septate junction proteins in drosophila (Tait *et al.*, 2000). It is a single-pass transmembrane protein with an extensive extracellular domain containing multiple immunoglobulin-like repeats and fibronectin-type-III repeats. NF155 is produced by alternate splicing of the neurofascin gene, which also produces neuronal NF186. At septate junctions, the extracellular domain of NF155 interacts with axonal binding partners *contactin and Caspr* (Contactin associated protein, also called paranodin) on the axon surface (Charles *et al.*, 2002b; Einheber *et al.*, 1997; Menegoz *et al.*, 1997; Rios *et al.*, 2000; Tait *et al.*, 2000) (Figure 4.8a). Contactin is a 135-kDa neural Ig superfamily cell adhesion molecule that is anchored to the axonal surface through a glycosylphosphatidylinositol (GPI) link (Ranscht and Dours, 1988). Contactin interacts in *cis* with Caspr (Cross *et al.*, 1994; Einheber *et al.*, 1997; Menegoz *et al.*, 1997), which is a 180-kDa single-pass transmembrane protein. Caspr, Contactin and NF155 form a trimeric adhesion complex across the axo-glial space (Figure 4.8a). Axo-glial junctions are abnormal or missing in transgenic animals in which Caspr or contactin are absent (Bhat *et al.*, 2001; Boyle *et al.*, 2001) (Figure 4.8c). Protein 4.1B is a cytoskeletal protein that binds to Caspr and is required for normal paranodal structure (Denisenko-Nehrbass *et al.*, 2003; Gollan *et al.*, 2002), suggesting that it acts as an intracellular scaffolding protein.

Juxtaparanodal regions

This region is defined as the 10–15 μm of the myelin internode that lies adjacent to the paranodal loops. Undistinguished by transmission

EM, freeze-fracture EM identified clusters of intramembranous particles in the juxtaparanodal axolemma. By immunostaining, these correspond to the location of shaker-type delayed rectifier K^+ channels. K^+ channels in myelinated axons include $K_v1.1$, $K_v1.2$ and their associated subunit β_2 (Rasband *et al.*, 1998). Some evidence suggests that an additional axo-glial complex may participate in localizing K^+ channels there. *Transient axonal glycoprotein-1 (TAG-1)* is a GPI-anchored Ig superfamily protein related in structure to contactin (Furley *et al.*, 1990) that co-localizes with K^+ channels. TAG-1 is present at juxtaparanodal membranes in both axons and oligodendrocytes (Figure 4.8a) and appears to interact homotypically in *trans* between the membranes. Within the axolemma, TAG-1 interacts with another Caspr isoform, Caspr2, which is also restricted to the juxtaparanodal region (Poliak *et al.*, 1999; Traka *et al.*, 2002). In TAG-1-deficient mice (Traka *et al.*, 2003), Caspr2 failed to localize to juxtaparanodal regions and K^+ channels were reduced in concentration and had a less restricted, paranodal distribution. K^+ channels in the juxtaparanodal region are thought to play a role in saltatory conduction by rectifying the membrane potential after Na^+ channel opening during action potential propagation, thus facilitating rapid, repetitive firing of the action potential. They may also prevent retrograde propagation of the action potential. Topologically, the juxtaparanodal oligodendrocyte membrane is the paranodal margin of the adaxonal inner tongue process and may also contain MAG.

Adaxonal membrane and internodal axolemma

The innermost tongue of the oligodendrocyte of CNS internodes ensheathes the axolemma for the entire internode. It includes the inner mesaxon and is uncompacted with its cytoplasm containing occasional organelles. In developing CNS fibers this inner wrap of the oligodendrocyte process extends around the entire circumference, but in mature CNS fibers much of the inner myelin wrap forms a major dense line with the spirals of the compact myelin lamellae. The inner surface of CNS myelin internodes is separated from the axon by a periaxonal space of 12–14 nm. The inner tongue process is also enriched for CNP and microfilaments (Trapp *et al.*, 1988) but is best characterized by the presence of MAG (Figures 4.4, 4.8a) (Sternberger *et al.*, 1979; Trapp *et al.*, 1989).

Myelin-associated glycoprotein (MAG) is a type I integral membrane glycoprotein consisting of a single transmembrane domain, a cytoplasmic carboxy-terminal, and five immunoglobulin-like domains. MAG is alternatively spliced to generate two developmentally regulated polypeptides of MW 72 kDa (L-MAG) and 67 kDa (S-MAG) (Arquint et al., 1987) which differ at the carboxy-terminal. Glycosylation increases the mass of the mature proteins to about 100 kDa. L- and S-MAG differ in their cytoplasmic domains which, as discussed in the section entitled "Molecular mechanisms of myelin membrane formation", likely contain protein targeting or sorting sequences. In the CNS, L-MAG is more abundant than S-MAG during the early stages of myelination, whereas L- and S-MAG are present at approximately equal amounts in mature CNS myelin internodes. MAG-containing uncompacted oligodendrocyte membranes are characterized by 12–14 nm apposition with other membranes and by the absence of an MDL. Thus MAG is positioned to interact with the axon and participate in maintaining the periaxonal compartment. Structurally MAG is a cell adhesion molecule of the Ig superfamily (Salzer et al., 1987). It is also a member of the siglec family of sialic acid binding proteins (Kelm et al., 1994) and designated as siglec-4. MAG has been shown to recognize sialylated glycans (Kelm et al., 1994) and to bind axonal gangliosides. Experiments with MAG-null mice (Li, C. et al., 1994; Montag et al., 1994) produce modest morphological changes and little initial phenotype. The periaxonal collar is lost from MAG-null CNS internodes except at the inner tongue process, and some myelin internodes develop aberrant overlapping morphologies (Bartsch et al., 1995b; Li, C. et al., 1994; Montag et al., 1994). Interestingly, mice lacking neuronal GM2/GD2 synthetase, an enzyme necessary for ganglioside GD1a and GT1b production, have similar defects of myelination (Sheikh et al., 1999). MAG may participate in establishing or maintaining intermembranous spacing.

The underlying internodal axolemma is enriched for Na^+/K^+ ATPases $\alpha 1$ and $\alpha 3$ (Figure 4.8a) (Mata et al., 1991; Young et al., 2008). On axons from MS lesions, the Na^+/K^+ ATPase distributions become continuous along the entire demyelinated segment, suggesting that oligodendrocytes play a role in restricting ATPase from nodal axolemma. Na^+/K^+ ATPases are essential for normal neuronal functioning. By exporting three Na^+ ions and importing two K^+ ions from the extracellular environment, they restore the gradients of Na^+ and K^+ across the plasma membrane following action potential firing. Internodal localization places them, like juxtaparanodal K^+ channels, beneath compact myelin. K^+ released into the periaxonal space can be efficiently recovered through Na$^+$/K$^+$ ATPase exchange, with Na$^+$ entering the axoplasm at the node. What happens to the Na$^+$ pumped into the periaxonal space is unclear, however, and may suggest active roles for the oligodendrocyte in Na$^+$ clearance.

The abaxonal membrane and outer tongue process

Central nervous system myelin internodes have a single external cytoplasmic channel, within the outer tongue process, which occupies 5–20% of the outer (abaxonal) myelin internode circumference (Figures 4.2, 4.4) and runs longitudinally the length of the internode (Figure 4.4). The remaining circumference of the outer myelin spiral appears identical to all other compact myelin lamellae, including a major dense line. In addition, the outer membrane can form an intra-period line with closely apposed neighboring internodes (evident in Figures 4.2, 4.7). This arrangement contrasts markedly with the Schwann cell outer membrane, which secretes and attaches to the basal lamina and collagen-rich extracellular matrix. Oligodendrocyte myelination thus achieves a substantial saving in extracellular space compared with peripheral nerve myelination. Oligodendrocyte outer tongue processes contain gap junction proteins, and these are assembled into junctions between the oligodendrocyte and astrocyte processes (Kamasawa et al., 2005; Orthmann-Murphy et al., 2008). Outer tongue processes contain no compact myelin proteins, para-nodal proteins (NF155) or MAG.

The myelin oligodendrocyte protein (MOG) is present in the abaxonal membrane (Figure 4.8a). MOG is a ~25-kDa glycoprotein that has an extracellular amino-terminal Ig-like domain, a transmembrane domain and a hydrophobic domain close to the carboxy-terminal domain, which may also interact with the membrane (Kroepfl et al., 1996; Linnington et al., 1984). Originally discovered, like many myelin proteins, as an autoantigen and immunogen for inducing demyelination, MOG is still widely used to induce experimental autoimmune encephalomyelitis (EAE). MOG is concentrated on the outer surface of the myelin internode (Figures 4.4, 4.8) (Brunner et al., 1989), almost mirroring the internal distribution of MAG, and it is not present in paranodal loops. MOG-null mice have no phenotype and exhibit little evidence of morphological dysfunction (Delarasse et al., 2003). Consequently, the role of MOG remains elusive.

MOLECULAR MECHANISMS OF MYELIN
MEMBRANE FORMATION

During peak periods of myelination, oligodendrocytes produce myelin components at a prodigious rate and incorporate them into an estimated $>10^4 \mu m^2$ myelin membrane surface area per cell per day (Pfeiffer et al., 1993). Myelin formation is much more than simple protein and lipid synthesis, however. Molecular mechanisms that mediate spiral and lateral membrane growth and localize proteins to specific myelin membrane domains are as fundamental to myelination as the structural proteins. Myelin protein structure may also partly reflect requirements to interact with protein localization machinery. Within oligodendrocytes, the backbone of myelination is provided by development of a large and specialized microtubule (MT) network, which organizes the Golgi apparatus and provides transport routes for both secretory and mRNA trafficking pathways (Figure 4.9). Spiral growth is likely to be actin-dependent and regulated locally at sites of contact with each axon. A robust process, spiral growth does not appear directly dependent on the insertion of most myelin proteins into the extending membrane. How spiral growth and myelin membrane assembly at each developing internode are regulated remains a crucial question for understanding myelination in development and disease.

Premyelinating oligodendrocytes have non-polarized membranes

Initial differentiation of oligodendrocyte progenitor cells (OPCs) into oligodendrocytes produces a cell capable of myelin protein gene expression but lacking the necessary machinery to assemble myelin components into functional internodes. The transition from OPC to premyelinating oligodendrocyte entails downregulation of OPC-related proteins, including the NG2 proteoglycan and growth factor receptors such as PDGFRα, and upregulation of myelin proteins and proteins associated with the oligodendrocyte cytoskeleton (see Chapter 3). At this stage, myelin proteins are inserted into oligodendrocyte membranes in a non-polarized fashion, such that immunostaining for PLP/DM20, MBP and MAG labels the cell body and radial processes (Trapp et al., 1997). Other proteins are not expressed prior to axonal wrapping, including PLP and MOG. Differentiating to the premyelinating stage is intrinsic to oligodendrocytes and not

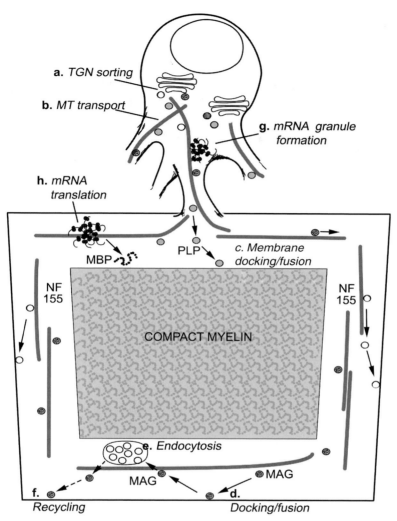

Figure 4.9 Summary diagram of protein trafficking to different myelin
domains through (a–f) the secretory pathway and (g,h) by mRNA
trafficking. MAG, myelin-associated glycoprotein; MBP, myelin basic
protein; MT, microtubule; TGN, trans Golgi network.

dependent on the axon, as it occurs in neuron-free cultures and in
the absence of axons in vivo (Ueda *et al.*, 1999). The switch to targeted
delivery of myelin proteins to discrete myelin membrane domains
involves axonal interaction and development of a specialized
cytoskeleton.

Establishment of a specialized microtubule network underlies oligodendrocyte polarization

Microtubules are fundamental to the cell biology of most cells, and expansion, reorganization and specialization of the MT network underlie the production of complex shapes in many large cells. MTs provide essential "railways" through the cytoplasm along which Golgi-derived and recycling carrier vesicles and organelles are transported (see reviews by Goldstein and Yang, 2000; Schliwa and Woehlke, 2003). MTs are polar filaments, with a fast-growing "plus" end, at which dimers of α and β tubulins are added or removed, and a slow-growing "minus" end. Classical kinesin motors propel vesicles and other cargos toward MT plus ends, while dynein-family motors mediate minus-end-directed transport. The Golgi apparatus endoplasmic reticulum, intermediate filaments and endosomes also become polarized via motor-mediated interactions with the MT network. The importance of the MT network to oligodendrocyte differentiation is amply demonstrated by myelin dysfunction following drug-induced MT depolymerization (Jacobs et al., 1972) and in taiep (tremor, ataxia, immobility episodes, epilepsy, paralysis) mutants (Song et al., 1999), which have disorganized MTs due to a genetic defect. Substantial changes in the molecular composition of the oligodendrocyte MTs adapt the network for myelination.

Migrating cells have a dynamic MT network typically organized with minus ends anchored at a central MT organizing center (MTOC) and plus ends uniformly oriented toward the cell periphery. Migrating OPCs share this kind of astral MT organization (Simpson and Armstrong, 1999). During differentiation, many complex cells generate a MT network that features highly stable MTs that may not remain attached to the centrosome. During Madin–Darby canine kidney (MDCK) cell differentiation, for example, MT minus ends relocate to beneath the apical surface (Bre et al., 1987), and this establishes an apico-basal network that forms the basis for site-specific apical and basolateral protein targeting. Schwann cells also radically reorganize their MTs into a non-centrosomal network during myelination (Kidd et al., 1996) that relocates and divides the perinuclear Golgi apparatus and provides transport pathways along the internode. Following axonal transection, Schwann cells again remodel their MT network to form multiple MTOCs (Kidd et al., 1996), which serve to localize lysosomes and endosomes to sites of degradation through association with MT minus ends. The oligodendrocyte MT network undergoes substantial transformation during differentiation (Kachar *et al.*, 1986; Wilson and Brophy, 1989), and in culture this includes development of a dispersed non-centrosomal MT network (Lunn *et al.*, 1997; Song *et al.*, 2001). MTs in the larger oligodendrocyte processes have a mixed polarity (Song *et al.*, 2001), similar to Schwann cells and dendrites. Confirmation of these observations in vivo was hampered by the difficulties in distinguishing oligodendrocyte MTs from those in nearby cells. Discovering that oligodendrocyte MTs are selectively enriched for β_{IV} tubulin, however, permitted confocal examination and provided evidence that, in vivo, oligodendrocytes also utilize a disseminated network of MTs that do not radiate from a common MTOC (Terada *et al.*, 2005). Consistent with a non-centrosomal MT organization, the minus-end-tethered Golgi apparatus appeared as scattered "biosynthetic stations" throughout the perinuclear cytoplasm and proximal processes (Sternberger *et al.*, 1979).

β_{IV} *tubulin expression*

β-tubulins are obligatory components of all cells, but cell-specific enrichment for some classes characterizes particular cells (reviewed by Cleveland, 1987; Luduena, 1998). β_{III} tubulin is enriched in neurons and identifies them (TuJ1 staining) in vivo and in cultured cells. Fortuitous cross-reactivity of a commercial antibody identified class IV β tubulin as an oligodendrocyte-enriched cytoskeletal marker (Terada *et al.*, 2005). Both β_{IVa} and β_{IVb} isotypes exist, but β_{IVa} mRNA is enriched in oligodendrocytes (Schaeren-Wiemers *et al.*, 1995), making it the likely isotype. Immunohistochemical staining of neonatal rat brains for β_{IV} tubulin produced prominent labeling of premyelinating oligodendrocytes and their processes (Terada *et al.*, 2005), and cyto-skeletal staining for β_{IV} tubulin could be traced to the developing myelin internodes and along the external surface of the compact myelin internode in the outer tongue process of actively myelinating cells. The functional significance of β_{IV} tubulin enrichment during oligodendrocyte myelination is enigmatic. Cell-specific use of particu-lar isotypes may reflect the evolutionary history or promoter prefer-ences of the individual cell type (Cleveland, 1987), rather than structural differences in MTs produced. Nevertheless, enrichment for β_{IV} tubulin is often a characteristic of MT networks that are stable or highly specialized, such as in cilia, retinal rod cells and neurites. Each β tubulin polypeptide is highly conserved, suggesting that structural differences are functionally important (Luduena, 1998). Isotype-specific carboxy-terminals interact differentially with some MAPs and may alter rates of MAP-promoted MT assembly. In oligodendrocytes, increased expression of β_{IV} tubulin accompanies process outgrowth and establishment of myelin internodes, which is thought to require increased stability. Oligodendrocytes also upregulate several MAPs (below) during differentiation, and it is possible that enrichment for β_{IV} tubulin and these MAPs may promote formation of a MT network with the stability and transport characteristics necessary for myelination.

Tau protein (MAP-T) is probably the best characterized MT-binding protein and is enriched in oligodendrocytes. Tau promotes MT stabilization in vivo and in culture. Tau is distributed throughout oligodendrocyte processes and co-localizes with MTs (LoPresti *et al.*, 1995). Levels of tau mRNA and protein increase in oligodendrocytes coincident developmentally with myelination (Gorath *et al.*, 2001; Richter-Landsberg and Gorath, 1999). Alternative splicing of a single tau transcript produces six tau isoforms ranging from 45 to 65 kDa, including isoforms that contain four (rather than three) MT-binding domains (4R-tau) (Gorath *et al.*, 2001; Richter-Landsberg and Gorath, 1999). These changes correlate with increased MT stability, and anti-sense inhibition of tau expression inhibits oligodendrocyte process outgrowth (Gordon *et al.*, 2008a). Tau is not indispensable to oligodendrocytes or neurons, however, as tau-null mice are viable with minor phenotypes (Harada *et al.*, 1994). Studies of tau biochemistry in human diseases have documented numerous signaling pathways by which tau modulation of MT stability can occur (Hasegawa, 2006; Schneider and Mandelkow, 2008). One consequence of oligodendrocyte utilization of tau is that they are vulnerable to tauopathies, including in familial frontotemporal dementias with parkinsonism linked to chromosome 17 (FTDP-17) (Spillantini *et al.*, 1997).

Oligodendrocytes express several other MAPs and MT-modulating proteins that are also developmentally regulated and can contribute to oligodendrocyte MT assembly, stabilization and organization during myelination. These include MAP1B (Fischer *et al.*, 1990), MAP4 (Vouyiouklis and Brophy, 1993) and MAP2C (Richter-Landsberg and Gorath, 1999; Vouyiouklis and Brophy, 1995), which are developmentally regulated in oligodendrocytes. Oligodendrocyte-specific STOP (stable tubule only polypeptide) isoforms have also been described (Galiano *et al.*, 2004), which like tau and other MAPs may promote MT stabilization. The MT-destabilizing protein stathmin-1 is expressed early in myelinogenesis and has been suggested to destabilize MTs at paranodal sites (Southwood *et al.*, 2007). Sirtuin 2 is a deacetylase enriched in myelin membranes (Roth *et al.*, 2006; Southwood *et al.*, 2007), including paranodal loops, and is also speculated to reduce MT acetylation. Acetylated α-tubulin is common in stable MTs and may enhance MAP and motor binding (Fukushima *et al.*, 2009).

It has also been postulated that oligodendrocytes may utilize unique molecules or mechanisms for stabilizing MTs. Dysmyelination in the mutant rat *taiep* results from MT abnormalities selectively in oligodendrocytes (Lunn *et al.*, 1997; Song *et al.*, 2001) that promote accumulation, bundling, and misorientation of MTs in oligodendrocytes (Song *et al.*, 2001). Oligodendrocyte-autonomous and autosomal recessive, the taiep gene has yet to be identified but may reflect genetic defects in an oligodendrocyte-specific MAP or tubulin-associated molecule.

Secretory pathway proteins are targeted to different oligodendrocyte membranes

More than half of the proteins in myelin are synthesized in the endoplasmic reticulum (ER) and processed through the Golgi apparatus. Precise pathways by which the integral membrane proteins, including PLP, MAG, MOG, claudin-11 and NF155, become localized to different myelin membrane domains are not known, although, as summarized in Figure 4.9, parallels with the secretory pathways in smaller polarized cells such as MDCK have provided some direction. Domain-specific targeting begins within the terminal Golgi compartment, called the trans-Golgi network (TGN), where different protein subsets are segregated into separate carrier vesicles (Figure 4.9a). In oligodendrocytes in vivo, it is not known which proteins are segregated into vesicle subsets, although PLP and MAG appear likely to be segregated (Trapp *et al.*, 1989).

Proteins are sorted in the TGN based on sorting signals embedded in their structure. In MDCK cells, a prototypical cell for studying molecular sorting and targeting machinery, such signals include small peptide motifs of two to ten amino acids (basolateral targeting), N- and O-linked carbohydrate moieties on the extracellular domain, presence of a glycosylphosphatidylinositol (GPI) lipid anchor to the plasma membrane and association with cholesterol-rich, glycolipid-rich lipid membrane microdomains called rafts (apical targeting). Often a hierarchy of signals is present in the same protein to affect targeting. PNS myelin glycoprotein P0, for example, contains dual overlapping basolateral targeting peptide motifs (Kidd *et al.*, 2006), and can also be targeted through the presence of carbohydrate in the extracellular peptide domain. Studies of CNS myelin proteins transfected into MDCK cells have confirmed that several have targeting sequences that do operate in polarized epithelial cell lines. S-MAG was targeted to apical domains (Kidd *et al.*, 2006; Minuk and Braun, 1996). MOG was targeted to basolateral domains and a potential basolateral sorting signal was identified at its carboxy-terminus (Kroepfl and Gardinier, 2001). PLP, a compact myelin component, was transported to the apical MDCK domain (Kroepfl and Gardinier, 2001). PLP has been suggested to associate with membrane rafts, and in transfected MDCK cells this may mediate apical delivery. The PLP aminoterminal (13 amino acids) is sufficient to transport LacZ to the myelin sheath (Wight *et al.*, 1993). L-MAG was localized to both apical and basolateral domains. Paranodal protein NF155 was specifically enriched in the lateral membranes of polarized MDCK cells (Maier *et al.*, 2006), which may result from basolateral targeting with selective stabilization in lateral membranes through homotypic interactions between adjacent membranes. The identity of most targeting motifs in myelin proteins is unclear at this stage, and the relevance of these motifs to targeting in oligodendrocytes in vivo remains to be fully characterized.

From the TGN, myelin proteins may traffic along MTs (Figure 4.9, b) directly to the target plasma membrane or follow indirect routes involving insertion into one membrane, recovery and retargeting via the endosomal compartment to another surface (transcytosis). Such pathways are well described in epithelial cells (Mostov *et al.*, 2000; Weimbs *et al.*, 1997). Docking and vesicle fusion at the plasma membrane ("exocytosis") may be tightly regulated or the protein may be selectively retained at some locations through protein–protein interactions in *cis* and *trans* (Mostov *et al.*, 2000). In oligodendrocytes, PLP is thought to be targeted directly to compact myelin (Figure 4.9, c). L-MAG was detected by immunocytochemistry in endosomes during early stages of CNS myelination (Trapp *et al.*, 1989) and in *quaking* mutant mice (Bo *et al.*, 1995). Endosomes enriched for L-MAG were present in inner tongue processes, paranodal loops, outer tongue processes, oligodendrocyte processes extending to myelin internodes and oligodendrocyte perinuclear cytoplasm, indicating that L-MAG is deposited in target membranes (Figure 4.9, d) and then endocytosed (Figure 4.9, e). Endocytosis and transcytosis utilize peptide motifs similar to those mediating basolateral targeting in MDCK cells. L-MAG (but not S-MAG) contains three consensus motifs (tyrosine-based, dileucine and diacidic), all located in the L-MAG-specific 44-amino-acid sequence (Bo *et al.*, 1995). As yet none has been tested for endocytic activity. As MAG is not detected in any other myelin membrane domains and was detected in endosomes that were transported back to the oligodendrocyte cell body, it seems unlikely that L-MAG is transcytosed. The most likely explanation is that endocytosed L-MAG is taken up during spiral growth of the periaxonal membrane and recycled back to growing MAG-containing regions (Figure 4.9, f) or degraded in the endosomal/lysosomal system. In vivo, PLP was not detected in endosomes (Bo *et al.*, 1995), indicating that MAG enrichment in endosomes is not simply part of a mechanism for bulk removal of non-polarized delivery of myelin proteins to the early oligodendrocyte plasma membrane.

Specific classes of molecules facilitate each stage of vesicle budding transport and fusion, including the coat proteins (e.g. COPs), small GTP-binding proteins (e.g. Rab proteins), tethering complexes such as the sec6/8 complex and docking/fusion proteins including soluble N-ethylmaleimide-sensitive factor attachment protein receptors (SNAREs; e.g. synaptobrevins/VAMPs) (see reviews by Low *et al.*, 1998; Weimbs *et al.*, 1997). Cognate pairs VAMP-2/syntaxin-4 and VAMP-7/syntaxin-3 are upregulated in oligodendrocytes (Madison *et al.*, 1999), syntaxin-4 is localized to myelin-like membranes, low levels of syntaxin-3 are detected in the cell body and syntaxin-2 appears ubiquitous (de Vries and Hoekstra, 2000). A number of Rab family GTPases have also been identified (Anitei *et al.*, 2009; Kramer *et al.*, 2001; Madison *et al.*, 1996) which may participate in protein targeting. Which combination of factors participates in the different targeting pathways of in vivo myelination has only just started to be addressed.

Unfolded protein response

When conditions such as mutant protein expression interfere with protein folding in the ER lumen, the accumulation of unfolded or misfolded intermediates results in ER stress. To alleviate ER stress, cells activate a complex signaling pathway termed the "unfolded protein response" (UPR), which affects nearly every level of the secretory pathway (reviewed by Schroder and Kaufman, 2005). If these mechanisms fail to decrease the unfolded protein load, however, cells enter into apoptosis. Mutations in the human PLP gene involving missense point mutations, deletions and duplications result in Pelizaeus–Merzbacher disease (PMD) in humans. Carboxy-terminal truncation of PLP in *Jimpy* (JP) mice (Macklin *et al.*, 1987b), a PLP point mutation in *Jimpy^{MSD}* (MSD) mice (Gencic and Hudson, 1990) and *rumpshaker* (*rsh*) mouse mutants (Griffiths *et al.*, 1998b) all trigger oligodendrocyte apoptosis. Comparisons of the behavior of wild-type (WT) and mutant proteins in transfected COS cells showed that mutant proteins were retained in the ER rather than transported to the plasma membrane (Gow *et al.*, 1994, 1998). In vivo, the intracellular accumulation of PLP is not prominent but may be sufficient to cause apoptosis of oligodendrocytes via an unfolded protein response. Overexpression of PLP can also kill oligodendrocytes by a similar mechanism (Kagawa *et al.*, 1994; Readhead *et al.*, 1994).

Myelin basic protein is localized via RNA translocation

Vesicular transport is not the only mechanism by which myelin proteins are selectively targeted to the myelin internode. Oligodendrocytes were among the first cells in which a mechanism for specifically transporting select mRNAs into the cell periphery was described (Colman *et al.*, 1982; Trapp *et al.*, 1987). Biochemical studies demonstrated post-translational incorporation of MBP into compact myelin within minutes of its synthesis. This contrasted with delays of 30 min or more observed between PLP synthesis and assembly into compact myelin (Benjamins *et al.*, 1978; Colman *et al.*, 1982). MBP mRNA was selectively enriched in isolated myelin fractions (Colman *et al.*, 1982) and was subsequently detected by *in situ* hybridization throughout white matter (Trapp *et al.*, 1987). This distribution was markedly different to that of other myelin protein mRNAs (e.g. CNP and P_2 protein), which are retained in the perinuclear region and translated on free polysomes (Gillespie *et al.*, 1990; Trapp *et al.*, 1988). Since those studies, several other mRNAs have also been localized to myelin internodes, including: myelin oligodendrocytic basic protein, tau and carbonic anhydrase II RNAs (Carson *et al.*, 2008; Ghandour and Skoff, 1991; Gorath *et al.*, 2001; Gould *et al.*, 2000).

Several factors may contribute to mRNA transport. Translocated transcripts contain *cis*-acting elements that mediate their localization by binding to specific *trans*-acting factors. With a few exceptions, these *cis*-acting sequences reside in the 3' untranslated regions (UTRs) of the transported mRNA. In MBP mRNAs, an 11-nucleotide RNA transport signal is sufficient to direct MBP mRNA recognition and transport out of the oligodendrocyte cell body into peripheral processes (Ainger *et al.*, 1997; Munro *et al.*, 1999). The *trans*-acting factor is a heterogeneous nuclear riboprotein, hnRNP A2 (Hoek *et al.*, 1998). hnRNP A2 is a 36-kDa protein with two RNA recognition motifs and a nuclear localization sequence. hnRNP A2 binds to the RNA signal sequence (Hoek *et al.*, 1998) which is called the A2 response element (A2RE). The A2RE is both necessary and sufficient for MBP mRNA targeting in culture.

Intracellular movement of MBP mRNA has been visualized in cultured oligodendrocytes (Ainger *et al.*, 1993). MBP mRNA is incorporated into loosely organized macromolecular complexes termed "granules" (Figure 4.9, g). Granules contain hnRNP A2, ribosomal RNA, the elongation factor EF1-α and arginyl-transfer RNA synthetase (Barbarese *et al.*, 1995). Granules often contain multiple transported mRNAs (Ainger *et al.*, 1997; Carson *et al.*, 2008) but not non-transported transcripts. The molecular basis for granule formation is not clear. One component may be a large (218 kDa) protein termed "tumor overexpressed gene" (TOG). This large flexible filamentous protein is identified in RNA granules and is proposed to crosslink hnRNP A2 molecules between different RNA strands (Carson *et al.*, 2008). Granule particles move at an average translocation rate of 12 μm/min, which is consistent with MT-mediated transport (Carson *et al.*, 1997). Translocation of the MBP mRNA granules is inhibited by MT depolymerization and treatment with kinesin heavy chain and hnRNP A2 antisense oligonucleotides (Carson *et al.*, 1997; Munro *et al.*, 1999). Available data support the plus-end anterograde MT-based translocation of MBP mRNA in translational competent ribonucleoprotein granules. Trafficking of mRNAs implied translational silencing of the message during transit. Although MBP appears in the cell body during early myelination (Sternberger *et al.*, 1978; Trapp *et al.*, 1987), translation predominantly occurs close to sites of incorporation (Figure 4.9, h) (Colman *et al.*, 1982). hnRNPA2 may regulate MBP mRNA translation, and complex interactions between multiple elements in the mRNA and their *trans*-acting factors have been proposed (Carson *et al.*, 2008).

Why are mRNAs translocated to the myelin internode? One explanation for MBP mRNA trafficking is that MBP is a sticky protein and translation close to sites of incorporation prevents potentially noxious accumulation in the cell body (Colman *et al.*, 1982). This idea does not explain the transport of other mRNAs encoding carbonic anhydrase II (CAII) and tau. Synchronous translation of multiple different mRNAs could also provide a mechanism for regulating the stoichiometry of different protein constituents in the developing myelin internode (Carson *et al.*, 2008). Oligodendrocytes continue to provide an important model system for elucidating mechanisms and functions of mRNA translocation that are utilized by all cells.

Spiral growth extends the oligodendrocyte plasma membrane around axons

Initial outgrowth of cellular processes from the oligodendrocyte cell body and their spiral and longitudinal growth around/along axons are likely to depend on actin-based mechanisms. Actin is abundant in the growing oligodendrocyte processes and in non-compact regions of the growing internode. Dynamic assembly of actin filaments underlies many modes of cellular shape change including lamellipodia and filopodia protrusion and phagocytosis (see review by Disanza *et al.*, 2005). Actin filaments (f-actin, microfilaments) assemble spontaneously from free actin in the cytoplasm (g-actin), and a large repertoire of actin-associated proteins direct and modulate actin assembly in several ways. Some promote actin filament nucleation (e.g. Arp2/3 complex and the formins), while others initiate filament depolymerization, including the actin-depolymerizing factor (ADF/cofilin) family and filament-severing proteins such as gelsolin. Other actin-binding proteins scavenge monomeric actin and regulate its availability for filament assembly (e.g. profilin). Proteins such as the WAVE complexes serve to cap and protect the ends of filaments, impeding disassembly. Actin-binding proteins are targets of diverse signaling pathways. In the CNS, oligodendrocytes grown in culture express lamellipod-like actin assemblies and microspikes at the leading edge of myelin-like membranes (Kachar *et al.*, 1986; Wilson and Brophy, 1989). Many components associated with actin-mediated membrane outgrowth have been described in oligodendrocytes in culture, including integrins, signaling pathways involving fyn, focal adhesion kinase and growth cone-associated pathways (Chun *et al.*, 2003; Sloane and Vartanian, 2007a, 2007b; Vartanian *et al.*, 1997). How these molecules contribute to the axon-regulated outgrowth of myelinating processes in vivo, however, is just beginning to be elucidated.

An oligodendrocyte-enriched isoform (Kim *et al.*, 2006) of WAVE1 is present at the actin-enriched leading edge of cultured oligodendrocytes. Mice deficient in WAVE1 have "patchy" hypomyelination, which entails a reduction in the number of axons that are myelinated and in oligodendrocyte number. Where myelination occurs as well, internode thickness and length appear normal, however. This indicates that WAVE1 is not indispensable for spiral growth but suggests that WAVE1 is important for processing outgrowth prior to spiral growth and may also affect premyelinating oligodendrocyte survival.

Cytoplasmic myosin II is an actin motor that assembles into filaments upon phosphorylation of the regulatory light chain. These filaments pull against actin microfilaments in an ATP-dependent manner and provide tension at sites such as focal adhesion complexes. A relatively recent paper (Wang, H. *et al.*, 2008) indicates that activation of myosin II promotes Schwann cell myelin spiral growth. In myelinating co-cultures of oligodendrocytes and neurons, however, activation of myosin II regulatory light chain retarded oligodendrocyte process outgrowth and myelination. Inhibition of myosin II activation promoted extensive process outgrowth and increased the numbers of internodes formed three- to fourfold over control cultures (Wang, H. *et al.*, 2008). Myosin II regulatory light chain becomes less phosphorylated, and thus less active, during myelination in rat brain lysates (Wang, H. *et al.*, 2008), and the oligodendrocyte-enriched myosin isoform myosin IIB is also reduced in concentration. These data suggest that myosin II may act as a brake, preventing oligodendrocyte processes from selecting and myelinating axons. Thus signaling pathways that modulate myosin activation may be crucial to myelination.

Gelsolin is an 82-kDa microfilament-severing protein implicated in lamellipodial movement of many cells. Gelsolin is one of a family of actin-severing and actin-capping proteins which, upon Ca^{2+} binding, break actin filaments and cap the fast-growing end of the filament. Gelsolin also binds monomers to inhibit actin growth. Phosphoinositide binding releases gelsolin from the filament ends and promotes rapid actin reassembly. In oligodendrocytes, gelsolin is selectively enriched in the cell body, processes and in paranodal cytoplasm (Legrand *et al.*, 1986; Tanaka and Sobue, 1994) and is developmentally upregulated during myelination (Lena *et al.*, 1994).

The effects of gelsolin loss in oligodendrocytes are unclear. Transgenic gelsolin-null BalbC or C57/BL mice die around birth, but in mixed-background mice lack of gelsolin produces very subtle phenotypes affecting a variety of cell systems (Kwiatkowski, 1999). While in vivo roles for gelsolin in myelination have yet to be tested, its distribution in paranodal loops and its central role in actin cytoskeletal dynamics in cell movement make it a likely component of the spiral growth machinery. Gelsolin, like many actin-associated proteins, is also a likely target for signaling pathways that modulate myelination.

RECIPROCAL INTERACTIONS BETWEEN OLIGODENDROCYTES AND AXONS REGULATE MYELINATION AND PROMOTE AXONAL SURVIVAL

During myelination, oligodendrocytes and axons establish a complex physical relationship that promotes saltatory conduction and requires reciprocal signaling between the two cells. A good example of this interaction comes from considering the well-known g-ratio, which is the ratio of the axonal diameter to the fiber diameter (i.e. including myelin). The geometric relationship between axonal diameter and myelin thickness/internodal length is scalable, such that the g-ratio is typically 0.6–0.7 for CNS internodes across a wide range of axon sizes (Hildebrand *et al.*, 1993; Peters *et al.*, 1991). The same oligodendrocyte can make myelin internodes of different thicknesses along different axons, indicating that the axon is the major determinant of myelin thickness. At the same time, myelination is necessary for axons to achieve their ultimate internodal diameter and dysmyelination results in axons with reduced diameters (Brady *et al.*, 1999; Colello *et al.*, 1994; Kirkpatrick *et al.*, 2001). Thus g-ratio values reflect both molecular cues from the axon to the oligodendrocyte regarding the number of compact myelin lamellae to produce, and signals from the oligodendrocyte to the axon that promote axonal expansion.

Coordination of axonal and myelin dimensions is important to normal signal conduction (Arbuthnott *et al.*, 1980; Waxman and Ritchie, 1993), but other aspects of signaling between the oligodendrocyte and axon are vital to axonal survival. When coordination and signaling are impeded they become a source of progressive disability in myelin-related diseases in humans. Chronic loss of compact myelin or damage to the oligodendrocyte in diseases such as multiple sclerosis and leukodystrophies results ultimately in axonal degener-ation (see reviews by Nave and Trapp, 2008; Trapp and Nave, 2008). Axonal survival requires more than simply the physical presence of the compact myelin lamellae, as considerable myelin production continues in the absence of myelin proteins PLP and CNP, but axonal pathology is progressive and substantial (Edgar *et al.*, 2004; Garbern *et al.*, 2002; Lappe-Siefke *et al.*, 2003). Understanding the molecular mechanisms underlying control of axonal diameter and axonal survival is central to current oligodendrocyte/myelin research, as identifying critical molecules and pathways offers possible novel therapeutic targets for treating demyelinating diseases.

Axonal signaling modulates myelin thickness

The neuregulin-1 (NRG1) family of growth factors has been directly implicated in axonal signaling to both Schwann cells and oligoden-drocytes in myelination. Three principal NRG1 forms exist (types I–III) and all contain an epidermal growth factor domain that interacts with their receptors, which are members of the ErbB family of recep-tor tyrosine kinases. NRG1 can bind to ErbB4 and ErbB3, and either receptor may also heterodimerize with ErbB2, although NRG1 is not a direct ligand for ErbB2. In the PNS, NRG1–ErbB interactions mediate initial Schwann cell-axon ensheathment and the production of myelin [(Michailov *et al.*, 2004; Taveggia *et al.*, 2005) and see reviews by (Corfas *et al.*, 2004; Nave and Trapp, 2008)]. Roles for NRG1 and ErbB receptor signaling in myelin thickness in the CNS may be more modest than for the PNS. In-culture and in-vivo evidence sug-gests that NRG1 enhances the proliferation and survival of oligoden-drocytes precursors (see Nave and Trapp, 2008). In vivo, transgenic reduction of type III NRG1 expression in the CNS through haploinsuf-ficiency resulted in fewer compact myelin lamellae (Taveggia *et al.*, 2008). This effect was restricted to the forebrain, however, and did not affect other CNS sites such as optic nerve or spinal cord. ErbB4 and ErbB2 are expressed by oligodendrocytes in culture (Vartanian *et al.*, 1997). Transgenic expression of a dominant-negative ErbB4 in oligodendrocytes resulted in a very modest CNS myelin thinning, i.e. fewer compact myelin lamellae (Roy *et al.*, 2007). NRGs are synthe-sized as single-pass transmembrane proteins but are released from the membrane by proteolytic cleavage; NRG1 types I and II are secreted or shed from the axon via enzymes including the tumor-necrosis factor alpha-converting enzyme (NRG1 type I). NRG1 type III

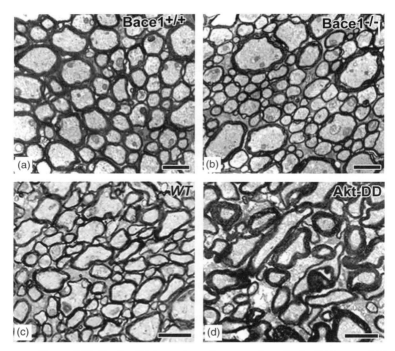

Figure 4.10 Myelin thickness in optic nerves from (a,c) wild type and (b) transgenic mice lacking BACE1 or (d) expressing constitutively active Akt (Akt-DD). Scale bars 1 μm. Reproduced from Hu *et al.* (2006) and Flores *et al.* (2008) with permission.

is activated through cleavage by the beta-amyloid converting enzyme (BACE1) (Hu *et al.*, 2006) but retains membrane association through a cysteine-rich domain. BACE1-null transgenic mice exhibited reduced rates of NRG1 cleavage in the CNS (Hu *et al.*, 2006) resulting in less secreted/cleaved NRG1 and higher levels of NRG1 tethered to the transmembrane domain. Compared with wild-type mice (Figure 4.10a), Bace-null mice exhibited fewer myelin lamellae, resulting in aberrant g-ratios, and had reduced levels of myelin proteins (Figure 4.10,b)(Hu *et al.*, 2006). These results implicate BACE1 substrates in regulating myelin thickness and are consistent with a role for NRG1.

Modulation of myelin thickness has also been described for signaling pathways utilizing other receptors. Oligodendrocytes express insulin-like growth factor 1 (IGF-1) (Carson *et al.*, 1993) and IGF has been implicated in OPC proliferation in culture. One of the first transgenic mice overexpressed IGF-1 under a metalloprotease promoter (Ye *et al.*, 1995) and produced an increase in myelin lamellae in the CNS. MBP-driven constructs yielded similar results (Luzi *et al.*, 2004). IGF-binding protein (IGF-BP) expression resulted in modestly fewer myelin lamellae (Ye *et al.*, 1995). Whether IGFs are acting locally as a secreted axonal factor regulating myelination, however, is unclear. Integrins have also been implicated in CNS myelination. Comprising α and β subunits, integrins are cell surface receptors that recognize extracellular matrix components and promote intracellular signaling cascades mediated by the β subunit. OPCs express several integrins in culture (Milner and Ffrench-Constant, 1994). In vivo, expression of a dominant negative β1 integrin under the PLP promoter (Lee *et al.*, 2006) resulted in abnormally thinly myelinated internodes in spinal cords and optic nerves and fewer myelinated axons. However corpus callosum axons were myelinated normally. The axonal ligand for oligodendrocyte integrins has not been identified.

Thus far, the greatest and most sustained increase in myelin thickness comes from transgenic overexpression of a constitutively active form of the signaling kinase Akt (Figure 4.10c,d) (Flores *et al.*, 2008). Akt is a frequent downstream component of receptor tyrosine kinase signaling and is implicated in several signaling pathways. ErbB receptors, IGF receptors and integrins all mediate their intracellular effects by initiating signaling cascades of kinase activation, particularly through phosphoinositide-3 (PI3) kinase activity. Culture studies suggested Akt signaling was invoked by NRG1 activation of the PI3 kinase pathway and served to enhance oligodendrocyte survival. In vivo, transgenic mice expressing constitutively active Akt in oligodendrocytes showed an increase in myelin lamellae throughout the CNS, both in corpus callosum and optic nerve (Flores *et al.*, 2008). Overstimulation of Akt signaling pathways resulted in oligodendrocytes with larger cell bodies, but there was no increase in total oligodendrocyte number relative to the number of axons myelinated, in contrast to culture models of Akt action. Oligodendrocytes in these mice continue actively increasing myelin thickness throughout life, resulting in enlarged optic nerves and white matter areas (Figure 4.10). Oligodendrocytes overexpressing constitutively active Akt had elevated levels of activated mTOR (mammalian target of rapamycin) and its downstream substrates (p70S6 kinase and S6 ribosomal protein) (Narayanan *et al.*, 2009). Rapamycin treatment of these mice during active myelination reduced myelination to approximately wild-type levels. Treatment of wild-type animals with rapamycin during active postnatal myelination resulted in reduced myelination. Elucidating the precise role of Akt and its upstream and downstream pathways in oligodendrocytes is likely to be a key to unraveling the mechanisms regulating myelination.

Oligodendrocytes modulate axonal diameter and survival

Effects of myelination on axon caliber have been recognized for some time. Changes in axonal diameter with Schwann cell myelination have been equated to increases in axonal intermediate filament packing density (deWaegh et al., 1992; Hsieh et al., 1994). Increased phosphorylation of NF-M and NF-H modulates neurofilament (NF) sidearms into an extended conformation that increases the distance between NFs. Loss of MAG results in minor myelin defects but substantial changes in PNS axonal diameter and NF spacing (Yin et al., 1998). Similarity in axonal defects in MAG-null mice and mice unable to synthesize certain complex axonal gangliosides (Pan et al., 2005; Sheikh et al., 1999) suggests that MAG–glycoplipid interactions may be involved. Dashiell et al. (2002) implicated decreased activities of extracellular-signal-regulated kinases (ERK1/2) and cyclin-dependent kinase-5 (cdk5) in reduced NF phosphorylation and decreased axon diameters in MAG-deficient axons. Effects of myelin protein loss on axonal diameter appear less dramatic in the CNS compared with the PNS, although this may reflect the overall smaller sizes of CNS axons. X-irradiation of the optic nerve to remove OPCs and oligodendrocytes resulted in axons of significantly smaller diameter (Colello et al., 1994). In shiverer mice, a deletion in the MBP gene resulted in optic nerve axons having reduced axonal diameters (Kirkpatrick et al., 2001), reduced NF concentration and reduced NF phosphorylation. Partial rescue of the shiverer phenotype by transgenic expression of MBP, which produces 25% normal MBP levels, resulted in thin myelin and a partial restoration of axonal diameter (Kirkpatrick et al., 2001). These results suggest that, in the CNS, oligodendrocytes also modulate axonal caliber, although this possibly also involves both NF concentration and phosphorylation.

While axonal diameter is important to axonal electrophysiology, far more devastating changes occur in axons following demyelination and in some myelin mutants. In diseases such as multiple sclerosis, exposure of the axon to the acute inflammatory environment is likely to directly promote axonal damage (Trapp and Stys, 2009). However, long-term degeneration of axons that are chronically demyelinated or dysmyelinated (Nave and Trapp, 2008; Trapp and Nave, 2008) indicates that ongoing interactions between oligodendrocytes and axons are essential for continued axonal survival. The precise nature of this interaction is unclear, but some clues come from transgenic animals in which expression of myelin proteins is impaired. PLP-null mice have initially little or no phenotype. Axons initially appear unremarkable, but a late-onset (>12 months) progressive loss of axons throughout the CNS affects particularly small caliber axons in long spinal tracts and eventually results in premature death (Griffiths *et al.*, 1998b). Axonal transport is impaired (Edgar *et al.*, 2004) and beginning at about 3 months pronounced swellings occur in myelinated axons, particularly at paranodal regions. Disrupted mitochondria and other organelles are common components of these swellings, which suggests impairment of axonal transport. Changes in microtubule motor components associated with impaired axonal transport were observed in the optic nerve of 60-day-old PLP-null mice (Edgar *et al.*, 2004). This effect was localized to the PLP-null internodes. Hemizygous mice had PLP-null and PLP-expressing oligodendrocytes myelinating adjacent segments of the same axon, and swellings were only detected in internodes lacking PLP (Edgar *et al.*, 2004). Interestingly, replacement of PLP with the PNS myelin glycoprotein P0 resulted in PNS-like compact myelin but accelerated axonal defects, and also resulted in shorter life spans (Yin *et al.*, 2006). Targeted disruption of the Cnp1 gene did not affect myelination but did induce a severe and early-onset axonal degeneration char-acterized by similar axonal swellings (Lappe-Siefke *et al.*, 2003) and early death. As discussed above, MBP-null mice also exhibit substantial changes in the axonal cytoskeleton and rates of axonal transport and die at about 6 months of age. These results suggest that oligodendrocytes modulate the axonal cytoskeleton and that some of the axonal defects in demyelinating and dysmyelinating diseases may result from misregulation or deregulation of the axonal cytoskeleton and axonal transport. In PLP-null mice, axonal swellings were frequently associated with the paranodal regions, suggesting that molecules in these regions may be espe-cially important.

SUMMARY AND CONCLUSIONS

Oligodendrocytes are complex cells that generate prodigious expanses of well-ordered spiraled membrane around multiple axons and participate dynamically in organizing the axonal surface and its cytoskeleton, yet they retain little cytoplasm or extracellular space. Investigating how molecules of the oligodendrocyte and its myelin achieve these functions has contributed greatly to our understanding of what myelination is and its importance. Far from being simple structural components of myelin membranes, oligodendrocyte proteins are ultimately as important to the structural organization of the axon and promotion of its function as they are to the provision of molecular building blocks for myelin membrane production and maintenance. Current advances in high throughput technologies, genomics studies and proteomics approaches are identifying new pieces in the molecular puzzle of myelination and are likely to provide new and unanticipated challenges to current concepts of how myelination occurs.

JOSEPH A. NIELSEN, PIERRE LAU
AND LYNN D. HUDSON

5

The genetics of oligodendrocytes

INTRODUCTION

Over the past decade, there has been tremendous progress in our understanding of oligodendrocyte biology. Many of the factors that are important for the specification of oligodendrocytes during development have been identified (Kessaris *et al.*, 2008). In addition, the emergence of genomic technologies has greatly improved our understanding of the factors that affect oligodendrocytes during development and in disease. In this chapter, we highlight some of the significant discoveries that have advanced our understanding of the genetic factors that are important in oligodendrocytes, and we identify some of the contributions that were made to this field using genomic technologies.

OLIGODENDROCYTE SPECIFICATION

A great deal of progress has been made in understanding the earliest events of oligodendrocyte specification. The spinal cord has received the most attention, and soluble signaling molecules such as sonic hedgehog (Shh) (Cai *et al.*, 2005) and bone morphogenic proteins (BMPs) are key early regulators of oligodendrocyte development in this part of the central nervous system (CNS). Shh is secreted from the ventral floor plate and is required for the specification of oligodendrocytes (Orentas *et al.*, 1999). Shh signaling induces the expression of the basic helix-loop-helix (bHLH) transcription factors Olig1 and Olig2 in a region of the ventral spinal cord referred to as the motor neuron progenitor (pMN) domain (Lu *et al.*, 2000; Zhou *et al.*, 2000). Shh and Olig gene expression is required for oligodendrocyte specification in the spinal cord and brain (Zhou and Anderson, 2002). As

The Biology of Oligodendrocytes, eds. Patricia J. Armati and Emily K. Mathey. Published by Cambridge University Press. © Cambridge University Press 2010.

development proceeds, the Olig2 expression domain eventually over-laps with an Nkx2.2 expressing domain in the ventral spinal cord, and the co-expression of Olig2 and Nkx2.2 in the pMN is required for oligodendrocyte specification (Zhou *et al.*, 2001). The co-expression of Olig2 and Nkx2.2 signals a switch from motor neuron production to oligodendrocyte specification in the pMN domain. The switch from neurogenesis to gliogenesis involves not only the induction of Olig2 expression, but also the downregulation of neurogenin 1 (Ngn1) and neurogenin 2 (Ngn2) via Notch signaling (Zhou *et al.*, 2001). In addition to positive ventral Shh signaling, negative signaling arising from the dorsal spinal cord has been identified. This negative signaling invo-lving BMPs inhibits oligodendrocyte specification by suppressing the expression of Olig2 (Mekki-Dauriac *et al.*, 2002). In summary, oligoden-drocyte specification can be viewed as taking place within gradients of both positive and negative inductive signals. These gradients set up transcription factor expression domains that generate oligodendrocyte progenitor cells (OPCs). Once oligodendrocytes have been specified, they proliferate and migrate to populate the white matter tracts throughout the spinal cord and brain.

In addition to ventral production of oligodendrocytes, a slightly later generation of oligodendrocytes has been identified in the dorsal region of the spinal cord that is independent of Shh signaling (Cai *et al.*, 2005). In the brain, multiple sources of oligodendrocyte generation have been identified using fate mapping studies (Kessaris *et al.*, 2006). In this study, multiple waves of oligodendrogenesis were identified with different spatial and temporal characteristics and, interestingly, not all sources of oligodendrocytes remain in the adult mouse.

There are numerous other transcription factors and signaling pathways that are expressed by oligodendrocytes at different stages of development, but many of these await functional studies to deter-mine their role in regulating oligodendrocyte development (Nicolay *et al.*, 2007; Wegner, 2000).

GENOMIC APPROACHES TO OLIGODENDROCYTE BIOLOGY

The complete sequencing of genomes has opened up new and powe-rful approaches to study oligodendrocytes. Technologies such as DNA microarrays have become increasingly sophisticated, with cur-rent microarrays capable of simultaneously assaying over 30 000 transcripts in a single experiment. Experimental approaches using microarrays have been applied to oligodendrocytes since their development in the late 1990s, but a series of papers that came out in 2006 took advantage of the latest microarray technology to address basic questions about oligodendrocyte development (Dugas *et al.*, 2006; Nielsen *et al.*, 2006; Sohn *et al.*, 2006). The first paper to come out used the CNP-EGFP mouse and flow cytometry to isolate oligodendrocyte lineage cells at different points during development. In this study, the transcription factor Sox17 was found to display an expression pattern that correlated with known myelin genes; moreover, Sox17 promoted oligodendrocyte differentiation (Sohn *et al.*, 2006). A second paper published by our laboratory took a slightly different approach by sorting A2B5$^+$ OPCs and O4$^+$ pre-myelinating oligodendrocytes from postnatal day seven (P7) rat whole brain using flow cytometry (Nielsen *et al.*, 2006). The global analysis of this dataset identified a large change in gene expression as O4$^+$ cells are preparing to myelinate. The upregulation of myelin structural genes, cholesterol biosynthesis genes and actin cytoskeleton regulatory genes demonstrated the commitment that O4$^+$ cells make towards acquiring a myelinating phenotype. A third paper used immunopanning to purify O4$^+$ oligodendrocytes and DNA microarrays to assess changes in gene expression at different time points post-differentiation (Dugas *et al.*, 2006). This group identified multiple different temporal transcription factor expression patterns occurring during oligodendrocyte differentiation. Comparison of these last two datasets reveals extensive overlap between the genes that are differentially regulated during oligodendrocyte differentiation. In a comparison of transcription factors, 70% of the upregulated transcription factors identified by Dugas *et al.* (2006) were also identified by Nielsen *et al.* (2006) (Table 5.1). These kinds of genomic comparisons strengthen the confidence placed in differentially regulated gene lists, and suggest that the transcription factors identified in Table 5.1 are likely to play a role in regulating oligodendrocyte differentiation. Moreover, since one dataset was derived from cultured oligodendrocytes while the other originated from oligodendrocytes plucked from the brain, the differences between the two datasets may point future research to genes regulated through axon-derived signaling.

Another important use of the genomic technologies has been genome-wide association studies (GWAS). These studies take advantage of current DNA microarray technology and the ability to identify millions of single nucleotide polymorphisms (SNPs). By comparing healthy people with those with disease, it is now possible to perform large-scale genetic association studies by following the SNPs and the disease phenotype. This technology has been applied to a number of

Table 5.1 *Transcription factors upregulated during oligodendrocyte differentiation*

Probe set ID	Gene symbol	Gene title
1371550_at	–	Similar to TSC22 domain family protein 4
1392592_at	–	Similar to transcription factor 7-like 2, T-cell specific, HMG-box
1374494_at	–	Similar to testes-specific chromodomain Y-like protein
1382647_at	–	Similar to selenoprotein SELM
1383013_at	–	Similar to BTEB3 protein (Woodward *et al.*, 2005)
1371572_at	App	Amyloid beta (A4) precursor protein
1388659_at	Carhsp1	Calcium-regulated heat stable protein 1
1377713_at	Ches1	Checkpoint suppressor 1 (Woodward *et al.*, 2005)
1370057_at	Csrp1	Cysteine and glycine-rich protein 1
1372668_at	Limd1	LIM domains containing 1 (Woodward *et al.*, 2005)
1370928_at	Litaf	LPS-induced TN factor
1367943_at	Nfkbib	Nuclear factor of kappa light chain gene enhancer in B-cells inhibitor
1374503_at	Pbx3	Pre B-cell leukemia transcription factor 3
1375205_at	Pcaf	p300/CBP-associated factor
1379369_at	Prickle1	Prickle-like 1 (*Drosophila*)
1374425_at	Tle1	Transducin-like enhancer of split 1
1392840_at	Zfp536	Zinc finger protein 536

different diseases including multiple sclerosis (MS). The etiology of MS remains unknown, but there is a strong immune component to the disease and many believe MS is an autoimmune disease in which the immune system inappropriately targets the CNS (McFarland and Martin, 2007). A recent GWAS study identified the interleukin-2 receptor alpha gene (IL2RA) and human leukocyte antigen (HLA) loci as being linked to MS (Hafler *et al.*, 2007). These studies demonstrate the power of the new genomic experimental approaches, offer tremendous potential for candidate gene identification and open up the discovery of therapeutic interventions.

GENETIC DISEASES AFFECTING OLIGODENDROCYTES

Only a handful of genes have been identified that, when mutated, cause myelin diseases in human (Table 5.2). This is somewhat surprising

Table 5.2 *Gene mutations associated with CNS myelin diseases*

Gene	Gene locus (humans)	Human disease	Mouse model	Reference
Proteolipid protein 1 (Warshawsky et al., 2005)	Xq22	Pelizaeus–Merzbacher disease (PMD)	jimpy, jimpy[msd], rumpshaker, plp1 knockout	(Garbern, 2007)
Myelin basic protein (MBP)	18q22-qter	18q- syndrome (hypomyelination detected by MRI)	shiverer mbp knockout	(Gay et al., 1997; Loevner et al., 1996)
Connexin 47 (Uhlenberg et al., 2004)	1q41-42	Pelizaeus–Merzbacher-like disease, autosomal recessive	cx47 knockout	(Henneke et al., 2008; Salviati et al., 2007; Uhlenberg et al., 2004)
Connexin 32	Xq13.1	Charcot–Marie–Tooth CMT1X with central conduction slowing	cx32 knockout	(Murru et al., 2006; Seeman et al., 2001)
Eukaryotic initiation factor 2B (eIF2B)	12q24.3 14q24 1p34.20 2p23.3 3q27	Vanishing white matter; childhood ataxia with CNS hypomyelination (Labauge et al., 2007)		(Labauge et al., 2007; Leegwater et al., 2001; Maletkovic et al., 2008)
Aspartoacylase (ASPA)	17pter – p13	Canavan disease	tremor (rat) aspa knockout	(Moffett et al., 2007; Namboodiri et al., 2006)
Galactocerebrosidase (Gard et al., 1995)	14q31	Globoid cell leukodystrophy (Krabbe's)	twitcher	(Suzuki, 2003)
ABCD1	Xq28	X-linked adrenoleukodystropy (X-ALD)	abcd1 knockout	(Moser et al., 2007)
Quaking (Qk1)	6q25–27	Susceptibility to schizophrenia	quaking	(Aberg et al., 2006)
Nogo receptor (NGR) eticulon 4 receptor	22q11	Susceptibility to schizophrenia	ngr knockout	(Sinibaldi et al., 2004)

given the large number of transgenic animal models that have been made to study the function of individual transcription factors, signaling component proteins and myelin proteins expressed by oligodendrocytes; many of these engineered mice display measurable defects in oligodendrocyte specification, development and/or myelinating activity (Baumann and Pham-Dinh, 2001). The full spectrum of myelin diseases in humans may need to wait until personalized genome sequencing becomes routinely available – only then will the phenotypic consequences of subtle alterations in genes expressed by oligodendrocytes be assessable.

Of the structural proteins comprising compact myelin, mutations in proteolipid protein (PLP) have been the most visible in humans. The other abundantly expressed myelin protein, myelin basic protein (MBP), is only associated with hypomyelination in the extremely rare 18q- syndrome, where MBP along with neighboring chromosomal regions are deleted. No point mutations in MBP have been detected to date in humans, while over 30 different point mutations in the PLP gene have been identified as causative for Pelizaeus–Merzbacher Disease (PMD) and spastic paraplegia type 2 (SPG2) (Garbern, 2007; Hudson, 2003). Most PMD patients do not display point mutations but rather rearrangements of the PLP locus that lead to duplication or deletion of the PLP gene. PMD is a pleiotropic disease that can vary from mild to severe clinical symptoms and usually includes tremors and muscle weakness. These symptoms reflect the fact that this highly expressed PLP gene is key to the compaction and stabilization of myelin. In animal models such as the jimpy mouse, a point mutation in the PLP gene causes tremors, early postnatal lethality due to oligodendrocyte cell death and a reduction in the number of properly myelinated nerve tracts (Yool et al., 2000). Interestingly, in a genetic animal model that completely lacks PLP expression, there is a much milder phenotype characterized by loosely packed myelin lamellae and a normal lifespan (Boison and Stoffel, 1994). These data demonstrate that point mutations in the PLP gene can be far more deleterious than a complete absence of the gene, a phenomenon echoed in PMD patients. Additionally, a double mutant lacking PLP and the second most highly expressed myelin protein, MBP, displayed less severe defects than some of the PLP point mutations in mice (Stoffel et al., 1997). Oligodendrocytes may be especially sensitive to disruption of protein trafficking because of the staggering amounts of myelin proteins that are made by these cells during myelinogenesis. There is evidence that the secretory pathway is disrupted in PLP mutant oligodendrocytes, and this may be caused by a failure of the mutated PLP protein to fold and/or traffic properly to the membrane surface (Duncan *et al.*, 1983). The interaction of mutant PLP proteins with chaperones provides indirect evidence for protein misfolding (Gow and Lazzarini, 1996). Indeed, a collection of PMD mutations that map to the extracellular loop region of PLP block the formation of the correct intramolecular disulfide bridges, leading to abnormal cross-links and retention of the mutant proteins in the endoplasmic reticulum (ER) (Dhaunchak and Nave, 2007).

There are a number of other dysmyelinating and demyelinating genetic diseases that involve genes in pathways critical for myelin formation, such as lipid metabolism: Krabbe, X-linked adrenoleukodystrophy (ALD) and Canavan disease (Moser *et al.*, 2007; Namboodiri *et al.*, 2006; Suzuki, 2003). Krabbe disease is caused by a mutation in the galactocerebrosidase (GALC) gene that hydrolyzes the major myelin constituent galactosylceramide into ceramide and galactose. X-linked ALD arises from mutations in the ABCD1 protein, a member of the superfamily of ATP-binding cassette (Crespo *et al.*, 2007) transporters that facilitate peroxisomal import of fatty acids. Canavan patients have mutations in the gene for aspartoacylase, the enzyme that supplies acetate for fatty acid synthesis (Moffett *et al.*, 2007).

Perhaps the most unexpected finding in the hunt for genes that cause myelin diseases came from examining patients with vanishing white matter disease [also termed childhood ataxia with CNS hypomyelination (Labauge *et al.*, 2007)]. This disorder is linked to mutations in the five genes encoding subunits of the eukaryotic initiation factor eIF2B (Leegwater *et al.*, 2001; Maletkovic *et al.*, 2008). Why would mutations in an integral part of the translational apparatus, machinery present in every cell in the body, be selectively detrimental to myelin-forming cells? Probably because of the enormous protein synthetic capacity of oligodendrocytes, where any change that slows down the process would be magnified. Of note, eIF2B mutations are thought to disrupt the ER stress pathways, which would put them in the same class as a number of PLP mutations in PMD.

The detection of mutations in humans associated with myelin deficiencies has also brought us closer to defining a role for myelination in a host of psychiatric disorders. Ultrastructural changes in white matter tracts, fewer oligodendrocytes along with decreased expression of myelin-related genes have each been associated with schizophrenia, bipolar disorder, depressive disorder and some addiction disorders (Peirce *et al.*, 2006; Roy *et al.*, 2007; Segal *et al.*, 2007; Sokolov, 2007).

But these changes in white matter could reflect secondary events. What makes these associations more compelling is the finding of families where mutations in the Quaking (Aberg *et al.*, 2006) and Nogo receptor (NogoR) genes are each linked to a higher susceptibility to schizophrenia (Table 5.2).

Much progress has been made in the identification and characterization of genetic diseases that affect oligodendrocytes, but inroads into treatment have lagged. One encouraging direction is being taken in Canavan disease, where acetate supplementation therapy is being investigated as a way of compensating for the inactive aspartoacylase in these patients (Namboodiri *et al.*, 2006). The challenge remains to offer better therapeutic interventions for the spectrum of debilitating myelin diseases.

POST-TRANSCRIPTIONAL REGULATION OF MYELINATION

Post-transcriptional regulation of myelin gene expression is known to figure in myelination, as reviewed elsewhere (Wang *et al.*, 2007). Mostly, studies have focused on the trafficking of mRNAs such as MBP along microtubules to the periphery of oligodendrocytes (Carson *et al.*, 2001). The specific localization of myelin messages in the processes of oligodendrocytes and their translation outside the cell body remain a pioneering area of inquiry – one that revealed complex interactions with proteins such as hnRNP A2. Of note is the subcellular localization of these proteins in RNA-containing granules such as stress granules and P-bodies (Maggipinto *et al.*, 2004). Coincidently, an emerging field of research showed localization of microRNAs (miRNAs) in P-bodies (Parker and Sheth, 2007), pointing to an important role for miRNAs in post-transcriptional gene regulation during oligodendrocyte development. miRNAs are a class of small non-coding RNAs that regulate post-transcription processing of their mRNA targets by either repression of translation or degradation. The biogenesis of miRNAs and their mechanisms of actions have been described in excellent reviews (Bartel, 2004; Bushati and Cohen, 2007). Briefly, following transcription miRNAs are subjected first to cleavage by the RNAse III enzyme Drosha, then the precursor miRNA (pre-miRNA) is further processed by a second RNAse III enzyme, Dicer. The resulting mature form (Smirnova *et al.*, 2005) is loaded into the RNA-induced silencing complex (RISC) where binding of the miRNA to the 3′ untranslated region (3′ UTR) of its mRNA targets, through base pairing, results in post-transcriptional silencing. Mammalian miRNAs have been recently cloned from diverse tissues and particular attention has been focused on the characterization of miRNAs expressed in the brain.

The initial cloning from brain tissues and neuronal cells revealed that a high number of miRNAs are present in the CNS of multicellular organisms (Kim *et al.*, 2004a; Miska *et al.*, 2004). An estimated 60% of known miRNAs were found in the brain and, among those, enrichment in the brain was noted for only a few miRNAs, including miR-9, miR-124 and miR-128 (Lagos-Quintana *et al.*, 2002). Functional studies of miRNAs in neural cells are still sparse. Historically, miRNAs were discovered as regulators of cell fate determination in the nematode *Caenorhabditis elegans* (Lee *et al.*, 1993). A more recent study showed that disruption of the Dicer gene in zebrafish led to severe defects in the neural tube due to abnormal neuronal differentiation (Giraldez *et al.*, 2006). Another experiment supports the importance of miRNAs in brain homeostasis since knockout of Dicer in mouse Purkinje cells was associated with progressive neuronal degeneration (Schaefer *et al.*, 2007). Similarly, deletion of Dicer in the telencephalon led to a size reduction of the forebrain caused by apoptosis of neuronal cells (Makeyev *et al.*, 2007).

In light of their importance in regulating proliferation and differentiation of neuronal cells, the elucidation of the microRNAome – the entire complement of miRNAs expressed by neural cells (neurons, oligodendrocytes and astrocytes) – will be a crucial step toward understanding their functions in neural cell biology. Northern-blot experiments and DNA microarray technology are being profitably used to characterize the miRNA expression profiles of neural cells at diverse embryonic and postnatal time points. In mammals, miR-9 and miR-124 are restricted to the CNS and their expression levels are upregulated during embryonic neurogenesis (Krichevsky *et al.*, 2003). Later, several families of miRNAs, including let-7 and miR-224, are induced at embryonic day 17 and persist through adult life while other miRNAs, such as the miR-29, miR-101 and miR-137 families, are brain-enriched and limited to the adult (Thomson *et al.*, 2004). The dynamic regulation of miRNA expression suggests that some miRNAs have a developmental role in mammals. For example, miR-9 and miR-124 appear to induce a neuronal identity in cell culture by suppressing the expression of two anti-neural factors: REST and PTBP1. Further experiments are needed to determine whether these two miRNAs are downregulated during glial differentiation, an event which would support the idea that expression levels of miRNAs are also dynamically regulated during glial lineage progression and ensure the proper induction or maintenance of the balance between neuronal/glial identity. One notable difference between neurons and oligodendrocytes is illustrated by miR-128, which is expressed by cultured neurons but not by astrocytes or oligodendrocytes (Smirnova *et al.*, 2005). *In situ* hybridizations in embryonic and adult zebrafish support the idea that some miRNAs are indeed lineage specific and their expression is further restricted to neuronal cell populations. A clear example is miR-218, whose expression is confined to cranial motor nuclei and spinal motor neurons at embryonic stages (Kapsimali *et al.*, 2007). Examples of neuronal miRNA with specific localization also exist in mammals. Hence, miR-7 was shown to be expressed by neuronal cells of the hypothalamus and pituitary gland (Farh *et al.*, 2005). Overall, the limited examples of miRNA expression differences between neuronal cells and glial cells suggests that miRNAs may contribute to regulating their respective gene expression programs, although many miRNAs families, such as the let-7 family, are indeed shared by all neural cell lineages.

Unlike the neuronal microRNAome, few miRNAs have been characterized in glial cells. miR-23 was shown to be restricted to astrocytes, while miR-26 and mir-29 were preferentially expressed in astrocytes compared with neuronal cells. Due to their common origins from neural stem cells, oligodendrocytes may share a set of miRNAs with the astrocytic lineage, as well as an overlapping repertoire with neurons.

Aside from regulating gene expression in normal physiological conditions, miRNAs have also been implicated in a number of neuropathological conditions, from neurodegenerative and psychiatric diseases (e.g. Alzheimer disease and schizophrenia) (Perkins *et al.*, 2007; Wang, W. X., *et al.*, 2008) to cancer (e.g. glioblastoma) (Chan *et al.*, 2005). Of note, miR-21 was strongly expressed in several glioblastoma cell lines and knock-down of miR-21 led to apoptosis. The effect of miR-21 on cell death was counteracted by miR-335 in a fetal mouse cerebral cortex cell culture. Further experiments using glial cells such as oligodendrocytes should confirm the antagonistic actions of miR-21 and miR-335 in the regulation of apoptosis in glial cells. Several alternative mechanisms can explain how miRNAs can contribute to or cause human neural diseases: (1) abnormal expression levels of miRNAs, which would lead to the subsequent deregulation of their target mRNAs; (2) mutations in the miRNA binding sites of the targets, which would suppress the usual binding interaction with the miRNA or create de novo a new miRNA binding site; (3) mutations within the miRNA precursor or processed sequence that affect binding to mRNA targets. It is tempting to speculate that abnormal expression of miRNAs in oligodendrocytes can alter their differentiation potential, since several well-described oligodendrocyte genes are predicted targets of miRNAs by several widely available prediction algorithms. For example, galactocerebrosidase (GALC) is upregulated during oligodendrocyte differentiation and is predicted to be regulated by miR-218 and miR-124. Since miR-124 is mainly expressed in proliferating cells of the brain, this miRNA may affect the timing of differentiation induction by preventing the appearance of oligodendrocyte markers such as galactocerebroside. MBP is another example as it is a predicted to be a target of several miRNAs including miR-15a, miR-16, miR-195, miR-424 and miR-497. It is also remarkable that the same set of miRNAs is predicted to regulate the RNA binding protein Quaking (Aberg *et al.*, 2006), another key molecule influencing mRNA stability in oligodendrocytes. Of note, mutations in QkI have been linked to schizophrenia (Table 5.2). Genetic linkage studies and analysis of SNPs revealed a negative selection against polymorphisms in predicted miRNAs binding sites of targets (Chen and Rajewsky, 2006). Such conservation increases the probability that variations in these sites may result in a noticeable phenotype. In Tourette syndrome, sequence variations in the binding site of miR-189 in the SLITRK1 transcript were recently associated with the disease (Abelson *et al.*, 2005). The ongoing linkage analysis identified two miRNA loci associated with schizophrenia (Hansen *et al.*, 2007), suggesting that miRNAs may be associated factors in psychiatric diseases.

The implication of miRNA in diverse nervous system diseases involving neuronal and glial cells will thus remain an active area of study. Based on the plethora of roles currently attributed to miRNAs in regulating the complexity of brain development and maintenance, this brief overview underscores the importance of transcriptional and post-transcriptional mechanisms in the regulation of neuronal and glial cell identity.

PROSPECTUS

In the present era of oligodendrocyte genetics, researchers are putting together the parts list for this myelin-producing machine. Mutational analyses will remain the most revealing read-out of the work performed by individual parts, but network analyses will increasingly chip away at the complexity of the countless molecular interactions that result in myelin – both compact and non-compact. While the finishing touches will be made to the portrait of the oligodendrocyte genome, transcriptome, microRNAome and proteome, breakthroughs in the other "-omics" fields will reveal the glycome, lipidome and metabolome of these cells. A systems biology approach to myelination will not only unravel the inherent complexity of oligodendrocytes – perhaps surprising neuroscientists who view these cells as only a source of myelin – but, more importantly, also point to pathways where interventions can be targeted to alleviate myelin disease.

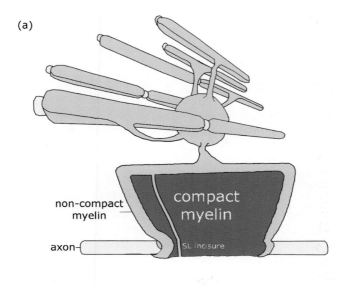

(a)

non-compact
myelin

compact
myelin

axon

SL incisure

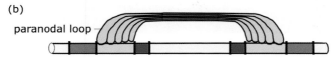

(b)

paranodal loop

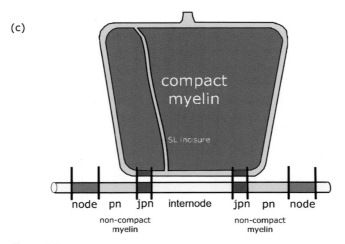

(c)

compact
myelin

SL incisure

node   pn   jpn   internode   jpn   pn   node

non-compact
myelin

non-compact
myelin

Figure 1.2a–c

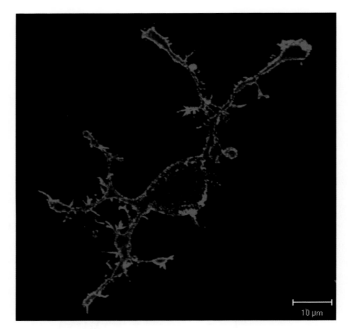

Figure 1.3

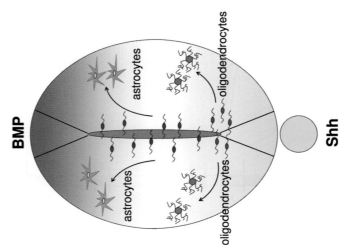

Figure 3.1

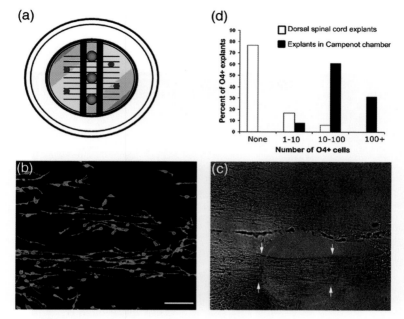

Figure 3.2

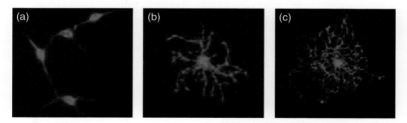

Figure 3.3

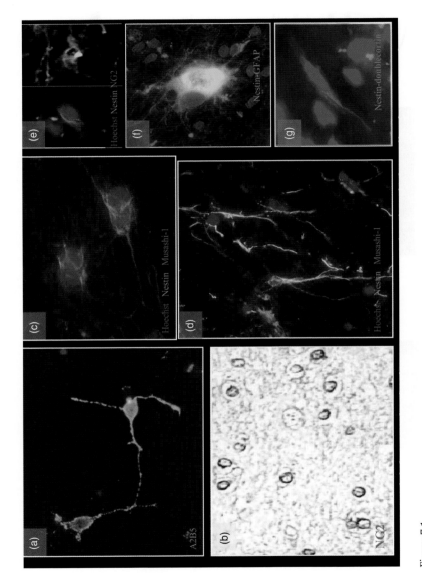

Figure 7.1

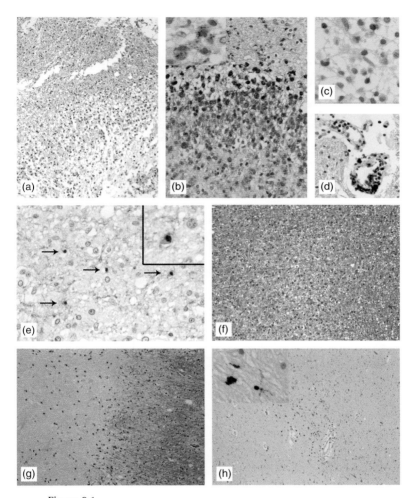

Figure 9.1

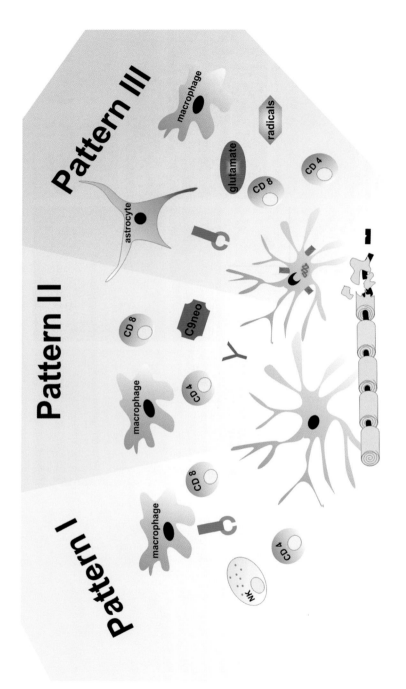

Figure 9.2

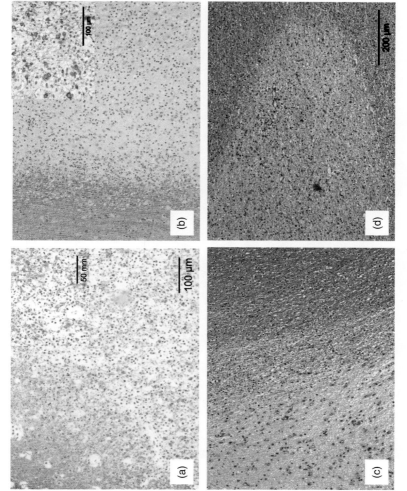

Figure 9.3

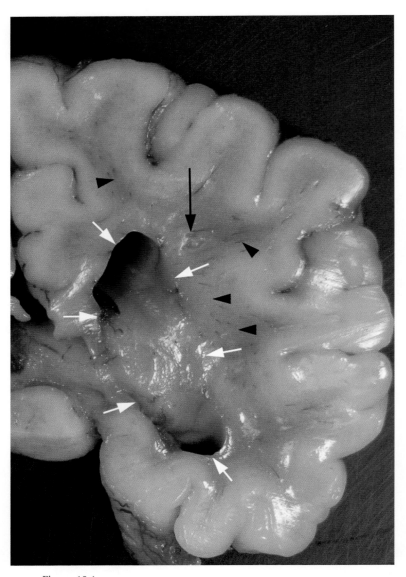

Figure 10.1

DAVID KREMER, ORHAN AKTAS,
HANS-PETER HARTUNG AND PATRICK KÜRY

6

Immunobiology of the oligodendrocyte

INTRODUCTION

Oligodendrocytes, as the myelin-producing cells of the central nervous system (CNS), are exactly what their Greek-derived name "oligodendroglia" suggests: they, alongside astrocytes, the non-neural microglia and ependymal cells, have been characterized as the "glue" that holds together the intricate apparatus of our brain. The fact that oligodendrocyte and astrocyte cells outnumber neurons by ten to one illustrates their importance, which is particularly highlighted by the oligodendrocyte's role in accelerating transmission of axonal action potentials. On the other hand, oligodendrocytes are involved in a number of serious diseases of viral, metabolic and immunological origin. This chapter tries to shed light on the immunobiological properties of oligodendroglial cells in the healthy and diseased CNS. We will begin with an overview of diseases featuring oligodendrocyte/immune system interactions and will then, in the second part, focus on the molecular repertoire that allows these cells to interact directly or indirectly with immune cells. Subsequently, we will discuss oligodendrocytes as antigen-presenting cells and finally we will present data on direct oligodendroglial/immune cell interactions.

IMMUNE-MEDIATED DISEASES AFFECTING OLIGODENDROCYTES

Multiple sclerosis

Multiple sclerosis (MS), which was first described by the French neurologist Jean-Martin Charcot in 1868 (Charcot, 1868), is a chronic inflammatory disease of the CNS of unknown etiology (Hemmer et al., 2006). Although an ideal system for the classification of different MS stages

The Biology of Oligodendrocytes, eds. Patricia J. Armati and Emily K. Mathey. Published by Cambridge University Press. © Cambridge University Press 2010.

does not yet exist (Van der Valk and De Groot, 2000) there is broad consensus that loss of myelin due to oligodendrocyte damage or death together with axonal degeneration leading to reactive glial scar formation are the key hallmarks of this disease (Trapp and Nave, 2008). In this context four different histopathological patterns of demyelination have been described (Lucchinetti *et al.*, 2000). Interestingly, these patterns are quite inhomogeneous, with patterns I and II showing close similarities to T-cell-mediated and T-cell- plus antibody-mediated autoimmune encephalomyelitis (EAE), respectively, while patterns III and IV are highly suggestive of a primary oligodendrocyte dystrophy, reminiscent of virus- or toxin-induced demyelination rather than primary autoimmunity. However, this classification system does not incorporate the common observation of axonal transection seen in MS, which is thought to be the pathological correlate of the irreversible neurological impairment in this disease (Trapp *et al.*, 1998). In summary, the data available thus far point to the still unclear nature of MS etiology, either primary autoimmune or neurodegenerative (Trapp and Nave, 2008), and suggest a polycausal disease process. The diversity of possible mechanisms of myelin damage is convincingly illustrated by adrenoleukodystrophy (ALD), where primary degenerative processes are amplified by subsequent autoimmune reactions. ALD is an X-linked inherited recessive disease characterized by the accumulation of saturated very long chain fatty acids (VLCFA) predominantly in the white matter of the brain and the adrenal glands. The disturbed breakdown of VLCFA due to mutations of the ABCD1 transporter gene family leads to myelin degeneration and secondary anti-myelin T lymphocyte autoimmunity. The resulting clinical picture is characterized by severe progressive MS-like symptoms and is usually fatal in childhood where it is often misdiagnosed as infantile multiple sclerosis (Moser *et al.*, 2005).

Histopathologically, the correlate of demyelination in MS is the so-called MS plaque. These lesions can primarily be found around small veins and venules, which show focal cuffs of perivascular inflammation. When perivenous lesions grow they can fuse with additional adjacent demyelinating areas forming large demyelinating plaques, which may reach several centimeters in diameter. MS lesions can also grow radially in which case active demyelination is observed at the periphery of the lesion, resulting in a gradual expansion of the plaque into the surrounding normal white matter. Interestingly, demyelinating lesions are not restricted to the myelin-rich white matter but can also occur in gray matter where they are difficult to identify (Brownell and Hughes, 1962). While in general lesions can be found in any

CNS region, certain neuroanatomical structures are affected more frequently than others such as the periventricular white matter, particularly the lateral angles of the lateral ventricles, the subcortical white matter, the optic nerves, the cerebellar peduncles and the spinal cord. As already pointed out above, all MS plaques feature a certain degree of axonal injury and loss, both of which can vary from plaque to plaque in the same brain and even more so between plaques of different individuals. It has been described that axonal density within plaques ranges 20–80% of that in the periplaque white matter and that within chronically demyelinated plaques the reduction of axonal density is on average 60–70% compared with that in normal tissue of the same area (Lassmann, 2003).

While there is no therapy available yet to directly reverse plaque formation in MS-affected brains, there are numerous approaches to alter the underlying (auto-)immune mechanisms leading to demyelination.

Besides the classical "ABC drugs" for MS, interferon-β1a (IFN-β1a), IFN-β1b and glatiramer acetate have emerged since 2000 as promising new treatments for MS.

Natalizumab, a humanized monoclonal antibody against the cellular adhesion molecule α4-integrin that interferes with leukocyte migration into the brain's parenchyma (Rice et al., 2005; Yednock et al., 1992), and fingolimod, a sphingosine-1-phosphate receptor 1 modulator causing lymphopenia by preventing egress of lymphocytes from lymph nodes (Matloubian et al., 2004), are two representatives of this new generation of MS drugs. In 2000, mitoxantrone, a type II topoisomerase inhibitor that disrupts both cellular DNA synthesis and DNA repair, was approved by the FDA as an effective treatment for worsening relapsing-remitting multiple sclerosis (MS), secondary progressive MS and progressive-relapsing MS (Hartung et al., 2002). Originally used to treat AML (acute myeloid leukemia) in adults, mitoxantrone suppresses the proliferation of T cells, B cells, and macrophages, impairs antigen presentation and decreases the secretion of proinflammatory cytokines (Neuhaus et al., 2006). It also enhances T cell suppressor function and inhibits B cell function and antibody production while it inhibits macrophage-mediated myelin degradation (Fox, 2004).

PROGRESSIVE MULTIFOCAL LEUKOENCEPHALOPATHY (PML)

Progressive multifocal leukoencephalopathy is a rare and mostly fatal viral disease characterized by progressive inflammatory damage to oligodendroglial cells occurring at multiple cortical locations (Tornatore *et al.*, 1992). PML is strongly associated with severe immune deficiencies such as immunosuppression after organ transplantation and, particularly, HIV/AIDS (Berger, 2003). In 1971, the pathogenic agent causing PML could be identified as a type of human polyomavirus similar to BK virus and SV40 (Padgett and Walker, 1973) and was thereafter named JC-virus (JCV) according to the initials of the index patient John Cunningham. Since then, the glial specificity of JC-virus has been the subject of numerous studies. One study suggests that the specificity of JC-virus for glia is based on a glial transcription factor that stimulates transcription of early and late viral genes (Wegner *et al.*, 1993). Other studies suggest that the specificity is a result of a combinatorial glial and viral promoter activation (Henson, 1994) or the specific expression of JC-virus receptor-type sialic acids on the cell surfaces of oligodendrocytes and astrocytes (Eash *et al.*, 2004). Interestingly, PML can also be triggered by the application of certain drugs such as the MS therapeutic natalizumab, particularly in combination with other immune-directed therapies (Chaudhuri, 2006). The drug was withdrawn from the market by its manufacturer, but was re-approved as monotherapy for severe forms of MS after a vigorous work-up of the participants of the large phase III trials (Yousry *et al.*, 2006). Recently, five new cases of PML were reported under natalizumab monotherapy (Hartung, 2009). The exact mechanism by which natalizumab triggers PML remains, however, poorly understood.

ACUTE DISSEMINATED ENCEPHALOMYELITIS

ADEM is an acute, inflammatory, demyelinating disease of the CNS. In most patients it has a sudden onset within days to several weeks after a viral exanthem or virus-like illness. However, ADEM is not specific to particular viruses such as measles, varicella zoster virus (VCV) or rubella virus (Scheld *et al.*, 2004) but has also been reported after several bacterial illnesses (Heick and Skriver, 2000), immunizations (Tsuru *et al.*, 2000), drug treatments (Schwarz *et al.*, 2000) and even allogenic bone marrow transplantation (Tomonari *et al.*, 2003). In the literature, ADEM can be found under a confusing variety of names which partly describe the clinical settings of the disease (e.g. post-infectious, para-infectious, post-exanthematous, post-vaccinal, post-measles, and post-influenza encephalomyelitis), the neuropathological features (acute disseminated encephalomyelitis, perivascular myelinoclasis, perivenous encephalitis, and acute demyelinating encephalomyelitis), or the possible underlying pathomechanisms (allergic encephalomyelitis, immune-mediated encephalomyelitis, hyperergic encephalomyelitis and disseminated vasculomyelinopathy). Histologically, ADEM is characterized by perivenous, macrophage-dominant, inflammatory infiltrations with a sleeve-like pattern of demyelination in the white matter. These lesions are, unlike MS lesions, poorly marginated (Alper and Schor, 2004). In AHL (acute hemorrhagic leukoencephalitis), a hyperacute form of ADEM, hemorrhages and necrotic venules can be observed (Love, 2006). Notably, EAE induced by myelin antigens such as myelin basic protein (MBP) or myelin oligodendrocyte glycoprotein (MOG), widely used MS models, results in a diffuse white matter encephalomyelitis that some authors describe as being more similar to ADEM than to MS (Chaudhuri and Behan, 2005).

NEUROMYELITIS OPTICA (NMO)

Neuromyelitis optica or Devic disease is a demyelinating process in the bilateral human optic nerves and the proximal spinal cord. It results in acute vision deficits and paretic symptoms, respectively. Recently, an NMO-specific IgG autoantibody binding to aquaporins-4 (AQP4), the predominant CNS water channel, was described (Lennon et al., 2004; Paul et al., 2007). Aquaporins are membrane-inserted water channel proteins engaged in osmotically driven water transport through cell membranes. In the CNS, AQP4 is expressed on astrocytic foot processes and ependymocytes which regulate osmoreception, potassium siphoning and cerebrospinal fluid (CSF) formation, and are therefore strongly implicated in the pathogenesis of cerebral edema. The histopathological findings in Devic disease range from modest perivascular inflammatory demyelination to complete hemorrhagic and necrotic destruction of gray and white matter (Wingerchuk, 2004). The inflammatory infiltrates in active NMO lesions are characterized by extensive macrophage infiltration associated with large numbers of perivascular granulocytes and eosinophils and few CD3[+] and CD8[+] T cells (Lucchinetti et al., 2002). The role of the eosinophils is unknown but may be a response to secondary activation by the C5a component of complement (Zeck-Kapp et al., 1995). In addition, immunopathological studies implicate humoral pathogenic mechanisms, particularly the disposition of IgG and C9 neoantigen in areas of myelin destruction similar to MS cases (Lucchinetti et al., 2002). In contrast to MS, oligoclonal CSF bands are mostly absent in NMO patients or disappear over time, an observation that is still not understood (Bergamaschi *et al.*, 2004).

The immune properties of oligodendrocytes as the myelinating cells of the CNS are of interest to not only developmental biologists but also – and in particular – researchers focusing on neuroinflammatory diseases of the brain. Given that oligodendrocyte loss and demyelination are common and widespread in the pathophysiological conditions presented above, a detailed understanding of how oligodendroglial cells (resident precursors of the adult brain as well as mature cells) interact with the immune system is imperative in order to generate novel therapeutic approaches that will protect and stabilize this glial cell population. It is therefore essential to study oligodendrocyte expression, presentation and secretion of immuno-relevant molecules in order to elucidate how they can induce, reinforce, inhibit and defend themselves against immune responses. In this regard, it seems appropriate to start with one of the molecular pillars of immunological cell identity and immunology: the MHC or HLA class of surface proteins.

Major histocompatibility complex (MHC)

Most studies investigating surface markers of oligodendrocytes state that there is next to no expression of MHC class II molecules on these cells (Bo *et al.*, 1994; Hayes *et al.*, 1987; Lee and Raine, 1989; Redwine *et al.*, 2001). This observation rather rules out the direct MHC class II-dependent activation of CD4[+] T lymphocytes by oligodendrocytes in neuroinflammatory paradigms such as MS. However, cell culture experiments have revealed that under certain immunological circumstances oligodendroglial MHC class II expression can be induced (Bergsteindottir *et al.*, 1992). On the other hand, CD4[+] T cells were described to mediate non-MHC-class-II-mediated cell death by upregulation of NK-cell-associated surface antigen CD56 (Antel *et al.*, 1998; Vergelli *et al.*, 1996). In contrast to MHC class II, MHC class I molecules, ubiquitously found on human cells, were shown to be expressed on oligodendrocyte cell surfaces as well. Here, they may be recognized by CD8[+] T cells which could then induce MHC-class-I-specific cytotoxicity, as has been suggested for MS (Babbe *et al.*, 2000; Hoftberger *et al.*, 2004).

Cytokines

Contrary to the long-standing belief that only immune cells such as CD4$^+$ or CD8$^+$ lymphocytes activated by APCs (antigen-presenting cells) can secrete proinflammatory cytokines, it is now well established that activated glia (i.e. oligodendrocytes, astrocytes, and microglia) can also release these factors. Cytokines then either cause direct myelin destruction or activate macrophages and plasma cells which in turn release reactive oxygen species (ROS), matrix metalloproteinases (MMPs), TNF-α and myelin-directed autoantibodies, respectively. On the other hand, the presence of cytokine receptors on oligodendrocytes suggests that glial-specific reactions might also be under the control of these signaling substances derived from either neural or immune cells.

Oligodendrocytes and their progenitor cells (OPCs) express interleukin-1β (IL-1β) and IL-1β receptor protein, and IL-1β was shown to inhibit proliferation of late progenitor cells (O4$^+$), but exerted no effect on early progenitor cell (A2B5$^+$) proliferation rates (Vela *et al.*, 2002). IL-1β is expressed at high levels in the CNS during pre- and postnatal development (Giulian *et al.*, 1988; Mizuno *et al.*, 1994) but only at low levels in adult CNS (Vitkovic *et al.*, 2000). However, a pathophysiological role of IL-1β is strongly suggested by the observation that in adult IL-1β knockout mice remyelination after brain injury no longer occurs (Mason *et al.*, 2001). Interleukin-6 (IL-6), on the other hand, can promote neuron and oligodendrocyte survival as a consequence of glutamate excitotoxicity, as seen, for instance, in MS (Pizzi *et al.*, 2004), and IL-6 receptor/IL-6 fusion was shown to enhance OPC differentiation (Valerio *et al.*, 2002). No immunoreactivity for IL-10 was observed in oligodendrocytes, ramified microglial cells, or perivascular lymphocytes (Hulshof *et al.*, 2002). However, oligodendrocytes were reported to express low levels of IL-18 and IL-18 receptor with the potential implication of this cytokine in the development of white matter injury (Cannella and Raine, 2004; Hedtjarn *et al.*, 2005). Apart from IL-1β and IL-18 receptors oligodendrocytes tested positive for expression of receptors for IL-3, IL-4, IL-6, IL-7, IL-10, IL-12, IL-13, IFN-γ, granulocyte macrophage colony-stimulating factor (GM-CSF) and macrophage colony-stimulating factor (M-CSF) (Cannella and Raine, 2004; Sawada *et al.*, 1993; Zeis *et al.*, 2008b).

Members of the interferon family of proteins are further important modulators of oligodendroglial behavior and migration. Since the early 1990s, IFN-β has been in use to treat MS patients (Paty and Li, 1993). Beside its immunomodulatory action, direct IFN-β effects on oligodendrocytes have been suggested, as it could be demonstrated that IFN-β knockout mice show accelerated remyelination in the cuprizone animal model of demyelination (Trebst et al., 2007). However, no protective effect of IFN-β on oligodendroglia exposed to H_2O_2, nitrous oxide (NO), complement or glutamate has been reported (Heine et al., 2006). Similarly, IFN-β appears to be ineffective with regard to oligodendrocyte survival, proliferation and migration as revealed by the use of the CG-4 cell line (Halfpenny and Scolding, 2003). Studies of IFN-γ functions yielded quite heterogeneous results. While Gao and colleagues reported that IFN-γ can protect against cuprizone-mediated demyelination (Gao et al., 2000), it was also shown to inhibit remyelination following cuprizone-induced demyelination through endoplasmic reticulum stress (Lin et al., 2006). In culture, IFN-γ was shown to inhibit OPC differentiation as well as oligodendrocyte progenitor proliferation (Baerwald and Popko, 1998; Chew et al., 2005) and in human oligodendrocyte cell lines IFN-γ was reported to induce apoptotic cell death (Buntinx et al., 2004). Overexpression of IFN-γ in transgenic mice can lead to demyelination (Geiger et al., 1994) which is in line with the observation that high levels of IFN-γ in serum and CSF of preterm infants correlates with white matter damage (Hansen-Pupp et al., 2005; Schmitz et al., 2007).

Tumor necrosis factor-α (TNF-α), another key player in neuroinflammatory paradigms, was suggested to limit the extent of inflammatory and demyelinating lesions as revealed by studies on TNF-α knockout mice (Liu et al., 1998). Immunizations with MOG led to increased mortality, brain inflammation and demyelination in these mutant mice. Complementary to that result, treatment with TNF-α antibodies increased inflammation in MS patients (van Oosten et al., 1996). However, in a certain variant of EAE induced by the adoptive transfer of MBP-specific T lymphocytes, administration of TNF-α antibodies prevented the appearance of inflammatory lesions (Selmaj et al., 1991b), an observation that supports results suggesting that TNF-α is implicated in oligodendroglial apoptosis (Hovelmeyer et al., 2005; Pang et al., 2005).

Members of the transforming growth factor-β (TGF-β) family, in particular TGF-β2, were found to be expressed by astrocytes and microglia in demyelinating MS lesions (Peress et al., 1996).

This is of interest as it was observed that cytotoxicity of activated microglia against oligodendrocytes in culture can be attenuated by TGF-β (Merrill and Zimmerman, 1991). Furthermore, TGF-β inhibits OPC proliferation while it promotes oligodendrocyte development (McKinnon et al., 1993) which suggests that TGF-β exerts an overall protective effect on oligodendrocytes. On the other hand, TGF-β1 expression (John et al., 2002) as well as upregulation by IL-1α could be confined to cultured oligodendrocytes (da Cunha et al., 1993) indicating that these cells apply paracrine or autocrine protective mechanisms.

Another modifier of oligodendrocyte behavior appears to be leukemia inhibitory factor (LIF). LIF receptor signaling enhances oligodendrocyte survival and limits demyelination in murine EAE (Butzkueven et al., 2006). When administered exogenously LIF limits cuprizone-induced demyelination while LIF knockout mice exhibit potentiated demyelination and oligodendrocyte loss following cuprizone treatment (Marriott et al., 2008). In addition, LIF was shown to prevent oligodendrocyte apoptosis through induction of JAK/STAT and Akt signaling pathways (Azari et al., 2006). LIF also promotes oligodendrocyte maturation, but directs differentiation of OPC into astrocytes in the presence of extracellular matrix derived from cultures of endothelial cells (Gard et al., 1995; Mayer et al., 1994). It thus appears to exert an overall protective effect on white matter and oligodendrocytes.

Chemokines

The human chemokine system comprises approximately 50 peptides and G-protein-coupled receptors (GPCRs) with the respective genes being highly conserved among mammalian species (Charo and Ransohoff, 2006; Tran and Miller, 2003). Chemokines can be grouped into subfamilies according to specific structural criteria, in particular the position of a pair of cysteine residues, located near the amino-terminus (Proudfoot, 2002; Rossi and Zlotnik, 2000). There is limited evidence that oligodendrocytes produce chemokines themselves, but it has been shown that astrocytic CXCL1 in the spinal cord enhances the proliferative response of OPCs to mitogen platelet-derived growth factor (PDGF) (Robinson et al., 1998), providing a possible explanation of why, in the dysmyelinating mutant jimpy mouse, increased numbers of OPCs are associated with elevated levels of CXCL1 (Wu et al., 2000). CXCL1 signaling through CXCR2 inhibits the directed migration of OPCs into the white matter, indicating that CXCL1 controls precursor cell recruitment to the presumptive white matter (Tsai *et al.*, 2002). Other data suggest that following stimulation with the proinflammatory cytokine IL-1β human fetal astrocytes produce high levels of CXCL1 while human oligodendrocytes express the CXCL1 receptor CXCR2. This may provide a model for astrocyte-mediated recruitment of oligodendrocytes to areas of damage as observed in MS (Omari *et al.*, 2006). The observations that CXCR2-ablated mice display reduced spinal cord white matter area and myelin thickness, and that these mutant mice show decreased conduction rates by spinal cord axons as well as lowered levels of myelin proteins (MBP, PLP) and astrocytic glial fibrillary acidic protein (GFAP) (Padovani-Claudio *et al.*, 2006) further support the importance of this receptor with regard to (re)myelination.

In contrast, CXCL12 (or SDF-1), acting through its receptor CXCR4, was shown to regulate oligodendrocyte proliferation (Maysami *et al.*, 2006b) as well as survival and chemotactic migration during embryonic and postnatal CNS development (Dziembowska *et al.*, 2005). It was furthermore shown to promote MBP synthesis in primary myelinating cell cultures (Kadi *et al.*, 2006).

Besides CXCR2, oligodendrocytes of the normal adult human CNS were also shown to express CXCR1 and CXCR3. Interestingly, expression levels of all three receptors were upregulated in MS and other neurological diseases (OND) (Omari *et al.*, 2005). The respective ligands CXCL8 (or IL-8), CXCL1 and CXCL10 were absent in healthy CNS tissue and in subjects with OND, but were present at high levels on hypertrophic (reactive) astrocytes at the edge of active multiple sclerosis lesions. This simultaneous expression of chemokine receptors on oligodendrocytes and of their ligands on astrocytes around multiple sclerosis lesions suggests functional roles in the recruitment of oligodendrocytes and subsequent remyelination.

Investigations concerning the expression of CC chemokine receptors revealed that cultured primary rat OPCs express CCR3, while CCR1, CCR2, CCR4, CCR5, and CCR7 could not be detected (Maysami *et al.*, 2006a).

Pretreatment of oligodendrocytes with IFN-γ in culture had a protective effect against oxidative stress and the inhibition of proteasome activity and resulted in upregulation and expression of a number of chemokines, notably CXCL10, CCL2, CCL3, and CCL5 (Balabanov *et al.*, 2007). Together with the observation that, in PLP/SOCS1 transgenic mice, these mutants display reduced oligodendrocyte responsiveness to IFN-γ, EAE onset was accelerated with enhanced early inflammation and increased oligodendrocyte apoptosis, which might yet be another indication that chemokine receptor expression and regulation by oligodendrocytes could contribute to successful regeneration and remyelination. The conclusion that in this regard IFN-γ/ oligodendrocyte interactions might be beneficial is of interest but to a certain degree contradictory to the rather detrimental effect this cytokine appears to exert in the course of acute demyelination (see above).

Toll-like receptors

Toll-like receptors (TLR) are predominantly used by cells of the innate immune system to recognize pathogen-associated molecular patterns (PAMPs), structures expressed by various classes of microbes but not by eukaryotic organisms. Thus far, ten different TLRs have been identified in humans and nine TLRs in mice (Medzhitov and Janeway, Jr., 1997). TLR activation ultimately leads to the induction of NF-κB (see further below), the transcription of chemokines, proinflammatory cytokines and cell surface molecules all involved in the initiation of adaptive immune responses to pathogens (Olson and Miller, 2004). Oligodendrocytes have been found to express TLR2 and TLR3 (Bsibsi et al., 2002). In order to investigate TLR-specific effects on oligodendrocytes, mediated directly or indirectly via activated macrophages, the extent of oligodendrocyte loss and OPC (NG2$^+$) proliferation and differentiation was studied following intraspinal injection of TLR2 and TLR4 agonists. Lipopolysaccharide (as TLR4 agonist) injection sites displayed a significant rise in precursor cell proliferation rates and oligodendrocyte differentiation, which exceeded that of control and lysolecithin-injected animals. Zymosan (TLR2) injections, on the other hand, led to complete oligodendrocyte loss without stimulating NG2 cell proliferation or oligodendrocyte replacement (Schonberg et al., 2007). Whether these contrasting effects arise from differentially activated signaling cascades in macrophages or result from direct TLR2 activation on oligodendrocytes needs to be further examined.

Clusters of differentiation (CD)

Cluster of differentiation is a historical term that was created to define cell-surface molecules that are recognized by a given set of monoclonal antibodies. Although this was initially used to classify leukocytes into subsets, many CDs were revealed to have more widespread expression, such as for example on neural cells.

CD9 is expressed by oligodendrocytes in the CNS (Kagawa *et al.*, 1997), in particular on progenitor cells committed to oligodendrogenesis, and is involved in the formation of the tetraspanin web beneath the plasma membranes. However, it turned out not to be essential for oligodendrogenesis and myelination (Terada *et al.*, 2002a). CD9 is also expressed by Schwann cells of the peripheral nervous system (Anton *et al.*, 1995) where it affects migratory behavior. Low levels of CD13 (aminopeptidase N) expression were found on the oligodendrocyte cell line MO3.13 and might thus confer susceptibility to human coronavirus infection (Lachance *et al.*, 1998). CD15 is a carbohydrate epitope (3-fucosyl-*N*-acetyllactosamine) that was found within the cytoplasm of oligodendrocytes and on the cell surface of astrocytes (Gocht, 1992). Round cells at the edge of demyelinating lesions present in increased numbers, presumably oligodendrocytes, were found to be devoid of CD3, CD20 and CD68 (Openshaw *et al.*, 2000). Oligodendrocytes and microglia are immunonegative for CD38 (Yamada *et al.*, 1997) but two reports revealed that human oligodendrocytes in culture as well as in the brain express CD44, a family of cell surface glycoproteins involved in cell–cell and cell–extracellular matrix adhesion (Bouvier-Labit *et al.*, 2002; Moretto *et al.*, 1993). In the adult brain, $CD45^+$ myelinating oligodendrocytes were detected in the supraventricular corpus callosum (Nakahara *et al.*, 2005). The CD45, a protein tyrosine phosphatase, appears to be involved in the oligodendrocyte maturation process as dysmyelination was observed in CD45-deficient mice, which is in line with previously reported CD45 mutations observed in some MS patients (Jacobsen *et al.*, 2000). CD46 (membrane cofactor protein) is a regulator of complement activation that also serves as the entry receptor for human herpes virus 6 (HHV-6) and measles virus (MV), and is expressed at low levels in healthy human brains and may be confined to oligodendrocytes (Cassiani-Ingoni *et al.*, 2005; McQuaid and Cosby, 2002). CD56 encodes a neural cell adhesion molecule and was found on neurons and astrocytes as well as on oligodendrocytes and Schwann cells (Hatano *et al.*, 1997). Rat oligodendrocytes can spontaneously activate complement C but controversial reports exist regarding the presence of the C inhibitor CD59 (Gasque and Morgan, 1996; Scolding *et al.*, 1998b). This is of interest, as such an absence could result in susceptibility to lysis by autologous complement C. Human oligodendrocytes were shown to possess CD59 on their surface. CD59 is absent from the human CNS before myelination but is induced in areas of myelin production. Following this CD59 expression becomes down-regulated but it reappears in reactive astrocytes in diseases such as

MS (Zajicek *et al.*, 1995). TAPA (target of the antiproliferative antibody) also known as CD81 was found on all CNS glial cells including oligodendrocytes and levels of expression were correlated with cellular maturation (Sullivan and Geisert, 1998) whereas CD88 (receptor for complement C5a) is expressed constitutively by astrocytes, microglia and fibroblast-like cells but not by oligodendrocytes (Gasque *et al.*, 1997). The cell death receptor CD95 (Fas/Apo-1) (Beattie, 2004; Krammer, 1999) was reported to be constitutively expressed on oligodendrocytes (Ricci-Vitiani *et al.*, 2000) as well as in MS lesions (D'Souza *et al.*, 1996) which makes these cells susceptible to Fas-ligand-dependent apoptosis induction (Aktas *et al.*, 2006). CD100, the transmembrane semaphorin 4D which acts as an inhibitor of axonal growth, is also expressed on oligodendrocytes and was moreover found to be upregulated after CNS lesion (Moreau-Fauvarque *et al.*, 2003). It might thus contribute to the myelin-dependent regeneration blockade of the adult CNS in this situation. CD140, known as platelet-derived growth factor receptor α (PDGFRα), is involved in OPC proliferation (Hart *et al.*, 1989; Richardson *et al.*, 1988). CD156, encoding the metalloprotease-disintegrin ADAM8, is present on neurons and oligodendrocytes and has been implicated in neuron–glia interactions during neurodegeneration (Schlomann *et al.*, 2000). CD181, CD182, CD183 and CD184 are synonyms for chemokine receptors CXCR1, CXCR2, CXCR3 and CXCR4, respectively, all of which were shown to be present on oligodendrocytes (see above). CD195 is the chemokine receptor CCR5, the expression of which is confined to macrophages and microglia but not oligodendrocytes in healthy and inflamed EAE spinal cords (Eltayeb *et al.*, 2007). Finally, the CD200-CD200R signaling pathway was demonstrated to play a critical role in the course of EAE in which neuronally expressed CD200 interacts with CD200R on micro- and macroglial cells (including oligodendrocytes). Axons of Wld(s) mice are protected from damage and degeneration and this was found to be a result of elevated CD200 levels (Chitnis *et al.*, 2007).

Glutamate

Magnetic resonance studies of the brains of human MS patients have demonstrated that altered glutamate metabolism may be important for the development of MS (Srinivasan *et al.*, 2005). In animal models, glutamate excitotoxicity mediated by the AMPA/kainate-type of glutamate receptors is known to damage not only neurons but also oligodendrocytes, which appear to participate in white matter glutamate clearance (Pitt *et al.*, 2000; Smith *et al.*, 2000). It has been shown that treating EAE with an AMPA/kainate antagonist ameliorates the disease course (Werner *et al.*, 2000). In another study it was shown that glutamate receptor expression and glutamate removal are defective in MS white matter, possibly mediated by TNF-α. Such deficiencies might underlie high extracellular glutamate concentrations and increase the susceptibility to glutamate excitotoxicity (Pitt *et al.*, 2003).

Corticosteroids and NF-κB

It has been shown that expression of NF-κB markedly prevents apoptosis of the oligodendroglial CG-4 cell line. This anti-apoptotic activity is repressed in culture by IκB-α, an inhibitor of NF-κB, which implies that NF-κB acts as a potent inhibitor of TNF-α-induced apoptosis in oligodendrocytes (Hamanoue *et al.*, 2004). In light of the fact that several apoptotic stimuli have also been shown to activate NF-κB in oligodendrocytes, this initial reaction may be part of a survival response rather than mediating cellular death signals. It was also demonstrated that the TNF-α effect on oligodendrocytes consists of not only induction of apoptosis but also the blockade of their differentiation (Mann *et al.*, 2008). Notably, co-treatment with corticosteroids at the time of TNF-α application improved survival as well as differentiation of oligodendrocytes. This was investigated at the level of morphological maturation, myelin protein expression and ion current maturation, suggesting that corticosteroids support or improve NF-κB-dependent survival. Thus, this observation provides a possible therapeutic approach for the functional restoration of cytokine-damaged immature oligodendrocytes. The question of exactly how corticosteroids interact with NF-κB is also of particular interest because corticosteroids are used for the treatment of acute bouts of MS. Activation of immune cells involves the targeted degradation of NF-κB's cytoplasmic inhibitor IκB-α and the translocation of NF-κB to the nucleus. It was shown that the synthetic glucocorticoid dexamethasone induces transcription of the IκB-α gene, which results in increased IκB-α protein synthesis (Scheinman *et al.*, 1995). Stimulation with TNF-α causes the release of NF-κB from IκB-α; however, in the presence of dexamethasone this newly released NF-κB quickly reassociates with newly synthesized IκB-α, thus markedly reducing the net amount of NF-κB that translocates to the nucleus. Immunosuppression is therefore the result of prevented NF-κB translocation, but the extent to which NF-κB-dependent oligodendrocyte survival is modulated similarly remains yet to be examined.

ADHESION MOLECULES

Oligodendrocytes express myelin-associated glycoprotein (MAG) initially described as a neural cell adhesion molecule involved in neuron-to-oligodendrocyte and oligodendrocyte-to-oligodendrocyte adhesions (Poltorak et al., 1987). MAG can promote neurite outgrowth from embryonic neurons, but blocks axon outgrowth from postnatal neurons, thus it qualifies as a myelin inhibitor of axonal regeneration (Mukhopadhyay et al., 1994). Oligodendrocytes also express the neural cell adhesion molecule (N-CAM) (Trotter et al., 1989) as well as ICAM-1, which can also be found on astrocytes and was furthermore shown to be upregulated upon immune mediator stimulation, an observation that might be relevant to lymphocyte–glial cell interactions at sites of inflammation in the CNS (Satoh et al., 1991). Oligodendrocyte pre-progenitors were also shown to express the polysialated form of N-CAM (PSA-NCAM), a post-translational modification the removal of which interfered with pre-progenitor cell migration, but has been reported to induce cellular differentiation (Decker et al., 2000). Apparently, oligodendrocytes are negative for VCAM-1 (Selmaj, 2000) but L-1, a molecule that has been described as important in the context of neuronal cell migration (Miura et al., 1992), can be found on oligodendrocytes (Takeda et al., 1996). Besides these molecules, oligodendrocytes can synthesize a variety of different GPI-anchored proteins. Among them is the cell adhesion molecule F3, one of the most prominent GPI-anchored proteins, which was previously thought to be exclusively expressed by neurons (Koch et al., 1997).

A number of integrin molecules have been shown to be expressed by oligodendrocytes such as integrin $\alpha1\beta1$ (CD49a/CD29), $\alpha6\beta1$ (CD49f/CD29), $\alpha8\beta1$ (CD-/CD29), $\alpha v\beta1$ (CD51/CD29), $\alpha v\beta3$ (CD51/CD61) and $\alpha v\beta5$ (CD51/CD-), indicating that integrins are not only involved in immune cell recruitment (Engelhardt, 2008) but may also mediate glial repair. This notion is further supported by the observation that in EAE TNF-α, as a potent mediator of CNS inflammation, leads to the expression of integrin $\alpha2\beta1$ (CD49b/CD29) (all reviewed in Archelos et al., 1999). In addition, integrin $\alpha6\beta1$ is expressed throughout development while αv-integrins show developmental regulation (Milner and Ffrench-Constant, 1994). While oligodendrocyte differentiation is accompanied by a loss of integrin $\alpha v\beta1$ and concomitant upregulation of integrin $\alpha v\beta5$, functional experiments reveal that OPC migration in culture is mediated primarily by the $\alpha v\beta1$ integrin, but not by $\alpha6\beta1$ or $\alpha v\beta3$ integrins (Milner, 1997).

Complement

Many studies have tried to define the relevance of complement/oligodendrocyte interactions in pathological paradigms such as EAE or MS. As outlined above the expression of complement-associated CD molecules has been demonstrated for oligodendrocytes. This is of interest as complement-activated oligodendrocytes (CAOs) were found to delineate miniature MS plaques of 300–500 μm in diameter (Schwab and McGeer, 2002). The plaques are devoid of myelin and are surrounded by a rim of activated microglia intermingled with the C4d-CAOs. In large MS lesions, C1q-C9 immunoreactive fibers were detected, indicating complete activation of the complement cascade in these more developed lesions. It was suggested that the miniature plaques, bordered by C4d-CAOs, represent the earliest stage of plaque development, preceding even the larger, transient plaques frequently observed in serial magnetic resonance imaging (MRI) studies.

Further evidence points to the possibility that MOG specifically binds C1q in a dose-dependent manner. This calcium-dependent interaction seems to be mediated by MOG's extracellular immunoglobulin-like domain, which contains an amino acid motif similar to the core C1q-binding sequence previously identified in IgG antibodies. These results demonstrate that MOG binds C1q near the IgG binding site and may be the protein responsible for complement activation in oligodendrocytes. Such a direct interaction has significant implications regarding CNS inflammation and provides a mechanism by which oligodendrocytes could subsequently be harmed (Johns and Bernard, 1997). Given that glutamate toxicity has been implicated in the generation of direct tissue damage in MS and EAE, the observation that a brief incubation with glutamate followed by exposure to complement can efficiently kill oligodendrocytes in culture and in freshly isolated optic nerves is of particular interest (Alberdi et al., 2006). The authors concluded that glutamate sensitization of oligodendrocytes to complement attack may thus contribute to white matter damage.

Beneficial effects might also relate to the expression of complement molecules. Oligodendrocytes and OPCs respond to serum withdrawal by a rapid decline of protective Bcl-2 expression resulting in caspase-3-dependent apoptotic death. However, sublytic assembly of membrane-inserted terminal complement complexes consisting of C5b, C6, C7, C8 and C9 proteins (C5b-9) was shown to inhibit caspase-3 activation through post-translational regulation of Bad

(Bcl2-antagonist of cell death). This mechanism may therefore be involved in the promotion of oligodendrocyte survival in inflammatory demyelinating disorders (Soane *et al.*, 2001). In addition, such sublytic complement activation was found to downregulate expression of myelin genes in culture and to induce the oligodendrocytes to enter the cell cycle (Badea *et al.*, 1998).

OLIGODENDROCYTES AS ANTIGEN-PRESENTING CELLS

Oligodendrocytes, as the axon-ensheathing myelinating cells of the CNS, produce a multitude of different myelin components which all show specific patterns of subcellular distribution. Myelin basic protein (MBP) is associated with microtubule organization and $Ca^{2+}/$ calmodulin-regulated microtubule stabilization in culture (Harauz *et al.*, 2004) and is detectable at high density over the compact myelin lamellae, but not in regions of the paranodal loops, cell body or other non-compacted regions of the oligodendrocyte plasma membrane (Brunner *et al.*, 1989). CNP (2′, 3′-cyclic nucleotide 3′-phosphodiesterase), an early myelin marker, links myelin-related proteins to the cytoskeleton (Dyer and Benjamins, 1989) and interacts with membrane lipids during the extension and wrapping of the oligodendroglial process around the axon (Barradas *et al.*, 2000). CNP reactivity is reported to be highest at the myelin/axon interface, and is found in lower concentrations over the outer lamellae of the myelin and throughout the compact myelin as well as at the cytoplasmic face of non-compacted regions of oligodendrocyte membranes. MOG, which has been reported to play a role in cell adhesion, microtubular stabilization and complement activation (Johns and Bernard, 1999), can be preferentially detected on the extracellular surface of oligodendrocytes but only in low amounts in the lamellae of compacted myelin and the oligodendrocyte/axon border zone. Probably due to MOG's exposed position on the extracellular surface of myelin on the one hand and MBP's abundance on the other hand, MOG and MBP are potent immunogenic agents used to induce EAE in a variety of mammals. In both MS and EAE, T-cell reactivity and antibody generation against MOG are considered to be predominant autoimmune mechanisms (Kerlero de Rosbo *et al.*, 1997). As to whether anti-MOG antibodies are directly involved in the demyelinating pathology or only amplify T-cell-mediated damage reactions (Linington *et al.*, 1988) is currently a matter of controversial discussions. However, doubts about the role of MOG as one of the most important MS-associated epitopes (Lampasona *et al.*, 2004) could be countered by the results of a more recent study which revealed a clear-cut pathogenic antibody response to native MOG protein (Zhou *et al.*, 2006). In this regard it is of interest to note that opsonization of oligodendrocyte surfaces by antibodies was found to promote Fc receptor-dependent cell lysis by macrophages (Scolding and Compston, 1991) and that the membrane attack complex (MAC) has also been implicated in demyelination (Mead *et al.*, 2002). An orchestrated pattern of epitope recognition appears to exist throughout the course of MS. According to our current knowledge, the epitope spectrum is rather restricted to certain myelin antigens in early phases of disease, and undergoes a dynamic expansion (coined "epitope spreading") in response to repeated inflammatory CNS attacks (Vanderlugt and Miller, 2002).

OLIGODENDROGLIAL/IMMUNE CELL INTERACTIONS

Macrophages

Brain-invading macrophages are active participants in all kinds of inflammatory myelin disorders, thus rendering their interactions with oligodendrocytes important to investigate. Early studies demonstrated that macrophage depletion by treatment with silica dust or dichloromethylene diphosphonate (Cl2MDP) can delay the onset of clinical signs and improve the EAE disease course (Brosnan *et al.*, 1981; Huitinga *et al.*, 1990). In order to determine how the deleterious effect of macrophages on oligodendrocytes is mediated it was important to discern intercellular relations. Of note, no adherence of macrophages to homologous oligodendrocytes can be observed when they are simply co-cultured. However, it could be demonstrated that antibodies against galactocerebroside or MOG specifically triggered attachment of macrophages to oligodendrocytes (Griot-Wenk *et al.*, 1991; Scolding and Compston, 1991), revealing yet another mechanism by which myelin antibodies can mediate damage to oligodendrocytes. After CD4[+] T cell-dependent activation, macrophages are thought to mediate damage to oligodendrocytes by means of TNF-α, reactive oxygen species (ROS) or reactive nitrogen species (RNS) secretion or by expression of the Fas death ligand (D'Souza *et al.*, 1996).

Microglia

Microglia of the CNS which are of macrophage lineage have recently been described as highly active cells in their presumed resting state, continually surveying their microenvironment with extremely motile processes and protrusions (Nimmerjahn *et al.*, 2005). Nevertheless, older studies have already stated that, under resting conditions, microglia show only minimal contact with oligodendrocytes, neither conferring cytotoxic effects nor producing TNF-α (Zajicek *et al.*, 1992). However, upon activation with interferon-γ (IFN-γ), either alone or in combination with the TLR4 agonist lipopolysaccharide (LPS), microglial cells increase their interactions with oligodendrocytes and produce TNF-α, which leads to oligodendroglial damage and degeneration. When complement was present such activated microglia even showed significant phagocytosis of MBP, indicating that the interplay of cytokines and complement can turn friendly neighbors into an oligodendrocyte's personal nightmare. In addition, high effector to target cell ratios were shown to increase natural microglial cytotoxicity against oligodendrocytes in culture (Merrill and Zimmerman, 1991), whereas in this case oligodendrocyte death was not mediated by the release of soluble factors. The observation that in MS lesions microglia express FasL (D'Souza *et al.*, 1996) indicates that oligodendrocytes might also be depleted via CD95 activation. Such cell/cell interactions may therefore underlie the microglia-mediated killing of oligodendrocytes in MS lesions – an effect which, however, might be counteracted by TGF-β, as this cytokine can inhibit the generation of nitric oxide (NO), the suspected effector of oligodendrocyte death (Merrill *et al.*, 1993).

Lymphocytes

Lymphocyte/oligodendrocyte interactions should mainly be seen in the context of target recognition, as myelin proteins and other oligodendrocyte-derived, myelin-associated molecules represent an important immunological stimulus to the adaptive immune system. This has been convincingly shown for EAE, where immunization with myelin-derived proteins or selected myelin peptides results in autoimmune demyelination. Thus, EAE serves both as a model for organ-specific harmful autoimmunity and as a key model for testing MS therapies.

Interestingly, mechanistic studies investigating the direct and immediate impact of T cells on oligodendrocyte integrity suggest that

T cells are rather orchestrating the immune attack by activating and attracting other immune cells such as macrophages, microglia and B cells (Steinman, 1996). For example, cultures of human oligodendrocytes were not susceptible to damage by activated autologous T cells, rather ruling out a direct cell-to-cell impact of T cells on oligodendrocytes in the course of autoimmune demyelination (Giuliani *et al.*, 2003). The same holds true for B cells and plasma cells, antibody-producing lymphocytes derived from B cells. On the other hand, several studies have shown that immune mediators such as pro-inflammatory cytokines belonging to a Th1-type or Th17-type immune response (IFN-γ, TNF-α, IL-12 and IL-17, IL-21, IL-22, respectively) may indeed exert deleterious effects on myelin integrity and affect oligodendrocyte survival (reviewed by Giovannoni and Hartung, 1996). However, cultured oligodendrocytes have been shown to be susceptible to CD8+ T-cell-mediated lysis (Jurewicz *et al.*, 1998), which is in agreement with the observed involvement of this lymphocyte population in EAE (Huseby *et al.*, 2001), and γ/δ T cells were also reported to mediate oligodendrocyte lysis indicating that these cells might mediate demyelination in an MHC-independent manner (Freedman *et al.*, 1991). On the other hand, the lack of MHC class II expression makes it unlikely that CD4+ T cells exert direct effects on oligodendrocytes; these are presumably mediated via activated microglia and macrophages instead.

In addition, B cell-derived anti-myelin antibodies have been shown to augment pre-existing EAE, by both activation of complement and attraction of Fc receptor-guided immune cells such as macrophages and microglia (Racke, 2008). On the other hand, one should note that certain antibodies may even have a regenerative impact on the injured CNS, as shown for selected antibodies of the IgM subtype reacting to specific myelin components and inducing remyelination, especially in the Theiler-virus-induced model of viral demyelination (Warrington *et al.*, 2000). It is believed that such antibodies may facilitate the opsonization of myelin debris, allowing repair (i.e. spontaneous remyelination by resident OPCs) to proceed. However, the recently reported clinical efficacy of B cell-depleting treatments such as the therapeutic anti-CD20 antibody rituximab indicates that net inhibition of B cell activity and function constitutes a promising therapeutic approach for MS (Hauser *et al.*, 2008).

Besides these models of CNS autoimmunity, investigations regarding the role of the human endogenous retrovirus HERV-W family (also multiple sclerosis-associated retrovirus, MSRV; recently reviewed by Dolei and Perron, 2009) indicate that oligodendrocytes could indeed represent targets of T lymphocytes. This is based on the observation that HERV-W ENV and GAG proteins were found to be upregulated in MS lesions (Perron *et al.*, 2005). Surprisingly, MSRV particles as well as recombinant ENV proteins were shown to induce a T cell response regardless of the immunological MHC class II background, suggesting non-conventional activation with polyclonal T cell expansion. It, thus, appears that MSRV structures can trigger an abnormal immune response with characteristics similar to that of superantigens, and that such an activation may have the capacity to induce and sustain a myelin-directed immune attack (Perron *et al.*, 2001).

Regarding the well-documented neurodegenerative features of MS first described by Charcot in 1868, it turns out that axonal trans-ection and neuronal death may occur in the course of autoimmune demyelination as well, mediated by rather unspecific collateral damage mechanisms. Moreover, immunization with primary neuronal proteins may induce CNS pathology (Mathey *et al.*, 2007; Pellkofer *et al.*, 2004) but it is apparently not sufficient for induction of a full-blown CNS-specific destructive autoimmune reaction, as compared with immunization with myelin antigens.

CONCLUSION AND PERSPECTIVES

Although the CNS has been regarded as an immune-privileged organ (Bechmann *et al.*, 2007), the large number of studies demonstrating that oligodendrocytes either synthesize immuno-relevant proteins or respond specifically to their exposure implies that in pathological situations, particularly upon blood–brain barrier breakdown, these cells actively participate in humoral and cellular interactions. It must therefore be concluded that these neuroglial cells cannot be regarded as exclusively passive target cells but must be re-evaluated as potent (local) modulators of the immune response. This notion is increasingly accepted and is in agreement with findings regarding the induction of genes involved in ischemic preconditioning and neuroprotection in MS normal-appearing white matter (NAWM) (Graumann *et al.*, 2003; Zeis *et al.*, 2008b). It is nevertheless clear that, due to their elaborate morphology and their numerous cell/cell interactions, mature oligo-dendrocytes remain among the most vulnerable cells of the CNS, unable to cope with sustained immune attacks. The fact that oligoden-drocyte damage and loss is in most cases the ultimate consequence of such interactions might therefore result mainly from their inability to respond adequately to lesion and insult, e.g. their failure to redifferentiate and regenerate. In order to increase our understanding of the molecular mechanisms underlying inflammatory demyelinating diseases it will therefore be necessary to investigate production of and response to immune-related molecules by oligodendrocytes, both in culture as well as in vivo, by means of large-scale systematic screenings. It is hoped that such results will then help to discriminate between harmful and beneficial processes taking place in oligodendrocytes themselves as well as in their vicinity.

7

Oligodendrocytes and disease: repair, remyelination and stem cells

INTRODUCTION

In many diseases of the CNS, oligodendrocytes are damaged and lost, and the related demyelination and consequent conduction block play a major role in producing neurological disability. In some, oligodendrocyte injury is secondary to non-specific insults, such as trauma or ischemia. In others, more specific or targeted oligodendrocyte damage occurs. Amongst the latter, multiple sclerosis (MS) is perhaps paradigmatic.

In MS, however, partial remyelination is conspicuous in many lesions, and is thought to contribute significantly to lasting recovery from acute relapse; it is also likely to contribute to the preservation of axons, and in this way to help reduce the accumulation of permanent neurological dysfunction. However, the progression of the disease, with relentlessly accumulating disability and handicap seen in the majority of patients with long-standing disease – and all with primary progressive MS – implies that reparative processes are overwhelmed or in some other way ultimately fail.

In this chapter, the biological background to oligodendrocyte and myelin repair in MS is briefly considered, and the reasons for the failure of more widespread and lasting tissue repair are explored. Experimental studies provide clear evidence that cell therapies to replace oligodendrocytes can be highly successful in promoting remyelination, but whether these can realistically translate into clinical management remains open to serious question. This said, few areas of emerging technology have commanded as much excitement in the past few years as that of stem cells and their potential therapeutic exploitation in an enormous range of currently incurable diseases. Here, the clinical approaches that might allow the

The Biology of Oligodendrocytes, eds. Patricia J. Armati and Emily K. Mathey. Published by Cambridge University Press. © Cambridge University Press 2010.

translation of these laboratory studies into neurological practice, together with some of the remaining problems and difficulties to be overcome, will be discussed.

OLIGODENDROCYTE DAMAGE IN DISEASE: DEMYELINATION

Since the principal function of oligodendrocytes is the synthesis and maintenance of myelin in the CNS, it is to be expected that the pathological hallmark of oligodendrocyte disease is the loss of myelin – demyelination. Indeed historically demyelination was recognized as a pathological change in diseased brain and spinal cord tissue well before oligodendrocytes were even discovered: only later did their description and the discovery of their role in myelin synthesis emerge.

Demyelination as a feature of disease may be primary or secondary: primary, where myelin or oligodendrocytes (or both) appear to be the primary target, or (if inherently disordered) cause, of the disease process; secondary, where the oligodendrocyte–myelin unit is the innocent and accidental victim of non-specific disease or damage, or indeed of specific disease processes primarily directed at other targets – neurons or astrocytes. MS, where oligodendrocytes and their myelin appear to be targeted in what many would view as a cell-specific autoimmune disease, is perhaps the paradigmatic illustration of an acquired primary demyelinating disease, whereas genetically determined hypomyelinating leukodystrophies such as Pelizaeus–Merzbacher disease constitute the inherited primary demyelinating diseases. "Bystander" oligodendrocyte damage and myelin loss is prominent in stroke and also in central nervous system (CNS) trauma, as examples of secondary demyelination. However, the distinction, while remaining useful in many ways, is less absolute and clear than it may superficially appear. In Alexander disease, for example, commonly considered to be an inherited primary demyelinating disease, myelin loss in fact is thought to occur as the result of defects in astrocytes and consequent loss of crucial trophic support for oligodendrocytes. In acquired neuromyelitis optica, classified as a variant of MS, antibodies that are targeted against an astrocyte foot-process surface protein (aquaporin) are suggested to cause a demyelinating pathology again through disrupting astrocyte function (Takano *et al.*, 2008; Vincent *et al.*, 2008).

Regardless of its primary or secondary nature, demyelination naturally has important functional consequences. Normal saltatory

conduction is blocked, and neurological function in the affected path-
way(s) is therefore disturbed. Persistent demyelination is followed
by adaptive or plastic change in the demyelinated axon, namely the
redistribution of sodium channels from their normal (in myelinated
axons) arrangement – clustered at the nodes of Ranvier – to a more
even distribution along the course of the axon (Waxman, 2006).
This facilitates the restoration of conduction along the axon, but not
saltatory conduction – the speed of conduction is therefore reduced
and normal overall function not fully restored. A normal conduction
velocity can, however, be attained, but requires restoration of the
myelin, or remyelination.

REPAIR OF DEMYELINATION; OLIGODENDROCYTE REGENERATION

We are fast approaching the fiftieth anniversary of the first description of the phenomenon of spontaneous myelin repair by Dick and
Mary Bunge, studying a feline model of demyelination (Bunge et al.,
1961). Later it became clear that remyelination also occurs in the
human nervous system, specifically in MS (Perier and Gregoire,
1965). However, spontaneous remyelination does not result in the
reinvestment of denuded axons with myelin that is morphologically
normal (or with myelin that is identical to that formed during
development); repaired myelin is thinner in relation to the axon
diameter compared with "normal" myelin, and the internode length
is shorter (Blakemore, 1974). This characteristic and distinctive structure is retained even in the long term (Ludwin and Maitland, 1984),
conveniently offering means by which the phenomenon of myelin
repair may be identified and studied (though the distinction is less
clear in relation to small diameter axons; Stidworthy et al., 2003).
The key point from a functional perspective, however, is that
normal saltatory conduction is successfully restored by remyelination
(Smith et al., 1979), and neurological function likewise improved
(Jeffery and Blakemore, 1997) (though it should be mentioned that
while the precise mechanisms of neurophysiological restoration
are not fully elucidated, careful studies show the reappearance of
saltatory conduction temporally precedes remyelination; Smith
et al., 1982).

Using these characteristic morphological features of repaired
myelin to explore MS, it has become clear that spontaneous remyelination is hardly a rare event in MS. Recent studies have in fact shown

extensive and widespread remyelination across the whole spectrum of the disease – in one important study of almost 170 demyelinated lesions, taken significantly from post mortem samples from patients with very long-standing MS, only 5% of lesions were found to be completed demyelinated with no repair, while the average extent of remyelination was some 47% (Patani *et al.*, 2007). Comparable studies of cortical lesions in MS also reported "extensive" cortical remyelination, indeed suggesting there was more remyelination in the cortex than in white matter lesions (Albert *et al.*, 2007). These findings have important implications for the use of cell-based approaches for therapeutic repair (see below).

WHAT CELLS ARE RESPONSIBLE FOR SPONTANEOUS MYELIN REPAIR?

While oligodendrocytes are the cells responsible for the synthesis and maintenance of myelin, it does not necessarily follow that the mature oligodendrocyte is the cell responsible for repairing myelin. Experimental studies rather suggest it is not. Mature oligodendrocytes – which have already been through one cycle of developmental differentiation, contact with a non-myelinated segment of axon, elaboration of a myelin membrane, enwrapment of the axon followed by myelin formation and then compaction – have an extremely limited capacity for recapitulating this complex sequence and resynthesizing new myelin following demyelination, even if they do survive the injury causing myelin damage. Such mature oligodendrocytes can be identified within areas of experimental demyelination but do not appear capable of remyelination (Kierstead and Blakemore, 1997). Rather, new oligodendrocytes appear in areas of myelin damage, and these are responsible for myelin repair.

There are, however, several potential sources of such new oligodendrocytes. Two of these have little experimental support and, like the above possibility, are considered improbable: the migration of mature oligodendrocytes from areas unaffected by injury, and re-engagement in myelination; and the de-differentiation of mature oligodendrocytes to form proliferative oligodendrocyte progenitors better able to remyelinate. Transplanted mature (human) oligodendrocytes achieve very little, if any, compact new myelin formation in the demyelinated rodent CNS, though they are able to elaborate membranes, engage with axons and enwrap them in one or two uncompacted loops of myelin (Targett *et al.*, 1996).

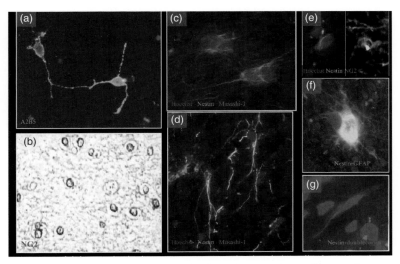

Figure 7.1 Adult human oligodendrocyte progenitor cellss may be identified in cell culture (a) and in the lesions of multiple sclerosis (MS) (b). The latter also contain increased numbers of cells with immunophenotypic properties compatible with neural precursors. Nestin-positive cells in MS lesions co-stained for musashi-1 (c), NG2 (e), GFAP (f) and doublecortin (g). Control spinal cord stained with nestin and musashi-1 (d). Reprinted with permission from Snethen et al. (2008). See color plate section for color version of this figure.

Rather, the overwhelming consensus of opinion is that new oligodendrocytes responsible for remyelination are formed from proliferative oligodendrocyte precursor cells. That such cells are present in the adult CNS was first demonstrated in the rodent more than two decades ago, (Ffrench-Constant and Raff, 1986) and in the human brain (Figure 7.1) some years later (Scolding et al., 1995, 1999). Similar to, but by no means identical with, the intensively studied perinatal oligodendrocyte progenitor (Wolswijk et al., 1991; Wolswijk and Noble, 1989), the adult progenitor may be derived from its developmental counterpart (Wren et al., 1992). It appears to play a major role in repair of myelin – but is likely to have a number of other functions, exhibiting as it does a number of complex electrophysiological properties contingent upon the expression and function of a range of glutamate receptors allowing direct cross-talk with the neuron–axon unit (Karadottir et al., 2005, 2008; Luyt et al., 2004). The "normal" function of the adult oligodendrocyte progenitor (i.e. when there is no local damage and demyelination) is still very actively under exploration, and is beyond the scope of this text (Levine et al., 2001).

In contrast to mature oligodendrocytes, mitotic oligodendrocyte progenitors are capable of extensive remyelination following transplantation into areas of experimental myelin damage (Nunes et al., 2003; Warrington et al., 1993; Zhang et al., 1999), with some evidence that adult progenitors achieve remyelination more rapidly than their embryonic counterparts (Windrem et al., 2004). There is good evidence also that endogenous oligodendrocyte progenitor cells are responsible for spontaneous experimental remyelination (Carroll and Jennings, 1994; Carroll et al., 1998; Gensert and Goldman, 1997), and cells with comparable immunophenotypes have been identified in the lesions of MS (Chang et al., 2000; Maeda et al., 2001; Reynolds et al., 2002; Scolding et al., 1998a; Wolswijk, 2002) (Figure 7.1; and see below).

A supplementary (additional, rather than alternative) possibility concerns the origin of these remyelinating progenitors. Whilst they are clearly present in the normal adult CNS parenchyma and responsive to disease processes (Fancy et al., 2004; Levine and Reynolds, 1999), it is also possible that endogenous neural stem cells or precursor cells proliferate and act as a source of oligodendrocyte progenitor cells (Picard-Riera et al., 2002). Indeed (and to complicate matters further) there is significant evidence that cells in the adult CNS previously considered oligodendrocyte progenitors in fact possess neural precursor properties, with the capacity to generate astrocytes and/or neuronal cells in addition to oligodendrocytes (Belachew et al., 2003; Kondo and Raff, 2000; Nunes et al., 2003). Endogenous neural precursors also appear to respond to disease processes in MS (Figure 7.1), though whether their progeny can contribute to remyelination is difficult if not impossible to prove in human disease tissue (Nait-Oumesmar et al., 2007; Snethen et al., 2008).

Finally, there is yet one further possible contributor to CNS myelin repair – the Schwann cell. This was indeed the first cell type shown to be capable of exogenous "therapeutic" CNS remyelination in experimental animals (Figure 7.2) (Blakemore, 1977), other studies showing that Schwann cells make a clear but quantitatively minor contribution to spontaneous myelin repair in MS, perhaps most particularly in the spinal cord (Ghatak et al., 1973; Itoyama et al., 1983, 1985; Ludwin, 1988; Ogata and Feigin, 1975).

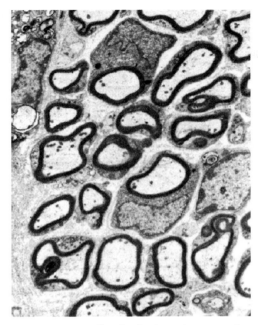

Figure 7.2 Remyelination in the rodent central nervous system by exogenous Schwann cells.

WHY IS SPONTANEOUS REMYELINATION NOT MORE EXTENSIVE?

Remyelination in MS is evidently much more extensive than originally thought, although it is far from complete. Historical pathological studies would hardly have granted MS its place as the paradigmatic demyelinating disease had myelin repair been complete, and recent studies emphasizing the success of spontaneous myelin repair, surprising in that they show the average extent of remyelination in lesions to be as much as 47%, still reveal that a larger percentage remain demyelinated. But given that a small proportion of lesions do remyelinate fully, why is myelin repair not even more complete? Again, there are a number of answers (and again these should in no way be seen as mutually exclusive) (Franklin, 2002).

Continuing disease processes in MS represent one obvious possibility. Perhaps surprisingly, however, there is evidence that repeated episodes of demyelination in fact fail to compromise spontaneous myelin repair (Penderis *et al.*, 2003) – although others have found that chronic demyelination does impair remyelination (Ludwin, 1980). Also, perhaps counterintuitively, the inflammatory environment may be conducive to remyelination rather than otherwise, both experimentally (Foote and Blakemore, 2005) and arguably in MS, where spontaneous myelin repair certainly seems most prominent in acute early lesions where there is notable inflammation (Prineas *et al.*, 1993a; Raine and Wu, 1993). The effect is only partly explained by the important role of macrophages in clearing myelin debris (Cuzner *et al.*, 1994; Kotter *et al.*, 2001), the latter being inhibitory to myelin repair (Kotter *et al.*, 2006); the release of pro-reparative neurotrophins and other growth factors by infiltrating inflammatory cells and local activated microglia may also play a role (Heese *et al.*, 1998; Kerschensteiner *et al.*, 1999; Nakajima and Kohsaka, 2001). Additionally, however, there are suggestions that oligodendrocyte progenitor-specific antibodies are found in patients with MS, and these of course could damage or at least inhibit the activity of progenitors in the CNS (Niehaus *et al.*, 2000; Trotter, 2005).

Other factors also contribute to the incompleteness of myelin repair in MS. Many studies have pointed to the presence of oligodendrocyte progenitors in lesions that are not remyelinated and concluded that these cells are self-evidently not functioning normally (or the lesions would be remyelinated). One possibility that has broad experimental support in the context of MS is that these cells have become blocked in differentiation before achieving functional maturity (Chang *et al.*, 2002; Kuhlmann *et al.*, 2008; Wolswijk, 1998). Myelin debris itself could contribute to this differentiation block (Kotter *et al.*, 2006), while the glycosaminoglycan hyaluronan also accumulates in MS lesions and this too inhibits oligodendrocyte progenitor maturation (Back *et al.*, 2005). Another possibility is that migration of progenitors into lesions is impaired (Williams *et al.*, 2007a), a possibility not incompatible with the above observations, firstly since not all demyelinated lesions contain significant numbers of progenitors (a significant proportion are depleted); and, secondly, because progenitors that only migrate into lesions in a delayed way, perhaps because of suboptimal semaphorin expression, may enter an environment no longer supportive of remyelination. Chronically demyelinated axons express molecules strikingly inhibitory to remyelination in MS, yet another contributory factor to impaired myelin repair in this disease (Charles *et al.*, 2002a; Coman *et al.*, 2005). Finally, the dense scar-like accumulation of hypertrophied and unreactive astrocytes in chronic MS lesions is also likely to present a profound barrier to myelin repair (Williams *et al.*, 2007b) – though arguably its appearance may reflect the consequence rather than the cause of failed remyelination.

THERAPEUTIC REMYELINATION: COULD THERAPY WITH MYELINATING CELLS REVERSE MS?

We are now close to a number of important anniversaries: the 50th of the discovery of spontaneous remyelination, the 40th of its demonstration in MS, and we have now also passed the 30th anniversary of Bill Blakemore's landmark report of therapeutic CNS myelin repair: Schwann cells isolated from rodent sciatic nerve, transplanted into the spinal cord, effected remyelination (Figure 7.2) (Blakemore, 1977). It is not insignificant that this study was part-funded by the (UK) MS Society: it has been a fundamental assumption ever since then that cell therapy in MS – the injection of myelinating cells into demyelinated lesions – offers the prospect of repairing lesions, restoring conduction and reversing disability in MS.

However, apart from one single trial in the USA (never published, to my knowledge), in which autologous Schwann cells were injected into non-lesional cerebrum in a small number of MS patients (later biopsy of the putative injection site unfortunately failing to strike the target and the study therefore proving uninformative), the concept of cell therapy in MS has yet to escape from the laboratory and trouble the patient community. Is this simply because the technical and clinical challenges are difficult, and the biology complex, but relentless scientific progress will eventually surmount these hurdles; or are there fundamental conceptual problems that undermine the rationale for cell injection therapies in MS? My personal view has always inclined strongly towards the former (Halfpenny *et al.*, 2002), although as the following suggests a strong case may be emerging for a fundamental reconsideration of this approach.

The likely solvable hurdles facing cell therapy in MS have been summarized elsewhere (Halfpenny *et al.*, 2002; Scolding and Dubois-Dalcq, 2008) but may be briefly rehearsed. First are the type and source of remyelinating cell. Schwann cells, the first studied in this context, would carry the advantage of relative accessibility and ease of expansion to large populations of high purity (Morrissey *et al.*, 1995; Rutkowski *et al.*, 1995); and purified human Schwann cells successfully lay down new myelin in the mouse (Levi and Bunge, 1994) and the rat spinal cord (Brierley *et al.*, 2001; Kohama *et al.*, 2001). In the macaque, highly successful large-scale spinal cord remyelination was achieved by autologous transplantation of expanded Schwann cells (Bachelin *et al.*, 2005). Finally, as mentioned above, this potentiality is given greater credence by repeated observations that Schwann cells make a certain contribution to spontaneous remyelination in MS (Ghatak *et al.*, 1973; Itoyama *et al.*, 1983, 1985; Ludwin, 1988; Ogata and Feigin, 1975) – findings that emphasize a further advantage, namely that Schwann cells and their myelin should be resistant to continuing MS-related immunological attack. The potential problems relating to Schwann cells, however, are serious. Tumor formation is described when rodent Schwann cells immortalized by growth factor expansion are transplanted (Langford *et al.*, 1988). Also, Schwann cell myelination is profoundly inhibited by the astrocyte scar, a core feature of the chronic MS plaque – although this may not be an insurmountable difficulty, and genetically modified Schwann cells might offer potential for therapeutic approaches in both MS and peripheral demyelinating diseases (Lavdas *et al.*, 2006).

Olfactory ensheathing cells, also relatively accessible and capable of expanding to form large and pure populations, represent another option. Again, autologous cells could be used; again, resistance to ongoing MS disease processes might be expected. Additionally, these cells appear far less vulnerable to inhibition of myelinating function by astrocytes; and olfactory glia are actively being explored in a number of preclinical and clinical settings (Franklin and Barnett, 2004; Raisman, 2004).

As outlined above, transplanted oligodendrocyte progenitor cells are an effective remyelinating population (Groves *et al.*, 1993; Windrem *et al.*, 2004; Zhang *et al.*, 1999), carrying the intuitive advantage of being the principal cell type responsible for spontaneous myelin repair in MS. Sourcing the cells, however, remains problematic – a brain biopsy for every patient needing such treatment if autologous adult cells were to be used, or a supply of human embryos if embryonic cells were considered suitable, with the added problems of immune rejection this would carry – quite apart from ethical considerations. Embryonic stem cell lines as a potentially limitless source of neural or more committed oligodendrocyte progenitors are currently the center of much attention, and can clearly accomplish successful remyelination in experimental settings (Brustle *et al.*, 1999; Keirstead *et al.*, 2005) – but again carry the immune problems of non-autologous tissue, present serious ethical difficulties and also offer the risk of tumor formation. Recent studies have shown that even when embryonic stem-cell-derived neuronal populations are pre-differentiated to more dopaminergic neurons before experimental implantation, the injected cells still exhibit tumorigenic properties (Roy *et al.*, 2006). Adult stem cells again offer the possibility of autologous implantation and ease of access, although bone marrow-derived stem cells, while offering a number of important advantageous properties (see below), have yet to be shown unequivocally to generate myelinating oligodendrocytes. Adult CNS neurosphere-derived cells have been shown clearly to offer this potential (Nunes *et al.*, 2003; Windrem *et al.*, 2004), but are of course not readily accessible. Others have suggested such cells may work largely by immune mechanisms (Pluchino *et al.*, 2005b) – or, perhaps surprisingly, that adult subventricular zone (SVZ) precursors remyelinate by differentiating into Schwann cells (Akiyama *et al.*, 2001; Oka *et al.*, 2004).

Aside from the cell source, other problems remain. What lesions to inject? Each patient is likely to have dozens. However, it is also the case that a disproportionate contribution to disability could be made by a very small number of awkwardly sited lesions, and so targeting these might at least offer proof of principal of this therapeutic approach (Compston, 1996) – though this will be returned to below.

Identifying remyelination to monitor outcomes, either clinically or by imaging, remains difficult, though multimodal neurophysio-ogical measures of conduction velocity have potential (Leocani *et al.*, 2006), while new MR imaging techniques – including the use of 3D MR with multiple contrast, radial diffusivity and MR tractography – offer improving sensitivity for disclosing remyelination (Behrens *et al.*, 2003; Deloire-Grassin *et al.*, 2000; Merkler *et al.*, 2005; Song *et al.*, 2002, 2005). Perhaps more important than these paraclinical tests, reproducible clinical measures of disability are also required, a beneficial clinical impact of these therapies of course representing the ultimate aim. The long-used Kurtzke score is not without prob-lems, but potentially more reliable measures are emerging (Hobart *et al.*, 2001, 2004). Last, and not least, there is the question of continu-ing inflammation and its effect on implanted cells – though again, as mentioned above, whether inflammatory cells have an unqualified negative effect on remyelination is more than arguable.

Clearly, therefore, significant problems remain to be solved, but much progress has been made, and in many instances solutions come to mind even where not yet achieved. But one or two questions may be less easily solved. As mentioned above, the extent of spontaneous remyelination in MS may have historically been underestimated. If, as now reported, the great majority of lesions show at least partial remyelination, would more myelin repair definitely offer therapeutic impact? If it is the case, as seems likely, that 70–90% of axons in any one area need to be demyelinated for conduction block to result in functional impact (because of the extent of luxury function in the CNS), then the mean of almost 50% remyelination reported (Patani et al., 2007) would surely be sufficient to restore normal function?

Also, and no less importantly, there is now considerable experimental evidence that oligodendrocyte progenitors are not deficient in lesions, but rather that the environment is not conducive to remyelination, again raising serious questions about the strategy of implanting remyelinating cells. Furthermore, both neuropathologists and MRI specialists have presented compelling evidence for significant abnormalities in MS in cortical and white matter tissue outside lesions (Filippi and Rocca, 2005; Kutzelnigg et al., 2005), or what has hitherto been called "normal-appearing white matter," which, if clinically eloquent, again would defy this therapeutic approach.

The very concept that individual lesions – so clearly the substrate for acute relapses – are also responsible for chronic disability can be questioned. Acute relapses in MS are of a different clinical nature to the features of chronic disability. Optic neuritis and sensory myelitis are not common features of chronic MS, while the common severe proximal tremor, cognitive and psychological change and central pain of chronic disease are very rare as acute relapse phenotypes. It is highly unlikely that these chronic features are explained pathophysiologically by individual and discrete lesions of the nature of those causing relapses, and attempts to identify individual plaques responsible for these chronic deficits (let alone inject them) are likely to prove futile. It should be recalled that the characteristic disabling neurological features of primary progressive MS, with no history of relapses, are not different from those of secondary progressive disease where relapses have occurred, again calling into question the relationship between individual relapse lesions and chronic disability in MS. Non-lesional disease may well be more relevant to chronic disability, and lesions "only" to the features of relapse.

Last and not least, and so far the elephant in the room in this whole discussion, is the question of axon loss. Before considering this, however, it is important to strike a more positive therapeutic note. While the author has labored perhaps to a fault the severe difficulties still facing cell therapy, and suggested some more profound problems of principle, it should be emphasized that "cell injection therapy" and "regenerative medicine" are by no means synonymous terms. The former is just one approach to the latter; and more subtle therapeutic interventions than the "simple" injection of a source of myelinating cells into MS lesions, namely interventions designed to promote and enhance endogenous repair (including but not exclusively myelin repair), remain to be considered and may well have clear future potential. Indeed, as will be shown, this circle may be close to being fully turned as it emerges that introducing some adult cell types may well have precisely the effect of stimulating local repair. But first, the crucial question of axon loss.

AXON DAMAGE AND MS

Although axon loss was very clearly described in the classical accounts of the histopathology of MS, over many generations (Adams and Kubik, 1952; Charcot, 1877; Dawson, 1916; Lumsden, 1951), there is no doubt that it had rather disappeared from the radar until neuro-pathologists in Oxford and in Cleveland re-focused attention on axon damage a decade ago and, importantly, reported considerable axon damage in acute MS lesions (Ferguson et al., 1997; Trapp et al., 1998). Although it seems rather unlikely that acute axon damage makes a major contribution to clinical deficits in acute relapse – the extent is less than the probable 80–90% required for functional impact and the commonly near-complete recovery from relapse difficult to explain – there is little doubt that axon loss makes a major contribution to chronic disability in MS (Bjartmar and Trapp, 2001).

At first glance, this would appear wholly to undermine the rationale for cell therapies in MS, whose aim of course is to reverse chronic disability, not treat relapse. However it is increasingly clear from a consideration of the mechanisms of axon and neuronal loss that this complexity of the pathophysiology of MS enhances, rather than diminishes, the potential importance of cell therapy.

There is little doubt that inflammation is a cause of axon damage in acute lesions; but, as mentioned, the functional consequences of this are not clear. More importantly, the evidence that inflammation is also the cause of the chronic progressive axon damage thought to underlie advancing disability in MS is far less compelling. Rates of disease progression are strikingly similar in patients with frequent, few, or even no inflammatory relapses (i.e. primary progressive disease) (Confavreux *et al.*, 2000), while even the most profound immune suppression, sufficiently potent to suppress acute relapses, fails to interrupt disease progression (Coles *et al.*, 1999).

If not inflammation, then what does cause axonal attrition in MS? The probable answer (or at least one answer) illustrates a second highly significant function of oligodendrocytes – not only do they make and maintain myelin, but they have a subtle and complex relationship with axons, which includes an important trophic effect on them.

Ben Barres and colleagues reported oligodendrocyte-derived trophic support for retinal ganglion cells in culture (MeyerFranke *et al.*, 1995). More recent cell culture studies disclosed distinct effects on neuronal survival and axonal length, and implicated glial-cell-derived neurotrophic factor (GDNF) and brain-derived neurotrophic factor (BDNF) secreted by oligodendrocytes as being among the mechanisms responsible (Wilkins *et al.*, 2001, 2003; Wilkins and Compston, 2005).

The importance in vivo of trophic support of axons by the oligodendrocyte–myelin unit has been powerfully demonstrated in transgenic rodent studies systematically exploring the effect of selectively "removing" individual myelin proteins. In PLP mutants, myelin may be laid down normally, but subsequently degenerates: axon degeneration is seen in previously myelinated axons, but not in those axons never developmentally ensheathed by compact myelin (Griffiths *et al.*, 1998b). In CNP mutants, myelin that appears structurally and functionally normal is laid down and sustained here, but still axon damage and widespread neurodegeneration are seen – the myelin-synthesizing and axonotrophic functions of oligodendrocytes having apparently been cleanly divorced (Lappe-Siefke *et al.*, 2003).

Aside from growth factor production, other mechanisms implicated in the neurodegenerative consequences of oligodendrocyte-myelin loss include sustained demyelination-induced conduction block and electrical silence (Lipton, 1986), disruption of axonal transport (Edgar *et al.*, 2004) and the increased vulnerability of exposed axons to injurious agents (Raine and Cross, 1989).

In MS, pathological studies show that chronic axon loss does not correlate with inflammatory cell infiltrate, or with tumor necrosis factor expression, nitric oxide expression, or demyelinating activity, but rather that it appears related to the overall extent of established myelin loss. Such findings are consistent with the proposition that axonal damage is, at least in part, a consequence of persistent myelin loss (Bitsch *et al.*, 2000b; Kornek *et al.*, 2000): it is seen in lesions that are demyelinated but that exhibit sparse or no inflammation, but it is rare in remyelinated lesions (Kornek *et al.*, 2000). More recent studies of experimental demyelination have clearly confirmed that "therapeutic" remyelination protects axons (Irvine and Blakemore, 2008).

These observations therefore add further impetus (and urgency) to the rationale for cell therapy in MS, and also shift the paradigm. Not only is remyelination an aim, but neuroprotection – using exogenous cells to deliver trophic support for axons and neurons and so prevent neurodegeneration – becomes a core component (Rodriguez, 2003; Wilkins and Scolding, 2008). Whilst oligodendrocytes undoubtedly exhibit both functions, the mission spread implicit in this consideration of axon loss, from the "mere" re-synthesis of the missing myelin to something more closely resembling regenerative tissue repair, perhaps helps draw a consideration of stem cells into our discussion.

STEM CELLS AND TISSUE REPAIR IN MS

As outlined above, initial interest in stem cells in relation to cell therapy in MS was stimulated by the prospect of an essentially unlimited source of oligodendrocyte progenitors. Considerations perhaps of the ethical problems implicit in the use of human embryonic tissue as a source of cells, and also of some of the risks (tumor formation not least amongst them) associated with the potential therapeutic use of embryonic stem cells helped focus attention on adult sources of stem cells. In point of fact, the ethical problems of human embryo research have now in all probability effectively been "solved" by the development of techniques that de-differentiate adult somatic cells to produce stem cells all but identical to embryonic stem cells, "induced pluripotent cells" (Dimos *et al.*, 2008; Huangfu *et al.*, 2008; Nakagawa *et al.*, 2008; Shi *et al.*, 2008; Takahashi *et al.*, 2007; Yu *et al.*, 2007). Nevertheless, an increasing appreciation of the full range and extent of the reparative properties of adult stem cells (Mimeault and Batra, 2008; Ting *et al.*, 2008) has led a number of groups to continue to concentrate their efforts on adult cells. Certainly a significant reason why embryonic stem cells have not yet been tested in patients relates to the hazards this would entail – not least infection and tumor formation (Braude *et al.*, 2005; Scolding, 2005). Recent studies have shown that even when (human) embryonic stem cells are pre-differentiated to form dopaminergic cells prior to injection (into rodents with experimental striatal damage), significant numbers of implanted cells still show potentially tumorigenic properties (Roy *et al.*, 2006).

What of adult stem cells? Those from the subventricular zone (SVZ) certainly have the capacity to significantly ameliorate experimental inflammatory demyelinating disease (Pluchino *et al.*, 2003), though it is suggested that while such cells undoubtedly infiltrate the CNS (Ben-Hur *et al.*, 2003; Pluchino *et al.*, 2003), the effect may principally be one of reducing damage through influencing the immune system rather than conferring a benefit depending on trans-differentiation (Einstein *et al.*, 2006, 2007; Pluchino *et al.*, 2005a, 2005b). Both adult and embryonic SVZ-derived neural stem cells remain under very active investigation, though practical problems concerning access to the former, if autologous transplantation were to be pursued (Oka *et al.*, 2004), and the above-mentioned medical hazards of embryonic cells remain to be fully solved.

Bone-marrow-derived mesenchymal or stromal stem cells also have pronounced immunosuppressive properties, which could of course be of potential benefit in MS. That these cells abrogate experimental forms of inflammatory demyelination has been repeatedly demonstrated, and an immunosuppressive contribution clearly shown (Gerdoni *et al.*, 2007; Gordon *et al.*, 2008b; Kassis *et al.*, 2008; Zappia *et al.*, 2005; Zhang *et al.*, 2005). However, beneficial effects are seen in other, non-immune, models of CNS disease (Chopp *et al.*, 2000; Li, Y. *et al.*, 2001a, 2001b) – and a pro-remyelinating effect is also clear in a non-inflammatory (toxic) demyelinating model (Akiyama *et al.*, 2002a, 2002b; Sasaki *et al.*, 2001). Nonetheless, the current consensus remains that transdifferentiation of bone-marrow-derived cells into myelinating oligodendrocytes has not been unequivocally confirmed, and indirect mechanisms are considered a more likely explanation for the enhancement of remyelination – perhaps especially the stimulation of local or endogenous neural precursors (Bai *et al.*, 2007; Rivera *et al.*, 2006).

The enhancement of local angiogenesis and also the reduction of scar formation (Li, Y. *et al.*, 2005) could contribute to the beneficial effects of mesenchymal stem cells. Additionally, neuroprotective properties of these cells have also been clearly described (Kassis *et al.*, 2008; Kim *et al.*, 2009; Park *et al.*, 2008; Simard and Rivest, 2006; Zhang, J., *et al.*, 2006), effects with important implications for MS and of course for other neurodegenerative diseases, and thought to occur principally through the synthesis and release of neurotro-phins (Chen *et al.*, 2005; Garcia *et al.*, 2004; Li, Y. *et al.*, 2002; Ye *et al.*, 2005).

However, more recently an important further potential means of neuroprotection has emerged. It is now clear that bone marrow stem cells can fuse with certain target cells, creating stable, fully integrated and apparently fully functional hybrid cells; and cerebellar Purkinje cells appear particularly amenable to such activity in the CNS (Johansson *et al.*, 2008; Nygren *et al.*, 2008). This process is stimulated by inflammation and may explain the appearance of donor-derived neural cells in the recipients of allogeneic, sex-mismatched bone marrow cell transplants (Cogle *et al.*, 2004; Weimann *et al.*, 2003) (though in fact the authors of both studies also presented evidence that transdifferentiation had contributed to these findings). Ironically therefore, although cell fusion was originally held to imply a lack of therapeutic potential of mesenchy-mal stem cells (Terada *et al.*, 2002b; Vassilopoulos *et al.*, 2003), these recent further studies have suggested precisely the opposite – that, as some predicted (Blau, 2002), fusion represents a further reparative property in the therapeutic armamentarium of particular relevance to neurological disease (Singec and Snyder, 2008).

The combination of these varied and several reparative proper-ties, together with their relative accessibility, known safety and their ability to "target" and infiltrate multiple areas of damage via the circulation (Korbling and Estrov, 2003; Rice and Scolding, 2004) has made bone marrow stem cells attractive as candidates for early clinical study in MS (Kassis *et al.*, 2008; Rice *et al.*, 2007; Rice and Scolding, 2008; Scolding and Rice, 2008). The rapid progress of com-parable studies in cardiac medicine, a recent overview concluding these cells were clearly of benefit in some forms of heart disease (Burt *et al.*, 2008), has provided further stimulation (and evidence of safety). The first indications of the effect – if any – of these cells in MS are likely to emerge very soon.

8

Glial progenitor cells and the dynamics of the oligodendrocyte and its myelin in the aged and injured CNS

INTRODUCTION

Louis-Antoine Ranvier first described myelin in 1878 (Ranvier, 1878); however it was not until 1928 that del Rio Hortega described the oligodendrocyte – the myelin-forming cell of the CNS (Hortega, 1928). Myelin pathology present in spinal cord injury was first mentioned in 1907 (Holmes, 1907) and had become more widely recognized by the 1960s (Bunge *et al.*, 1960). Today the oligodendrocyte with its compact and non-compact myelin components has become an avidly pursued therapeutic target, yet our understanding of the physical and functional changes in the oligodendrocyte myelin with injury are relatively understudied and misunderstood.

Spinal cord injury (SCI) is a devastating condition currently affecting 250 000 people in the United States, with 11 000 new cases recorded each year (2005). SCI is a complex neurological disorder with varied pathological patterns. The majority of injuries result in permanent anatomical and functional deficits. The most frequent type of injury – contusion injuries in the cervical and thoracic regions – is caused by a bone or disk displacement into the spinal cord due to bone dislodgement or fracture of the spinal column (Rothman and Simeone, 1992). Few injuries are caused by laceration or transection of the spinal cord. Contusion injury is typified by a necrotic core or cavity, which is partly surrounded by a rim of remaining white matter containing spared descending and ascending axons (Balentine, 1978a; Blight, 1983). SCI results in a loss of function due to the disruption of sensory and motor pathways and glial cell support. The functional impairment is approximately related to the extent of anatomical

The Biology of Oligodendrocytes, eds. Patricia J. Armati and Emily K. Mathey. Published by Cambridge University Press. © Cambridge University Press 2010.

damage incurred during and after the injury event (Fehlings and Tator, 1995; Noble and Wrathall, 1989).

Anatomically, SCI is characterized by primary and secondary damage, both contributing to the final functional outcome for the patient. As we describe later, both injury phases contribute to the pathology of the oligodendrocyte and its myelin. Primary damage occurs at the onset of the injury event and results in immediate mechanical damage to CNS tissue, including the vasculature (Tator, 1995). Immediate necrotic cell death results from mechanical and ischemic effects mostly affecting gray matter with a preserved ring of white matter. In addition, disruptions of blood flow result in vasogenic edema, thrombosis, hemorrhage and vasospasms that further exacerbate neural and glial damage (Hulsebosch, 2002; Schwab and Bartholdi, 1996). Furthermore, the intracellular and extracellular ionic environment is deregulated whereby Na^+, K^+ and Ca^{2+} concentrations abnormally increase causing yet more damage (Hulsebosch, 2002). Lastly, the acute SCI phase is characterized by toxic increases of excitatory amino acids such as glutamate released by lysed cells which further activate lipid peroxidation and free-radical formation (Hulsebosch, 2002) further discussed in Chapter 10. Such free radicals can harm lipid membranes so that they do not function normally as insulators. Demyelination or changes in the organization of the compact or non-compact myelin can create ionic leaks that result in incomplete saltatory conduction. Hence, oxidative damage to lipids and proteins essential for myelin compaction can lead to oligodendrocyte death but also subtle damage that inhibits the organization of the cell and its function (Figure 8.1a and b).

Secondary damage occurs days to months or even years after SCI. Reactive gliosis, defined by activated microglia and astrocytes, is the most prominent late response to the injury. Microglial processes increase in number and upregulate the expression of major histocompatibility complex (MHC) molecules and complement receptors, which can lead to their becoming phagocytic (Perry *et al.*, 1993). Astrocytes also undergo hypertrophy, increase their expression of glial fibrillary acidic protein (GFAP) and form a glial scar that becomes a major impediment for axonal regeneration (Reier, 1988). A second major response after SCI is inflammation marked by peripheral immune cell infiltration such as white blood cells and monocytes or macrophages, which increase the concentration of cytokines and chemokines that further damage the tissue. The inflammation resolves several days after the injury and a fluid-filled cyst forms in

Degenerating myelin

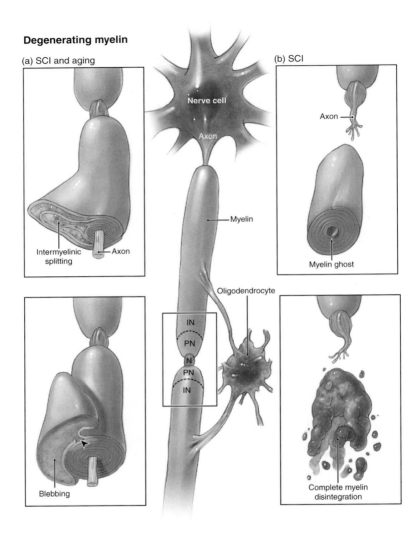

Figure 8.1 Similarities and differences between age-related and traumatic demyelination and remyelination. There are many similarities in the process of myelin degeneration as a result of injury such as trauma, infection, multiple sclerosis and that resulting from normal aging. In these divergent conditions, edema or inflammation of the myelin lamellae is seen as blebbing and intermyelinic splitting (a). However the rates and endpoints of these events may vary between direct axonal insults and aging. Direct axonal insults can lead to nerve degeneration with myelin sparing, resulting in a myelin "ghost" as well as complete myelin disintegration (b). Myelin disintegration and/or abnormal axon–oligodendroglial signaling results in the activation and proliferation of oligodendrocyte progenitor

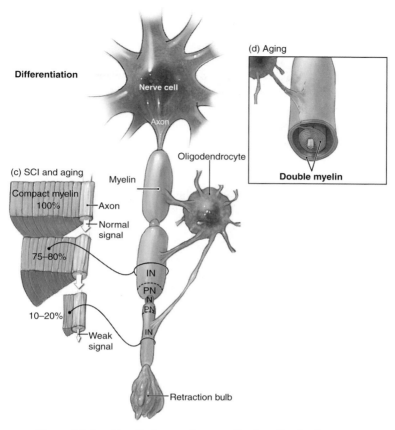

Figure 8.1 (cont.) cells that produce myelinating oligodendrocytes. Theoretical hallmarks of new myelin include shortened internodes (IN) and thinner myelin thickness, i.e. fewer lamellae (c). Myelin "ghosts" and myelin disintegration are less commonly reported in normal aging; however, myelin hypertrophy and the presence of double-wrapped internodes occur commonly in aging and are likely the result of abnormal axon–olidodendroglial signaling (d). Both in aging and injury, little is known about the dynamics of the remyelination process. Hence, in conditions where axonal ensheathment has been directly damaged or during aging, the presence of either fewer myelin lamellae or shortened internodes may be insufficient to verify that remyelination has occurred. Future work on the dynamism of myelin degeneration and regeneration may reveal that myelinated internodes can shrink or atrophy both in thickness and internodal length. Simultaneous measurement of multiple myelin indices is needed to understand the mechanics of normal and insult-derived myelin degeneration and assembly. N, node; PN, paranode.

the lesion epicenter, surrounded by a gliotic scar (Hulsebosch, 2002; Schwab and Bartholdi, 1996). Wallerian degeneration and demyelination are the last of the secondary responses to SCI. Cut axons degenerate distal to the site of their transection while the proximal stump usually forms retraction bulbs or active ends resembling growth cones (Tom *et al.*, 2004). We will discuss demyelination in detail later in the chapter.

Animal SCI models represent contusion, compression and laceration injuries present in human patients (Kwon *et al.*, 2002). The most commonly used animal SCI model is a contusion injury that yields trauma that is anatomically and functionally similar to that present in the human population (Stokes and Jakeman, 2002).

OLIGODENDROCYTE PATHOLOGY IN INJURY

The initial impact to the spinal cord tends to primarily damage central gray matter, most probably because this area is subject to greater shear forces and is more vascular (Wolman, 1965). The injury core size increases with time affecting not only central gray matter, but also white matter tracts (Grossman *et al.*, 2001). Oligodendrocyte death has been observed within 24 hours after SCI (Balentine, 1978a). At the ultrastructural level, damaged oligodendrocyte nuclei contain condensed clumps or aggregates of chromatin and their cytoplasm exhibits dark aggregates and swollen endoplasmic reticulum (Grossman *et al.*, 2001; Wakefield and Eidelberg, 1975) consistent with apoptosis. Many other oligodendrocytes have nuclei that appear to be swollen. During the first four hours after injury, 50% of oligodendrocytes are lost at the epicenter of the injury, with a further 25% lost in the surrounding 3 mm, but with no further significant loss 24 hours post injury (Grossman *et al.*, 2001).

The extent of oligodendrocyte and axonal damage depends on the type and severity of injury (Balentine, 1978a, 1978b). The cause of oligodendrocyte death in the acute phase after injury has not been explored in depth; nevertheless, some explanations have been proposed. First, decreased blood flow resulting in ischemia is thought to cause necrotic oligodendrocyte death (Ducker *et al.*, 1978; Lohse *et al.*, 1980; Sandler and Tator, 1976; Stokes *et al.*, 1981). Because of the considerable energy required to maintain the large lipid membrane of myelinated oligodendrocytes, they have high metabolic demands that would be significantly affected by oxygen depletion (Norton, 1984). Compression SCI causing extensive ischemia also increases apoptotic cell death as seen in the rat spinal cord (Hamamoto *et al.*, 2007).

Next, it is well documented that the accumulation of calcium in neurons and their axons, due to the great release of glutamate after injury, plays a crucial role in cell degeneration and death (Arundine and Tymianski, 2004; Balentine and Spector, 1977; Moriya *et al.*, 1994). Oligodendrocytes possess both glutamate-activated α-amino-3-hydroxyl-5-methyl-4-isoxazole-propionate (AMPA) and *N*-methyl-D-aspartate (NMDA) receptors, which makes them sensitive to calcium influx (Karadottir *et al.*, 2005; Stys, 2004). The excessive glutamate release after SCI damages oligodendrocytes by raising their intracellular calcium levels mainly through the AMPA receptors, which are primarily localized on the oligodendrocyte cell body (Karadottir and Attwell, 2007; Stys, 2004). The role of glutamate receptors is further discussed in Chapter 10. Abnormal build up of internal calcium not only activates a range of calcium-dependent enzymes such as calpains, proteases and lipases, but also triggers internal signaling cascades that can lead to irreparable cell damage (Stys, 2004).

Finally, apoptosis, as mentioned above, has been proposed as one of the major mechanisms of both initial and prolonged oligoden-drocyte loss (Crowe *et al.*, 1997; Li, G.L. *et al.*, 1996; Liu *et al.*, 1997). Cells that co-label with TUNEL and oligodendrocyte markers are observed as early as four hours after injury (Crowe *et al.*, 1997). There is a surprisingly delayed oligodendrocyte apoptosis extending away from the injury epicenter as late as three weeks post injury (Crowe *et al.*, 1997; Li, G.L. *et al.*, 1996). It has been postulated that FAS, p75 and tumor necrosis factor receptor (TNFR) pathways may be involved in initiating the apoptotic process in oligodendrocytes (Casha *et al.*, 2001; Yan *et al.*, 2003). In addition, excitotoxic insults such as increased levels of glutamate are also implicated in oligoden-drocyte apoptosis (Matute *et al.*, 2007; Park *et al.*, 2003). However, it is not exactly clear what causes prolonged oligodendrocyte death/apoptosis weeks after injury. Myelin gene expression changes have also been reported in chronically injured animal cords. The mRNA of the main compact myelin structural proteins such as proteolipid protein (PLP) and myelin basic protein (MBP) is decreased in spinal cords two months after injury even though the overall numbers of oligodendrocytes remain comparatively normal (Wrathall *et al.*, 1998). Other studies also confirm that oligodendrocyte numbers return to pre-injury levels after SCI (Rabchevsky *et al.*, 2007). These studies suggest that remyelination and the total production of myelin may be restricted after injury due to damage of the oligodendrocytes or the failure of new oligodendrocytes to form normal levels of myelin proteins.

MYELIN SHEATH PATHOLOGY IN INJURY

Compact myelin shows pathological changes as early as one hour post injury (Balentine, 1978b). The first abnormality is the appearance of a space between axon and the ensheathing first wrap of the oligodendrocyte process – predominantly at the paranodal loops (Balentine, 1978b; Griffiths and McCulloch, 1983) (Figure 1.2). The compact myelin then progressively breaks down, exemplified by a loss of lamellae progressing along the internode to node (Gledhill and McDonald, 1977; Griffiths and McCulloch, 1983). In earlier studies this was described as compact-myelin-forming small clusters of vesicles with later formation of intramyelinic vacuoles or "splitting" (Balentine, 1978b; Bunge et al., 1960). Initially myelin debris fills the extracellular space, but it is later cleared by phagocytosis (Bunge et al., 1960). Demyelination can be observed preceding or following axonal degeneration, sometimes without damage to the axon itself (Balentine, 1978b). Currently we do not understand the precise molecular signaling between the axon and the complex of compact and non-compact myelin at the onset of demyelination after SCI. Most studies reporting demyelination, especially chronically, have not correlated the breakdown of compact myelin or changes in the numbers of spirals or lamellae with the degenerative changes in the axon. This is a very important consideration as a single oligodendrocyte can myelinate up to 50 internodes, each on a different axon. Thus the conversation between the oligodendrocyte and its associated axon is extraordinarily complex and highly orchestrated. However, due to methodological challenges, axonal status (e.g. intact, cut or degenerating) and myelin indices are rarely measured simultaneously. Hence many theoretical tenets regarding measured changes in oligodendrocyte/myelin indices and their impact on axonal function are purely correlative.

In addition to the technically challenging aspect of collecting multiple oligodendrocyte/myelin and axon indices simultaneously, we must also consider the injury model when discussing and interpreting the myelin injury literature. For example, it is important to differentiate between the demyelination observed in traumatic contusion injury paradigms and that of spinal cord compression models. Traumatic contusion injury tends to produce extensive necrotic trauma with severe injury to axons and associated oligodendrocytes. Compression models, especially acute ones, exhibit better preservation of axonal integrity with clear demyelination around intact axons that are later extensively remyelinated (Balentine, 1978a, 1978b; Blight, 1983; Bunge *et al.*, 1961; Gledhill *et al.*, 1973a). These models demonstrate that myelin loss or oligodendrocyte damage can occur in a context of axon sparing depending upon the characteristics of the injury. The dynamics of myelin loss and remyelination will be explored later in the chapter.

In addition to morphological evidence of demyelination, there are also reports of molecular changes. On myelinated axons, sodium (Na^+) channels, mostly the $Na_{v1.6}$ type, are densely concentrated at the nodes of Ranvier, which mediate action potential propagation (Caldwell *et al.*, 2000; Waxman and Ritchie, 1993). The axonal membrane of the paranodal region (the termination of the non-compact myelin loops, Figure 8.1) contains contactin and contactin-associated protein (Caspr), which are part of the adhesion complex necessary for formation of the axon and myelin membrane junction or paranode (Rios *et al.*, 2000). Voltage-gated (shaker) potassium (K^+) channels, mainly responsible for maintaining internodal resting potential, are localized in the adjacent juxtaparanodal region (Poliak and Peles, 2003). Immunohistochemical studies show that after injury, demyelinated axons lose the positional configuration of the Na^+ and K^+ channels as well as Caspr distribution. $K_{v1.1}$ and $K_{v1.2}$ channels and Caspr disperse one hour after injury and on some axons such redistribution persists for up to six weeks post SCI (Karimi-Abdolrezaee *et al.*, 2004). The dispersal of the highly organized arrangement of these essential molecules is an accepted indicator of the loss or dysfunction of a myelinated internode.

The demyelination and resulting molecular reorganization of demyelinated axons leads to impaired electrophysiological function (Waxman, 1989). Electrophysiological impairment is typified by a decrease in conduction velocity or complete conduction block, associated with increased latency in transcranial magnetic motor-evoked potentials (Fehlings and Nashmi, 1995). The compact myelin and complex architecture of the myelinated internode not only potentiates axonal conduction, but also participates in axonal maturation and survival, and may influence the integrity of axonal transport mechanisms. Demyelinated axons show impaired retrograde and anterograde axonal transport as well as decreased neurofilament phosphorylation and decreased microtubule numbers and neurofilament density (Brady *et al.*, 1999; Edgar *et al.*, 2004; de Waegh *et al.*, 1992). Hence myelin disruption adversely affects the conduction of axons but may also adversely affect their ability to maintain organelle transport, as well as their structural and bioenergetic needs.

Demyelination is most evident in medial regions, rostral and caudal to the lesion site (Griffiths and McCulloch, 1983). Chronic demyelination has not been well established, but animal and human studies provide some evidence for persisting demyelinated axons long after injury (Kakulas, 1999; Norenberg *et al.*, 2004; Totoiu and Keirstead, 2005). We also do not know whether the oligodendrocyte itself is damaged first, prior to demyelination, or whether the myelin sheath can disintegrate independently. Recently, it was demonstrated that calcium entry not only affects oligodendrocyte cell bodies, but also that influx through activated NMDA receptors located directly on the myelinating processes leads to myelin damage (Micu *et al.*, 2006). The discovery of NMDA receptors on the oligodendrocyte as well as on its myelinated processes establishes that demyelination could occur without damage to the oligodendrocyte cell body. However, the molecular mechanisms of such demyelination and how it relates to oligodendrocyte/axonal damage remain to be elucidated.

RESPONSE OF OLIGODENDROCYTE PROGENITORS TO INJURY

As discussed earlier, about three weeks post injury, the number of oligodendrocytes increases to 80% of the level in uninjured cords at six weeks post SCI and to pre-injury levels at eight weeks post injury (Rabchevsky *et al.*, 2007; Wrathall *et al.*, 1998). The most probable source of new oligodendrocytes is not the replication of mature oligodendrocytes, as they have not definitively been shown to divide efficiently (Norton, 1996; Peters and Sethares, 2004). Polydendrocytes and cells expressing the cell surface proteoglycan NG2$^+$ (nerve/glial antigen 2) have been proposed as the likely candidates (Dawson *et al.*, 2000; Wilson *et al.*, 1981).

Before the NG2 marker was discovered (Wilson *et al.*, 1981), ultrastructural studies revealed the appearance of "reactive macroglia" after trauma that combined the characteristics of both interfascicular oligodendrocytes and fibrous astrocytes; they are most numerous before the onset of remyelination (Bunge et al., 1960; Schultz and Pease, 1959). "Reactive macroglia" were first described by the Bunges as cells with large, oval nuclei and enlarged nucleoli as well as many processes of variable length, embracing axonal lengths (Bunge et al., 1961). These cells were hypothesized to give rise to mature myelinating oligodendrocytes as well as fibrous astrocytes. In 1962 Adrian and Walker identified mitotically active cells by radioactively labeling DNA using tritiated thymidine injections in intact and injured cords (Adrian and Walker, 1962). Modern molecular markers and techniques confirmed and expanded these initial observations establishing the existence of a large pool of glial progenitors immunopositive for NG2$^+$ in the spinal cord that divide and differentiate into mostly oligodendrocytes after SCI as well as astrocytes (Peters and Sethares, 2004; Horky et al., 2006; Nishiyama 2007).

NG2$^+$ cells are not a homogeneous population; their roles and functions are still not fully understood (Nishiyama, 2007). NG2$^+$ cells represent up to 2% of the total cell population and 70% of all dividing cells in the spinal cord of adult rodents (Horner et al., 2002). NG2$^+$ cells proliferate slowly in the intact CNS, but their division rate increases significantly after SCI (Horky et al., 2006; Horner et al., 2000; McTigue et al., 2001; Yamamoto et al., 2001; Zai and Wrathall, 2005). These mitotic cells have been shown to proliferate in both ependymal and non-ependymal regions of the spinal cord after injury (Horky et al., 2006; Yamamoto et al., 2001). Cell proliferation is highest one to three days after SCI and declines after four weeks (Horky et al., 2006; McTigue et al., 2001; Zai and Wrathall, 2005). 5-Bromodeoxyuridine (BrdU) pulse and retroviral studies show that many dividing cells are NG2$^+$ positive immediately after injury, but that with time their numbers decline while oligodendrocyte numbers increase (Horky et al., 2006; Zai and Wrathall, 2005). The transcription factors Nkx2.2 and Olig1/2 are necessary for oligodendrocyte generation during development. In demyelinated lesions NG2$^+$ cells upregulate Nkx2.2 and Olig2 expression, which suggests that these cells can then differentiate into oligodendrocytes (Talbott et al., 2005; Watanabe et al., 2004). In addition, loss of Olig1 function delays progenitor maturation into oligodendrocytes (Arnett et al., 2004). Fifty percent of NG2$^+$ cells in mouse spinal cord co-express platelet-derived growth factor alpha (PDGFα) receptor, which is important during the development of oligodendrocytes (Diers-Fenger et al.,

2001). In addition, NG2$^+$ cells can co-label with the more mature oligodendrocyte marker O4, but rarely with mature oligodendrocyte markers MBP, RIP or CNP (Dawson *et al.*, 2000; Reynolds and Hardy, 1997).

NG2$^+$ cell proliferation and differentiation are guided by a number of molecular signals, yet not all of them are known. Even though PDGFα seems to play a bigger role during development in NG2$^+$ progenitor expansion, it also seems to be a mitogen for adult NG2$^+$ cells that express the PDGFα receptor (Woodruff *et al.*, 2004). Basic fibroblast growth factor (FGF2) increases cell division not only in culture, but also in vivo (Fortin *et al.*, 2005). Neonatal studies suggest that FGF2 increases the pool of dividing oligodendrocyte progenitor cells, arresting their differentiation (Naruse *et al.*, 2006). Furthermore, insulin-like growth factor-1 (IGF-1 has been linked to oligodendrocyte survival and differentiation (Goddard *et al.*, 1999). In addition to molecular cues, NG2$^+$ cell proliferation and differentiation may be affected by electrophysiological signaling. Recently it has been discovered that NG2$^+$ cells have AMPA and NMDA receptors that respond to glutamate and ATP release from axons in white matter tracts resulting in raised intracellular calcium levels (Kukley *et al.*, 2007; Ziskin *et al.*, 2007). A role has been proposed for glutamate and ATP in regulating NG2$^+$ cell differentiation, where adenosine and ATP released during action potential propagation stimulate NG2$^+$ cell differentiation into oligodendrocytes, while release of glutamate from axons via vesicular fusion prevents NG2$^+$ cell differentiation (Wigley *et al.*, 2007). In addition, it could be that after injury, high levels of glutamate mediate calcium influx, which plays a role in the observed increase in NG2$^+$ cell proliferation (Wigley *et al.*, 2007).

Hence, although some of the key regulators of oligogenesis in the adult CNS have been discovered there is much to be learned. Studies of development are now being utilized to describe the lineage and migration of adult progenitor cells (Meletis *et al.*, 2008; Sellers *et al.*, 2009). This is in part due to limited migration of adult progenitor cells in the absence of injury (Horner *et al.*, 2000). Without migration and the use of correlative BrdU studies several aspects of oligogenesis in the adult remain to be delineated. The creation of lineage marking tools such as retroviruses and genetic mutants that track lineage-specific genes will be needed to better understand oligodendrocyte genesis from the most immature stem cell to committed oligodendrocyte progenitors. Defining the lineages and regulatory components of each aspect of oligodendrocyte formation in the adult will be important for understanding how myelin homeostasis is achieved not only in normal aging but also under conditions where there is a challenge to the CNS, such as SCI.

REMYELINATION AFTER INJURY: HOW COMPLETE IS IT?

Numerous studies show that demyelination after either compression or contusion SCI is complete by seven days and new compact myelin is first seen 19 days post injury (Balentine, 1978b; Bunge *et al.*, 1960, 1961). There are three generally accepted criteria by which to determine whether such myelin is new and not old myelin in the state of degeneration. The first criterion is that new myelin should appear at a time after demyelination that allows for complete demyelination of "old myelin" and for the development of mature oligodendrocytes from a precursor population. Second, the new compact myelin lamellae should surround the axon in a spiral manner with the adjacent inner, i.e. cytoplasmic surface, membranes fused to form the major dense line. Typically, such compact myelin is seen as having only two major dense lines, i.e. two complete spirals of oligodendrocyte compacted plasma membrane. Third, newly formed myelin internodes should be significantly shorter than in developmentally formed myelin (Gledhill *et al.*, 1973a; Gledhill and McDonald, 1977).

Before myelination begins, axonal lengths (i.e. internodes) are ensheathed by oligodendroglial processes. At 19 days post injury, axons of varying diameters exhibit compact myelin seen as two or three lamellae. The number of lamellae increases up to the point at which myelin thickness, i.e. number of lamellae/spirals, is comparable with that of normal myelinated internodes, about a year after injury; however, most new myelin does not reach the thickness found in normal myelinated internodes (Bunge *et al.*, 1961). Electron microscopic studies reveal that after injury, the morphology of the nodal and paranodal regions resembles that of a normal node and paranode, respectively. Myelin lamellae terminate in non-compacted, i.e. cytoplasm-filled, loops of the spiraling oligodendrocyte process, attached to the axolemma (Gledhill *et al.*, 1973b). In normally myelinated axons each internodal length is predictably around 100–200 times the axon diameter as described in Chapter 1 (McDonald and Ohlrich, 1971). However, after injury, remyelinated internodes are significantly shorter, only about 10–80 times the axon diameter (Gledhill et al., 1973b; Gledhill and McDonald, 1977). In addition, there is also molecular reorganization of Na^+ and K^+ channels, and Caspr nodal/paranodal distribution is significantly altered (Black et al., 2006; Coman et al., 2006). Remyelination characterized by morphological and molecular myelin changes affects the electrophysiological functioning of axons. It has been shown that remyelination after chemical demyelination restores conduction and refractory periods to normal levels (Smith et al., 1981). Despite the abnormally thin myelin, i.e. very few lamellar spirals, and shortened internodes observed in this axon-sparing demyelination model, near-normal conduction properties are observed. This is likely due to the resolution of the physiological techniques, the small size of the lesion zone and the small organism size. Nonetheless, there are also direct correlations between the time of onset of remyelination in chemical lesions with improvements in locomotor function (Jeffery and Blakemore, 1997). These studies provide firm proof that endogenous remyelination under the appropriate conditions can be functionally complete. However, the full extent of the contribution of remyelination to axon function after more destructive insults such as SCI or stroke have not been investigated directly.

The extent of remyelination after SCI is therefore a very important aspect of discussion within the scientific community regarding functional improvements. As mentioned above, contusion and compression SCI result in demyelination. There is currently no satisfactory consensus on whether remyelination is functionally complete or whether endogenous oligodendrocytes are not capable of fully remyelinating intact axons. This controversial area has correlative anatomical data from both sides. For example, early reports of injury in humans and large animals have postulated that remyelination is surprisingly complete (Bunge et al., 1961; Gledhill et al., 1973a, 1973b; Gledhill and McDonald, 1977; Griffiths and McCulloch, 1983; Harrison et al., 1975; Harrison and McDonald, 1977). However, many studies report extensive and chronic demyelination after SCI (Blight, 1983; Cao et al., 2005; Totoiu and Keirstead, 2005). Neither set of data is able to correlate the state of myelination with the health of the axon and hence there is no definitive understanding as to the extent to which intact axons are remyelinated (Blight, 1983). Indirect proof of incomplete remyelination can however be gained from transplantation studies where myelin-forming cells, Schwann cells or oligodendrocytes, are transplanted into injured cords and anatomical and functional improvement follows (Akiyama *et al.*, 2002b; Cummings *et al.*, 2005; Keirstead *et al.*, 2005; Lepore and Fischer, 2005; Li, Y. *et al.*, 1997). Functional recovery can be achieved only if transplanted cells are delivered within three weeks after injury. If a cell therapy intervention is applied later than three weeks, there is no functional or anatomical improvement (Karimi-Abdolrezaee *et al.*, 2006; Keirstead *et al.*, 2005). These studies demonstrate that remyelination, particularly early after injury, can be improved beyond that produced by the endogenous oligodendrocyte. One explanation could be that if transplanted cells are delivered before endogenous remyelination programs are effective, the spinal cord will benefit from early remyelination by exogenous cells. Currently, the exact mechanism of transplant therapy potentiating functional recovery is not well understood, but remyelination as well as trophic and structural support have been proposed.

MYELIN PATHOLOGY IN INJURY AND NORMAL AGING: MANY COMMONALITIES?

The CNS during normal aging exhibits a lot of changes that are reminiscent of the traumatic injury environment. It is important to understand normal changes occurring during the lifespan especially if we want to understand chronic injury environment patterns. We will focus on oligodendrocyte and associated myelin changes during aging and how those changes are similar to SCI.

In the normal CNS, aging oligodendrocytes undergo a series of morphological changes. Many oligodendrocytes have been described in the primate cortex to develop bulbous enlargements along their processes and "lumpy" inclusions in their cytoplasm (Peters *et al.*, 1996). Such alterations could occur due to many factors known to change both in an aging CNS and after injury. First, activated microglia are observed in increasing numbers during aging to express markers usually associated with acute CNS injury such as MHC class II molecules, ED1 and CD4 (Conde and Streit, 2006; Duce *et al.*, 2006). Activated microglia are also a large source of nitric oxide (NO) to which oligodendrocytes are extremely sensitive (Merrill *et al.*, 1993; Sloane *et al.*, 2003). Similarly, after SCI, activated microglia and macrophages release cytokines, chemokines and NO, which participate in secondary nervous tissue damage affecting both neurons and oligodendrocytes (Bethea and Dietrich, 2002). Release of NO after SCI and in normal aging might generate toxic free radicals and cause lipid peroxidation (Bethea and Dietrich, 2002). In addition, oligodendrocytes in the aging CNS are sensitive to oxidative damage due not only to their high lipid and iron content, but also to an age-related increase in internal formation of free radicals by mitochondria (Back *et al.*, 1998; Husain and Juurlink, 1995; Juurlink, 1997; Squier, 2001). Finally, there is an age-related increase in iron levels. Oligodendrocytes may become damaged by iron toxicity due to their high internal iron stores and because their ferritin subunit composition makes iron easily available as an oxidizing agent (Connor and Menzies, 1996; Kress *et al.*, 2002). Correspondingly, it has been shown that SCI induces reactive oxygen species such as anions, hydrogen peroxide and hydroxyl radicals to participate in secondary tissue damage (Liu *et al.*, 1999, 2003). Together, these observations suggest that oligodendrocytes may be vulnerable to aging in a way similar to that occurring after SCI.

Myelin pathology is the most prominent feature in the aging CNS. Ultrastructural studies in aging primate cerebral cortices show degenerating compact myelin that resembles degenerating myelin after SCI (see earlier). The most common change seen in aging compact myelin is the splitting of the major dense line, usually on one side of the axon, so that electron-dense cytoplasm with vacuoles and dense bodies is enclosed (Peters and Sethares, 2002). The second common change is the formation of "myelin balloons" usually filled with fluid (Feldman and Peters, 1998; Peters *et al.*, 2000). Most interestingly, the aging brain and spinal cord show signs of myelin repair in ways that are similar to remyelination after SCI, with some exceptions. As we have seen, it has been demonstrated that myelin internodes are shorter after remyelination than in normal myelinated internodes (Gledhill and McDonald, 1977). In a similar way, internodes in the spinal cord become shorter with normal aging, possibly due to remyelination because there are no reports of spontaneous internodal shortening (Lasiene *et al.*, 2009). This is an interesting point as there is virtually no literature pertaining to oligodendrocyte turnover or remyelination in normal aging. Another corollary of myelin turnover is the observation that paranodal profile densities measured at the electron microscope level increase with age in primate cortex. Given that axon densities do not change significantly, this observation is consistent with shorter internodes and new myelin segments in at least some axons (Peters and Sethares, 2003). In addition to evidence of myelin turnover, there are unique myelin pathologies that have been described for the aging CNS. For example, in aged CNS, there are many myelinated axonal internodes which are larger in diameter than is found in normal mature internodes. This is due to a separation of the inner compact myelin lamellae from the outer lamellae (Peters *et al.*, 2001). Also, there is an increase in the frequency of "double" myelin sheaths, where a set of compact lamellae is surrounded by a second set (Peters and Sethares, 2002). Studies indicate that these abnormalities originate from a single oligodendrocyte (Figure 8.1d). Little is known about how the introduction of new myelin segments and myelin pathologies impact either the health of axons or the function of the aged brain and spinal cord. This is undoubtedly an important and fascinating area for future research.

CONCLUSION

We have recently come to appreciate that oligodendrocytes with their complex architecture of compact and non-compact myelin, i.e. the myelin sheath, exhibit a remarkably dynamic life cycle in the adult CNS. This is true both in the context of aging and in response to insult. Regenerated compact myelin was once thought to be abnormally thin, i.e. few lamellae, but we now know that new myelin varies greatly in its number of lamellae after a demyelinating challenge. We also know that there is a critical structure–function relationship between the oligodendrocyte, its myelin and the many axons it myelinates. This complicated and very precise relationship is disrupted when myelin is destroyed. However, there is a lack of knowledge as to the functional impact of changes in myelin indices. A key challenge in the future will be to develop techniques that combine quantitative myelin morphology with indicators of axonal status, form and physiological function. Such technologies will not only give rise to a clearer understanding of the role of the oligodendrocyte and its myelin in the health of aged or injured axons but also help to accurately identify therapeutic targets for restoring axon function. Research is accelerating in the field of oligodendrocyte replacement by both endogenous and ex vivo manipulation of stem and progenitor cells. However, many key issues are still to be resolved to improve the effectiveness of these approaches. These include fully defining the oligodendrocyte progenitor in the adult CNS and discovering the age- and injury-related signals that activate it. Also, factors that influence progenitor maturation into fully mature, myelinating oligodendrocytes are not well understood, and neither are the factors that influence myelin thickness and internode length. Furthermore, the extent and timing of de- and remyelination with SCI have still not been fully characterized. Many investigations into these questions are currently under way. The next decade should bring exciting new answers to the questions regarding modulators and the plasticity of the oligodendrocyte and its myelin.

TANJA KUHLMANN AND
WOLFGANG BRÜCK

9

Oligodendroglial pathology in multiple sclerosis

Multiple sclerosis (MS) is the most frequent demyelinating disease of the human central nervous system (CNS) with a prevalence of 100 per 100 000 in North America and Northern Europe. The histopathological hallmarks of MS lesions are demyelination, inflammation, astrogliosis and relative axonal preservation. Oligodendrocytes and their myelin are considered to be the major targets of the disease process. Oligodendroglial damage and cell death can be observed very early and may represent an initial event in lesion formation. In MS lesions of patients with a long disease duration oligodendrocytes are almost completely absent. The mechanisms underlying the oligodendroglial cell death are not well understood and may be heterogeneous among patients. Apoptotic, necrotic and lytic cell death are implicated in the disappearance of oligodendrocytes from MS lesions. Remyelination occurs in MS lesions, but is limited in the majority of patients. Oligodendroglial precursor cells (OPCs), which have the capability to form new myelin, can be found in early MS lesions, and in reduced cell numbers also late during the disease process.

Oligodendrocytes and their progenitors have been shown to be susceptible to a broad range of inflammatory and toxic mediators in vivo and in culture. This chapter gives an overview of the current concepts regarding demyelination, oligodendroglial damage and remyelination in MS lesions.

OLIGODENDROGLIAL PATHOLOGY IN EARLY AND CHRONIC MS LESIONS

The pathological hallmarks of MS are multifocal inflammatory demyelinating lesions in the white and gray matter of the CNS (Figure 9.1a).

The Biology of Oligodendrocytes, eds. Patricia J. Armati and Emily K. Mathey. Published by Cambridge University Press. © Cambridge University Press 2010.

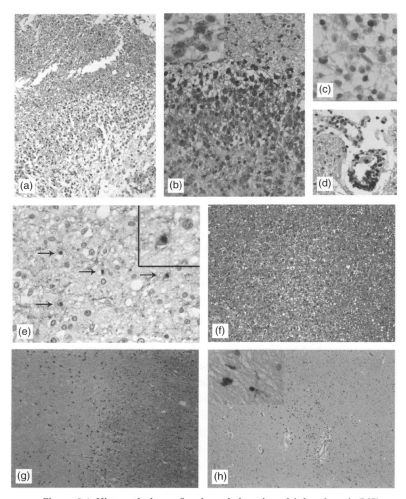

Figure 9.1 Histopathology of early and chronic nultiple sclerosis (MS)
lesions. (a–d) Early MS lesions are characterized by (a) demyelination and
(b–d) an extensive inflammatory infiltrate. (b) Macrophages form the
dominating cell population in early MS lesions (immunohistochemistry
for KiM1P). T cells are either diffusely distributed within the parenchyma
(c) or they form perivascular cuffs (d) (immunohistochemistry for CD3).
(e) In a subset of patients, dying oligodendrocytes with condensed and/or
fragmented nuclei – indicative of apoptosis – are observed in actively
demyelinating lesion areas as indicated by arrows and in the inset
(immunohistochemistry for CNP). These lesions have frequently ill-
defined lesion borders (LFB-PAS staining) (f). (g, h) Chronic MS lesions
have a sharp border and the extent of inflammation is markedly reduced

Early MS lesions are characterized by a prominent proinflammatory response from macrophages/microglia, T and B cells. In early disease stages macrophages/microglia are the dominant cell population and outnumber T cells readily by a factor of 10 (Figure 9.1b–d). The extent of oligodendroglial damage in early MS lesions varies between patients (Brück *et al.*, 1994; Ozawa *et al.*, 1994; Raine *et al.*, 1981). In a large histological study analyzing MS lesions from patients with a short disease duration, two different patterns of oligodendroglial pathology could be distinguished. While the first pattern is characterized by a relative preservation of oligodendrocytes within the lesions, the second pattern that has been found in about 30 % of the lesions showed a profound loss of oligodendrocytes (Lucchinetti *et al.*, 1999). In the latter, numerous oligodendrocytes with morphological signs of apoptosis, e.g. condensed/pyknotic and/or fragmented nuclei, have been found in the periplaque white matter (PPWM) and in areas of active demyelination defined by the presence of early myelin degradation products in the cytoplasm of macrophages (Figure 9.1e). A more recent study described the death of oligodendrocytes in the presence of activated microglia and few or no T cells, suggesting that oligodendroglial damage might be the initial event in MS lesion formation (Barnett and Prineas, 2004). Early MS lesions with a prominent loss of oligodendrocytes in actively demyelinating lesion areas and PPWM have ill-defined lesion borders (Figure 9.1f) and show as an additional characteristic the preferential loss of myelin-associated glycoprotein, while other myelin proteins such as myelin basic protein (MBP), proteolipid protein (PLP) and myelin oligodendrocyte protein (MOG) are still preserved or even overexpressed. Similar histopathological changes can be found in a variant of MS, Baló's concentric sclerosis (Stadelmann *et al.*, 2005). Baló's concentric sclerosis is characterized by alternating layers of demyelinated and normally myelinated white matter; this pattern might be caused by an upregulation of neuroprotective proteins involved in tissue preconditioning (Aboul-Enein *et al.*, 2003).

Caption for Figure 9.1 (cont.)
compared with early MS lesions. (h and inset in h) Many chronic MS lesions are hypocellular in the lesion center and display a rim of activated microglia separating lesions and periplaque white matter (immunohistochemistry for KiM1P). CNP, 2′,3′-cyclic nucleotide 3′-phosphodiesterase; LFB-PAS, Luxol Fast Blue and Periodic Acid Schiff. See color plate section for color version of this figure.

Ultrastructurally, a widening of the inner myelin lamellae and an accumulation and degeneration of organelles within the inner paranodal loops of the oligodendrocyte – areas of uncompacted myelin – have been described as the initial signs of myelin degradation in early inflammatory MS lesions, resulting in the concept of a dying-back oligodendrogliopathy (Rodriguez *et al.*, 1993).

In MS patients with a long disease duration and a progressive (primary or secondary) disease course, mature oligodendrocytes are completely or almost completely eliminated. The chronically demyelinated lesions are often hypocellular and the inflammatory reaction is limited to scant perivascular infiltrates (T cells, a few plasma cells, macrophages/microglia) (Figure 9.1g and h); a subset of chronic MS lesions (chronic active lesions) shows an accumulation of microglia/macrophages at the lesion border (Figure 9.1h).

These findings suggest that potentially heterogeneous mechanisms leading to demyelination and oligodendrocyte loss in early stages of lesion formation result in chronic lesions with a uniform histological appearance. However, the exact mechanisms resulting in demyelination, oligodendroglial injury and death are still unknown.

MECHANISMS LEADING TO OLIGODENDROGLIAL DAMAGE IN VIVO AND IN CULTURE

Apoptosis-related mechanisms

Apoptosis (also called programmed cell death) plays an important role in the elimination of cells during development as well as under pathological conditions. The apoptosis program is initiated either by cell death receptors of the extrinsic pathway (TRAILR1, TNFR1, FAS) or by factors such as reactive oxygen species (ROS), DNA damage and growth factor withdrawal via activation of the mitochondrial (intrinsic) pathway. Both pathways lead to the activation of initiator caspases (e.g. caspases 8 and 9) and effector caspases (e.g. caspases 3 or 7). Histopathologically, apoptotic cells are recognized by their typical morphology consisting of condensed and fragmented nuclei.

In human CNS and/or in MS lesions, oligodendrocytes displaying the morphological signs of apoptosis, as well as expressing apoptosis-related proteins, can be detected. In a subset of early MS lesions, the presence of oligodendrocytes with condensed and fragmented nuclei, morphological hallmarks of apoptosis, is a prominent feature as described above (Barnett and Prineas, 2004; Dowling *et al.*, 1997;

Lucchinetti *et al.*, 2000). Furthermore, in situ expression of FAS, TRAILR and tumor necrosis factor (TNF) receptors, as well as of proteins involved in the intrinsic pathway such as members of the bcl-2 family and p53, have been described (Cannella *et al.*, 2007; D'Souza *et al.*, 1996; Dorr *et al.*, 2002; Kuhlmann *et al.*, 1999; Wosik *et al.*, 2003). The ligands of the death receptors FASL, TRAIL and TNF have been observed in astrocytes, microglia/macrophages and infiltrating lymphocytic cells in MS lesions (Bitsch *et al.*, 2000a; Cannella *et al.*, 2007).

Experimental autoimmune encephalomyelitis (EAE), an animal model of MS, was exacerbated when the TRAIL receptor was blocked. These results suggest an overall beneficial effect of the TRAIL system in MOG-induced EAE, which might be caused by an impaired activation of encephalitogenic T cells (Hilliard *et al.*, 2001). In contrast, experimental studies using transgenic mice lacking TNF-R1 and FAS specifically in oligodendrocytes showed an almost complete absence of clinical signs – despite the presence of inflammation in the spinal cord – indicating that oligodendroglial cell death is mediated via both of these death receptors in EAE (Hovelmeyer *et al.*, 2005). Mice overexpressing the anti-apoptotic protein p35 in oligodendrocytes also demonstrated a reduced severity and incidence in EAE compared with wild-type (WT) controls, strengthening the hypothesis that apoptotic pathways play a major role in oligodendroglial cell death in EAE (Hisahara *et al.*, 2000).

Numerous culture studies demonstrated the susceptibility of oligodendrocytes to the death receptor-activating stimuli (Figure 9.2). Pro-apoptotic factors such as FAS, TNF or TRAIL are able to induce cell death of oligodendrocytes in culture (Benjamins *et al.*, 2003; Burgmaier *et al.*, 2000; Cudrici *et al.*, 2006). However, the vast majority of studies were performed in rodent glial primary cell cultures or cell lines. In human oligodendrocytes, TRAIL and TNF were found to induce cell death via AIF- or JNK-dependent pathways (Cannella *et al.*, 2007; Jurewicz *et al.*, 2003, 2005, 2006). FAS or the combination of FAS and IFN-γ has been shown to induce cell death in a human oligodendroglial cell line as well as in cultured primary human oligodendrocytes (D'Souza *et al.*, 1996; Lim W. *et al.*, 2002; Pouly *et al.*, 2000). Overexpression of p53 induced the upregulation of cell death receptors such as TRAIL and FAS, rendering the cells susceptible to caspase-dependent cell death (Wosik *et al.*, 2003).

Cell-mediated mechanisms

In EAE the injection of whole myelin, myelin proteins/peptides or myelin-reactive T cells is sufficient to induce a disease that mimics

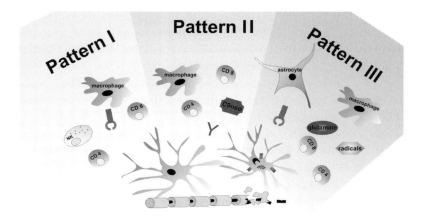

Figure 9.2 Multiple mechanisms have the potential to induce oligodendroglial cell death. A variety of different mechanisms have been shown to induce oligodendroglial cell death in cell culture or in vivo. Macrophages and T cells can be found in all early MS lesions. We hypothesize that in MS lesions characterized by relative oligodendroglial preservation (pattern I), demyelination might be induced by cytokines, cellular (NK cells, T cells) or humoral (immunoglobulins, complement) components of the immune system. In lesions with dying oligodendrocytes found in actively demyelinating lesion areas, oligodendroglial cell death might be induced either by interaction between death receptors and their ligands, resulting in the activation of the apoptotic cascade, or the presence of radicals or glutamate released by macrophages or astrocytes. Increased amounts of radicals or glutamate might lead via mitochondrial dysfunction to the upregulation of heat shock proteins and HIα (histotoxic hypoxia). See color plate section for color version of this figure.

histopathologically some aspects of MS. Additionally, T cells are an important, although not dominant, feature of the inflammatory infil-trate in MS and are found in all histopathological subtypes. Therefore, the presence and significance of T cells in the blood or serum of MS patients have been studied extensively. CD4 or CD8 T cells recognizing myelin proteins such as MBP, MOG, PLP or myelin-oligodendrocyte basic protein (MOBP) have been identified in serum or cerebrospinal fluid (CSF) (Burns *et al.*, 1983; Kerlero de Rosbo *et al.*, 1993; Martin *et al.*, 1992; Neumann *et al.*, 1996; Ota *et al.*, 1990; Trotter *et al.*, 1991; Zang *et al.*, 2004). Opposing results have been published regarding the differ-ences in frequency between myelin-specific T cells in MS patients and healthy controls. The role of myelin-reactive T cells in MS patients is therefore controversial (as reviewed in Martino and Hartung, 1999). They might either represent the trigger of the inflammatory cascade resulting in the human disease MS or be secondary to myelin damage induced by another as yet unknown disease mechanism.

Furthermore, CD8, γδ T cells and natural killer (NK) cells have been described as directly damaging or killing oligodendrocytes. Most T cells recognize their targets by antigen-specific T cell receptors (αβ chain of T cell receptor) in combination with major histocompatibility complex molecules (MHC I for CD8 and MHC II for CD4) and co-stimulatory molecules (CD80/86 and CD40, which bind to CD28/CTLA4 or CD154 respectively). Cultured human and rat oligodendrocytes have been described as expressing MHC I and/or II, depending on culture conditions and co-incubation with pro-inflammatory cytokines (Bergsteindottir *et al.*, 1992; Grenier *et al.*, 1989; Hirayama *et al.*, 1986; Kim *et al.*, 1985). The cytotoxic capabilities of CD8 T cells in relation to oligodendrocytes can be inhibited by MHC class-I-blocking antibodies, indicating an MHC-I-dependent injury mechanism (Jurewicz *et al.*, 1998; Ruijs *et al.*, 1990).

A minority of T cells whose T cell receptors consist of the γδ chains, so-called γδ T cells, are able to recognize antigens by an antigen-independent mechanism. γδ T cells have been detected in acute and chronic MS lesions and have been reported to lyse preferentially cells expressing high levels of heat shock proteins (hsp) (Raine, 1991; Wucherpfennig *et al.*, 1992). Oligodendrocytes upregulating hsp in MS lesions may therefore be lysed by γδ T cells in an hsp-independent, perforin-mediated mechanism (Freedman *et al.*, 1992; Scolding *et al.*, 1990; Selmaj *et al.*, 1991a; Stadelmann *et al.*, 2005).

NK cells form another cell population that has been shown capable of directly injuring oligodendrocytes, at least in culture. In culture IL2-activated NK cells are cytotoxic to human oligodendrocytes. NK-induced cell death may be mediated by an interaction of the co-activating receptor NKG2D located on the surface of NK cells and its ligand, which is expressed on oligodendrocytes but not on neurons, astrocytes or microglia (Saikali *et al.*, 2007). Binding of the ligand to its receptor leads to the secretion of cytokines and cytotoxic granules (Andre *et al.*, 2004; Rincon-Orozco *et al.*, 2005). NK cells have been detected in the CNS of rats with EAE and depletion of NK cells led to either an aggravation or an improvement of EAE symptoms, depending on the time point of depletion and targeted NK subsets (Jahng *et al.*, 2001; Matsumoto *et al.*, 1998; Singh *et al.*, 2001; Xu *et al.*, 2005). However the effects on EAE caused by depletion of NK cells are most likely due to modulation of encephalitogenic T cells. So far there are no studies demonstrating a direct toxic effect of NK cells on oligodendrocytes, in either EAE or MS tissue specimens in situ.

Antibody- and complement-mediated mechanisms

Complement and/or autoreactive antibodies have been implicated as playing a role in myelin and oligodendroglial injury in MS lesions. In a subset of MS lesions, depositions of immunoglobulins have been found on compact myelin and on myelin debris within the cytoplasm of macrophages (Lucchinetti et al., 2000). Also, macrophages with cap-like immunoglobulin deposits on the cell surface and myelin degradation products within their cytoplasm have been described (Prineas and Graham, 1981). These findings were interpreted as the participation of immunoglobulins in myelin breakdown and subsequent phagocytosis of the myelin debris by macrophages. Furthermore, myelin-specific antibodies or antibodies directed against antigens expressed by oligo-dendroglial progenitor cells have been detected in MS lesions and in the CSF and serum of MS patients (Cross et al., 2001; Genain et al., 1999; Niehaus et al., 2000; Zhou et al., 2006) (reviewed in Antel and Bar-Or, 2003). However, anti-myelin antibodies are found also in the CSF and serum of healthy controls (Iglesias et al., 2001) and the contribution of these antibodies to disease course and phenotype remains controversial (Berger et al., 2003; Rauer et al., 2006; Zhou et al., 2006).

In EAE, the addition of myelin-specific antibodies leads to more extensive demyelination, but does not induce disease (Aboul-Enein et al., 2004; Genain et al., 1995; Linington et al., 1988, 1992). Cultured anti-myelin antibodies have been shown to injure oligodendrocytes and their myelin (Griot-Wenk et al., 1991; Menon et al., 1997).

In addition to the detrimental effects of anti-myelin antibodies described above, antibodies may also have beneficial properties by enhancing remyelination (Miller and Rodriguez, 1995; Mitsunaga et al., 2002), either protecting oligodendrocytes against cell death (Howe et al., 2004; Soldan et al., 2003) or improving opsonization and removing myelin debris by macrophages (Kuhlmann et al., 2002).

In EAE and MS lesions, the membrane attack complex (C5b–C9), the final member in the complement cascade that can be activated by myelin in the presence or absence of myelin-specific antibodies, has been detected (Compston et al., 1989; Linington et al., 1989; Lucchinetti et al., 2000; Vanguri et al., 1982). The C9neo epitope was shown to cause demyelination and axonal loss in EAE (Mead et al., 2002), while complementary, complement-deficient mice show an attenuation of EAE (Nataf *et al.*, 2000). In culture, rodent oligodendrocytes are also susceptible to complement-mediated damage (Piddlesden and Morgan, 1993; Scolding *et al.*, 1989). However, there are no similar findings with regard to human oligodendrocytes (Zajicek *et al.*, 1995).

Cytokine-mediated mechanisms

Cytokine receptors such as for IL-4, IL-6, IL-10, IL12, IL-18 as well as IFN-γ are constitutively expressed on oligodendrocytes in healthy subjects and are upregulated in MS tissues (Cannella and Raine, 2004).

The effects of cytokines such as IFN-γ are complex. For example, transgenic mice displaying a suppressed oligodendrocyte responsiveness to IFN-γ have an accelerated onset of EAE associated with enhanced early inflammation and markedly increased oligodendrocyte apoptosis, while CNS delivery of IFN-γ before the onset of EAE ameliorates the disease course and prevents demyelination, oligodendrocyte loss and axonal damage (Balabanov *et al.*, 2007; Lin *et al.*, 2007). In culture experiments, IFN-γ induces either apoptotic or necrotic cell death in oligodendrocytes depending on exposure time, concentrations and maturation stages of the oligodendrocytes (as reviewed in Popko and Baerwald, 1999). In contrast, pretreatment of rat oligodendrocytes with low concentrations of IFN-γ resulted in a protective effect against oxidative stress but potentiated the toxic effects of anti-Fas antibody and staurosporine (Balabanov *et al.*, 2007). IFN-γ also induced the upregulation of different chemokines (CXCL10, CCL2, CCL3, CCL5), indicating that oligodendrocytes have the capability to actively participate in the immune network (Balabanov *et al.*, 2007). Exposure of the murine oligodendroglial tumor cell line MOCH-1 or primary rat oligodendrocytes to IFN-γ led to the upregulation of MHC I and II, rendering these cells more susceptible to T-cell-mediated injury (Bergsteindottir *et al.*, 1992). Little is known about the effects of other cytokines on oligodendrocytes. Importantly however is a clinical trial of IFN-γ in patients with relapsing and remitting MS, which resulted in an increase in frequency and severity of attacks (Panitch *et al.* 1987).

Histotoxic hypoxia

A subset of MS lesions (so-called pattern III lesions according to Lucchinetti *et al.*, 2000) is characterized by a profound loss of some myelin proteins such as MAG and CNP, while other myelin proteins such as MBP, MOG and PLP are still preserved or even upregulated. Additionally, oligodendrocytes showing morphological characteristics such as condensed and fragmented nuclei are observed in these lesions. Similar morphological changes have been noted in early ischemic CNS lesions and in viral CNS disease (herpes virus, cytomegalovirus, and JC virus) (Aboul-Enein *et al.*, 2003; Itoyama *et al.*, 1980). These observations have given rise to the suggestion that similar injury mechanisms may occur in early stages of stroke, viral CNS diseases and early MS lesions. At the penumbra of stroke regions, protective mechanisms (so-called hypoxic preconditioning) are active to limit hypoxic damage. Key proteins regulating these protective cascades are the transcription factors, hypoxia-inducible factors (HIFs) α and β and stress proteins such as HSP 70. However, these protective mechanisms are not specific to ischemic events and can also be observed in inflammatory conditions (Kimura *et al.*, 2000; Sharp and Bernaudin, 2004). Interestingly, in Baló's-type MS lesions an upregulation of HIF-1α and heat shock proteins has been observed at the edge of actively demyelinating lesions and in the PPWM (Stadelmann *et al.*, 2005). Gene expression studies comparing white matter from controls with normal appearing white matter from MS patients revealed an upregulation of genes involved in ischemic preconditioning, such as HIF-1α (Graumann *et al.*, 2003). However, despite the morphological similarities between some MS lesions and early stages of stroke, no stroke-like vascular pathology, such as vessel occlusion, has been observed in MS lesions. We therefore hypothesize that energy failure due to mitochondrial dysfunction may be the driving cause behind the specific pattern of oligodendrocyte loss and myelin damage in pattern III lesions.

Glutamate-mediated mechanisms

Like neurons, oligodendrocytes are susceptible to glutamate-induced damage (Matute *et al.*, 1997; McDonald *et al.*, 1998a; Oka *et al.*, 1993; Yoshioka *et al.*, 1995). Glutamate receptors can be divided into AMPA, kainate and NMDA receptors as well as metabotropic receptors (class 1–3). In rodents, mature oligodendrocytes and oligodendroglial progenitor cells express AMPA, kainate receptors and AMPA receptors, while metabotropic receptors are expressed only at low levels (Berger *et al.*, 1992; Karadottir *et al.*, 2005; Patneau *et al.*, 1994). However, contradictory results have been published regarding the expression of glutamate receptors in human oligodendrocytes.

Infusion of kainate in rodent optic nerves leads to the formation of MS-like lesions with numerous apoptotic oligodendrocytes (Matute, 1998). In contrast, administration of AMPA and kainate antagonists ameliorates the clinical symptoms of EAE significantly (Groom et al., 2003; Kanwar et al., 2004; Pitt et al., 2000; Smith et al., 2000).

Glutamate may be released by activated and resting microglia or astrocytes and may lead to excitotoxicity by increased cellular levels of Ca^{2+} (Domercq et al., 2007; Nedergaard et al., 2002). Mitochondrial overload of Ca^{2+} may trigger the activation of intrinsic apoptotic pathways or induce the production of oxygen radicals leading to necrotic cell death (Atlante et al., 2001; Luetjens et al., 2000). In addition to these direct toxic effects, glutamate may also mediate oligodendroglial damage by a more indirect way, e.g. by production and release of TNF-α from microglia cells upon activation of their AMPA or kainate receptors (Merrill and Benveniste, 1996). Activation of glutamate receptors by kainate in a non-toxic dose, followed by complement administration, induced caspase-independent oligodendroglial cell death accompanied by formation of the membrane attack complex as well as increased membrane conductance, calcium overload and an increased amount of intracellular reactive oxygen species in oligodendrocytes (Alberdi et al., 2006).

Reactive oxygen species- and reactive nitrogen species-mediated mechanisms

Reactive nitrogen and oxygen species have been implicated in oligodendroglial cell death. These reactive species have a half-life of a few seconds and cannot therefore be directly detected in human CNS tissue specimens. Instead, "footprints," such as the enzymes generating NO or nitrotyrosine residues formed as a degradation product of peroxynitrite, are used as markers. The inducible isoform of NO synthase is upregulated in astrocytes and macrophages in MS lesions (Bagasra et al., 1995; Bitsch et al., 2000b; Jack et al., 2007; Liu et al., 2001; Oleszak et al., 1998), but no correlation with the extent of oligodendroglial damage has been observed (Jack et al., 2007). Nitrotyrosine residues have been detected in macrophages and astrocytes as well as in dying oligodendrocytes in MS lesions (Cross et al., 1997; Jack et al., 2007; Oleszak et al., 1998).

Primary rodent oligodendroglial cell cultures derived from newborn rodents as well as rodent cell lines are highly susceptible to NO-mediated cell damage, while astrocytes and microglia are relatively resistant (Mitrovic et al., 1994). However, human adult CNS-derived oligodendrocytes are also relatively resistant to NO-induced damage (Jack *et al.*, 2007), indicating either a species difference or that the susceptibility of the oligodendroglial cell lineage to NO depends on maturation. NO can react spontaneously with superoxide to generate peroxynitrite, which is highly cytotoxic to primary rat and human primary oligodendrocytes and oligodendroglial cell lines (Jack *et al.*, 2007; Li, J. *et al.*, 2005; Scott *et al.*, 2003).

Peroxynitrite induces DNA strand breakage (Scott *et al.*, 2003), lipid peroxidation (Radi *et al.*, 1991) and protein nitration (Ara *et al.*, 1998; Crow *et al.*, 1997). In addition, peroxynitrite may activate a death cascade involving the release of intracellular zinc and activation of ERK42/44 and lipoxygenase, leading to the generation of reactive oxygen species such as shown in recent culture studies (Zhang, Y., *et al.*, 2006). In EAE, peroxynitrite scavengers or decomposition catalysts are beneficial (Brenner *et al.*, 1997; Hooper *et al.*, 1998; Scott *et al.*, 2002).

Reactive oxygen species such as superoxide anions, hydrogen peroxide or hydroxyl ions are capable of directly damaging oligodendrocytes and their progenitors in culture (Bernardo *et al.*, 2003; Mronga *et al.*, 2004). Reactive oxygen species are also released by IFN-γ-activated microglia (Liu *et al.*, 2006b). Uncoupling protein2 (UCP2) reduces the generation of reactive oxygen species, and mice lacking UCP2 suffer from more severe EAE (Vogler *et al.*, 2006). Relatively little is known about the presence of reactive oxygen species in human MS lesions due to the lack of markers. However, detoxification enzymes, such as NQO1, have been found to be highly expressed in astrocytes and macrophages, while only few NQO1-expressing oligodendrocytes have been observed (van Horssen *et al.*, 2006). The higher levels of NQO1 and other radical scavengers such as glutathione in astrocytes and microglia/macrophages may explain the relative resistance of these cell populations to injury and damage mediated by reactive oxygen and nitrogen species (Juurlink *et al.*, 1998; Thorburne and Juurlink, 1996).

REMYELINATION AND OLIGODENDROCYTE PROGENITOR CELLS IN MS LESIONS

Remyelination in MS lesions

Remyelinated axons are characterized by shortened internodes and a decreased ratio of myelin thickness to axon diameter (g ratio). These morphological changes have been identified in remyelinating animal models and in MS lesions (Lassmann, 1983). The light microscopic

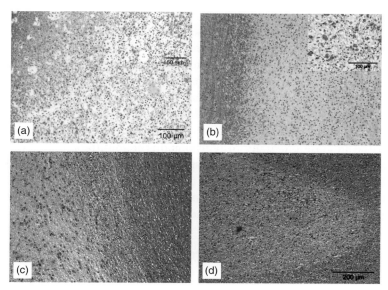

Figure 9.3 Remyelination in early and chronic MS lesions. Remyelination
is characterized by thin and irregularly compacted myelin lamellae. (a,
b) In early MS lesions the majority of lesions show signs of (a)
remyelination (immunohistochemistry for CNP). (Inset in b) However, a
few early lesions are observed which are completely demyelinated
despite the presence of numerous mature oligodendrocytes
(immunohistochemistry for Nogo-A) and preserved axons, indicating that
either the lack of certain factors (e.g. growth factor) or the presence of
inhibiting factors contributes to the lack of remyelination. (c, d) In
chronic MS lesions remyelination is limited in the majority of cases. (c)
The lesions are either completely demyelinated or limited to the lesion
border as shown (LFB-PAS staining). (d) A minority of chronic MS lesions
are completely remyelinated as shown (LFB-PAS staining). Due to the
thinner myelin sheaths, i.e. fewer compacted lamellae, the remyelinated
area appears pale compared with the surrounding normal-appearing
white matter. See color plate section for color version of this figure.

hallmark of remyelination is thin, irregularly formed compact myelin
which is readily detectable by staining (Figure 9.3a and b) and the
presence of remyelinated MS lesion areas has been described in a
variety of MS studies (Barkhof *et al.*, 2003; Lassmann *et al.*, 1997;
Prineas and Connell, 1979; Prineas *et al.*, 1993a). More recent studies
have revealed that in most MS lesions in chronic disease stages, remyelination was limited or completely absent; only a subset of about 20% of
the lesions showed extensive remyelination (Figure 9.3c and d) (Patani

et al., 2007; Patrikios *et al.*, 2006). The remyelinated MS lesion areas were frequently confined to the lesion border and the extent of remyelination varied from lesion to lesion (Patani *et al.*, 2007). Gray as well as white matter lesions are able to remyelinate (Albert *et al.*, 2007). However, recent animal experiments suggest that the time course of remyelination may differ between white and gray matter lesions (Merkler *et al.*, 2006). In MS remyelination is present early during the disease process and lesion areas of ongoing demyelination can be found in close proximity to remyelinating lesion areas (Lucchinetti *et al.*, 1996). Imaging studies support the hypothesis that remyelination occurs early during the disease process and that the decision of whether a lesion remyelinates or not takes place early in the formation of an individual lesion (Barkhof *et al.*, 2003; Chen *et al.*, 2007a).

Oligodendrocyte progenitor cells

A prerequisite for remyelination is the presence of myelinating cells and axons. Although the source of remyelinating cells is still a matter of debate, the generally accepted point of view is that the remyelinating cells are derived from oligodendroglial progenitor cells (OPCs) (for a review see Franklin, 2002). Animal studies have shown that the presence of dividing OPCs is essential for remyelination (Blakemore and Keirstead, 1999; Targett *et al.*, 1996). In demyelinating animal models, the number of OPCs increases quickly as a consequence of demyelination and decreases during remyelination, indicating that the OPCs remyelinate demyelinated axons and develop into mature oligodendrocytes. Increased numbers of progenitor cells as well as mature oligodendrocytes have been observed in MS lesions (Lucchinetti *et al.*, 1999; Raine *et al.*, 1981), suggesting that the increased number of mature oligodendrocytes is caused by a recruitment of OPCs followed by their development into mature oligodendrocytes, as observed in the remyelinating lesions of rodents. Recent publications report a reduction of OPCs in MS lesions over time (Chang *et al.*, 2002; Reynolds *et al.*, 2002; Wilson *et al.*, 2006; Wolswijk, 2002). In mice, repeated episodes of ethidium bromide-induced demyelination with intervening recovery did not affect the extent of remyelination or the numbers of OPCs (Penderis *et al.*, 2003). In contrast, mice that underwent chronic demyelination over an extended period of time showed lack of remyelination caused by a depletion of the OPCs (Mason *et al.*, 2004). Repeated events of demyelination within the same CNS lesions have been reported in MS (Prineas *et al.*, 1993b) and may contribute to the reduced numbers of OPCs found in MS lesions. However, progenitor cells are still present even in chronic and completely demyelinated MS lesions and have been found in close proximity to axons, indicating that a lack of neither OPCs nor axons is a major cause of limited remyelination in chronic MS lesions (Chang *et al.*, 2000). A failure of differentiation may therefore contribute to remyelination failure in chronic MS lesions. Potential causes of remyelination failure include the absence of factors promoting differentiation such as growth factors (IGF-1, TGF-β1, GGF2) (Carson *et al.*, 1993; Mason *et al.*, 2000; McKinnon *et al.*, 1993; Park *et al.*, 2001) or integrins (Blaschuk *et al.*, 2000; Relvas *et al.*, 2001) or the presence of inhibitory molecules such as the polysialylated form of the neural cell adhesion molecule, PSA-NCAM (Charles *et al.*, 2000, 2002a), Notch (Wang *et al.*, 1998) or Lingo1 (Mi *et al.*, 2005).

SUMMARY

In early MS lesions, heterogeneous patterns of oligodendroglial pathology are observed. A subset of lesions is characterized by dying oligodendrocytes and a differential expression of myelin proteins in lesion areas with actively ongoing demyelination, while in other lesions oligodendrocytes are mostly preserved. In some lesions the appearance of dying oligodendrocytes even precedes demyelination. In contrast, in demyelinated lesions from patients with a long disease duration, the oligodendroglial cell population is uniformly almost completely eliminated. Culture and animal experiments have identified a broad range of pathways that have the potential to damage oligodendrocytes; however which of these mechanisms is responsible for the loss of oligodendrocytes in MS lesions is unknown. Most likely not one but a combination of different noxious factors leads to oligodendroglial injury. Furthermore, the presence of a variety of noxious factors in MS lesions may render oligodendrocytes susceptible to other factors which by themselves would not be sufficient to cause oligodendroglial cell death. The different histological patterns observed in early MS lesions, which vary between but not within patients, suggest the existence of heterogeneous injury mechanisms in different patients.

Although remyelination is limited in the majority of chronic MS lesions, it does occur. Oligodendroglial progenitor cells that drive remyelination are present in early and chronic MS lesions and can be found in close contact with axons. Identifying the mechanisms responsible for the absence of remyelination may contribute to developing new neuroprotective therapeutic strategies in MS.

TARA M. DESILVA AND PAUL A. ROSENBERG

10

Glutamate receptors, transporters and periventricular leukomalacia

INTRODUCTION

Glutamate is the major excitatory neurotransmitter in the central nervous system (CNS). Glutamate exerts its role by activating ionotropic (Dingledine *et al.*, 1999) and metabotropic glutamate receptors (Conn and Patel, 1994). Ionotropic glutamate receptors are ligand-gated ion channels consisting of α-amino-3-hydroxyl-5-methyl-4-isoxazole-propionate (AMPA), N-methyl-D-aspartate (NMDA), and kainate receptors. Metabotropic glutamate receptors are not ion channels, but rather G-protein-coupled receptors that activate biochemical cascades that can indirectly influence ion channels. Glutamate transporters are responsible for regulating the concentration of glutamate in the vicinity of synaptic and extrasynaptic glutamate receptors (Tzingounis and Wadiche, 2007). Excessive accumulation of extracellular glutamate causes prolonged activation of glutamate receptors resulting in excitotoxicity (Lipton and Rosenberg, 1994). High levels of glutamate cause an excessive influx of calcium into the cytosol via glutamate receptors coupled to ion channels, resulting in the pathological activation of a number of enzymes including phospholipases, endonucleases and proteases, such as calpain. Increased glutamate levels also result in mitochondrial dysfunction (Choi, 1988). Excitotoxicity is a common pathway of injury in many neurological diseases leading to neuronal cell death. Excitotoxicity has also been implicated in oligodendrocyte death in disorders of cerebral white matter, including periventricular leukomalacia (PVL).

PERIVENTRICULAR LEUKOMALACIA

Periventricular leukomalacia (PVL) is the major brain pathology, in long-term survivors of prematurity. Approximately 5–10% of babies

The Biology of Oligodendrocytes, eds. Patricia J. Armati and Emily K. Mathey. Published by Cambridge University Press. © Cambridge University Press 2010.

born with a birth weight of less than 1500 g develop cerebral palsy. Nearly 5500 new cases of cerebral palsy in premature infants are diagnosed each year in the United States. With emerging advances in neonatal intensive care the severe focal cystic necrotic lesions that were formerly a prominent feature of PVL have become less common, and there is a greater incidence of less severe focal lesions and diffuse non-cystic changes in the cerebral white matter. These improvements in intensive care have increased the survival of infants born prematurely. However, the clinical sequelae in these children remain extremely complex including motor deficits in conjunction with cognitive, behavioral and sensory deficits (Volpe, 2009).

The pathology of PVL is focal necrosis accompanied by astrocytosis, reactive microgliosis and infiltrating macrophages in the white matter (Folkerth and Kinney, 2008) (Figure 10.1). The prevailing concept is that PVL represents primarily damage to the cerebral white matter. However, recent imaging studies show not only changes in cerebral white matter myelination but also atrophy in cerebral gray matter structures (Counsell et al., 2003; Hamrick et al., 2004; Inder et al., 2003; Miller et al., 2003). In a recent pathological study of gray matter injury associated with PVL, neuronal necrosis, neuronal loss and/or gliosis were found in the thalamus, basal ganglia, cerebellum and brainstem in approximately one-third of PVL cases with relative sparing of the cerebral cortex (Pierson et al., 2007). This gray matter injury may underlie the predominance of cognitive impairments in survivors of prematurity with or without cerebral palsy. In fact, learning disabilities and deficits in cognition affect 20–50% of very low birth weight preterm infants compared to the 5–10% that develop cerebral palsy (Ancel et al., 2006; Volpe, 2003; Woodward et al., 2005). These data support an emerging hypothesis that the complex clinical abnormalities resulting from prematurity do not arise from a single lesion, PVL, but rather are a consequence of combined gray and white matter insults.

During cerebral white matter development, oligodendrocytes arise from progenitor cells identified by the monoclonal antibodies NG2 (against chondroitin sulfate proteoglycan) and A2B5 (against polysialoganglioside) as well as by the expression of platelet-derived growth factor receptor (Dawson et al., 2003; Levine et al., 1993; Polito and Reynolds, 2005; Rivers et al., 2008; Zhu et al., 2008). Oligodendrocytes develop through stages characterized by their labeling with the monoclonal antibodies O4 (against a sulfatide) and O1 (against galactocerebroside) (Pfeiffer et al., 1993). Mature

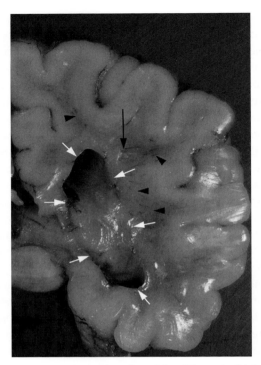

Figure 10.1 Coronal section of the right parietal lobe of an infant born at 30 weeks and surviving 2 weeks postnatally showing focal white matter necrosis – characteristic of PVL – with early cavitation (long black arrow) surrounded by diffusely injured white matter (black arrowheads) with pink-gray discoloration. Damage is localized to the periventricular regions (ventricular surface is outlined with white arrows). Note the relative sparing of the cerebral cortical ribbon. Courtesy Dr. R. Folkerth, Children's Hospital Boston. See color plate section for color version of this figure.

oligodendrocytes are recognized by their expression of myelin basic protein (MBP). The specific oligodendrocyte phenotype is defined by the expression or lack of expression of these specific cell markers, i.e. $O4^+O1^-MBP^-$ expression indicates a proliferating precursor cell, called the pre-oligodendrocyte; $O4^+O1^+MBP^-$ expression indicates a postmitotic, immature oligodendrocyte; and $O4^+O1^+MBP^+$ expression indicates a mature oligodendrocyte (Pfeiffer *et al.*, 1993). MBP$^+$ oligo-dendrocytes are myelin-producing cells of the CNS, and have up to 50 "arms" which spiral around individual axonal lengths and form the compact myelin lamellae that is required for saltatory conduction of the action potential (Sherman and Brophy, 2005) (see also

Chapter 1). The peak age of vulnerability to PVL is 24–32 gestational weeks, which coincides with the predominant expression of developing oligodendrocytes (pre-oligodendrocytes and immature oligodendrocytes), but not MBP-expressing oligodendrocytes (Back *et al.*, 2001). Death or injury to these developing oligodendrocytes is thought to be the most significant cause of hypomyelination documented by neuropathological and neuroimaging studies in the PVL brain. It is noteworthy, however, that when using the pan-oligodendrocyte marker olig2 (Rowitch *et al.*, 2002), no loss of cells was found in the white matter in PVL cases (Billiards *et al.*, 2008). The hypothesis is that oligodendrocytes are indeed injured and die, and are replaced by proliferating oligodendrocyte precursor cells. The dilemma is why, if there is no net loss in oligodendrocytes, is there hypomyelination? PVL also occurs in full-term (40 weeks) neonates with congenital cardiac or pulmonary disease within the first year of life (Kinney *et al.*, 2005; Kinney and Volpe, 2009). This finding is consistent with the vulnerability of immature (unmyelinated) oligodendrocytes to PVL. Expression of MBP similar to adult levels in the human normally occurs between six months and one year of age (Haynes *et al.*, 2005; Kinney *et al.*, 1988).

Clearly, to understand why the premature brain is prone to this age-specific vulnerability requires careful evaluation of the variables involved in predisposing the developing cerebral white matter to damage. Hypoxic-ischemic injury and/or perinatal infection have been implicated in the pathogenesis of PVL.

HYPOXIC-ISCHEMIC INJURY AND PERIVENTRICULAR LEUKOMALACIA

Hypoxia-ischemia (HI) is an important pathogenic mechanism contributing to PVL (Banker and Larroche, 1962). HI insults result in a deficit in oxygen supply to the perinatal brain by two major mechanisms: hypoxia, or diminished oxygen in the blood supply; and ischemia, or diminished blood flow to the brain. Lack of oxygen due to underdeveloped lung capacity and disturbances in cerebrovascular autoregulation in premature infants have been well documented (Volpe, 2008). Banker and Laroche (1962) originally correlated the vascular anatomy in the cerebral white matter with the pathology of PVL by demonstrating that focal necrotic lesions occurred near the end zones of the long penetrating arteries that provide blood supply to the periventricular white matter. Further evidence of ischemic insults producing PVL was found in a study of neonatal cardiac patients who developed cerebral white matter damage after cardiac surgery (Kinney et al., 2005).

EXCITOTOXICITY AND PVL

Elevation of extracellular glutamate as a consequence of HI has been demonstrated clinically in the CSF of full-term infants after perinatal HI (Hagberg, 1992), experimentally by in vivo microdialysis in a perinatal rat model of ischemia (Benveniste et al., 1984; Silverstein et al., 1991), and in an umbilical cord occlusion model in the near-term fetal sheep (Loeliger et al., 2003). More recent work has shown that both oligodendrocytes and axons in perinatal rat cerebral white matter contain high levels of glutamate, which decline significantly during HI. Comparatively, astrocytes had very little glutamate suggesting that both oligodendrocytes and axons are a major source of glutamate during HI injury (Back et al., 2007).

An alternate hypothesis regarding the pathogenesis of PVL holds that maternal infection is of critical importance, an idea based originally in epidemiological studies of Leviton and Gilles (1973) and subsequently on the experimental demonstration of white matter lesions in kittens given intraperitoneal injections of the endotoxin lipopolysaccharide (LPS) (Gilles et al., 1976). PVL has been associated with maternal intrauterine infection and chorioam-nionitis, known predisposing factors for premature delivery (Choi et al., 2000; Dammann and Leviton, 2000; Dammann et al., 2002). Several animal models have demonstrated cerebral white matter injury after Escherichia coli or LPS exposure in the preterm fetus (Cai et al., 2000; Yoon et al., 1997). More recent studies have also demon-strated the production of cerebral white matter lesions in utero with injection of LPS into ovine fetuses under conditions of cardiovascular monitoring (Dalitz et al., 2003; Duncan et al., 2002; Mallard et al., 2003; Peebles et al., 2003). These studies showed that cerebral ische-mia did not occur, although transient systemic hypotension and cerebral hypoxemia were produced by LPS exposure. The mechanism by which a maternal infectious process might affect the fetus is unclear. However, peripheral LPS blocks neurogenesis in the dentate gyrus (Monje et al., 2003), and so the idea of a systemic inflammatory state disrupting CNS myelination seems entirely plausible. In addi-tion, excitotoxicity has been shown to be produced by inflammation. As a consequence of inflammatory activation, astrocytes and microglia may produce nitric oxide which can inhibit cellular respiration causing energy failure and glutamate release, resulting in excitotoxicity (Bal-Price and Brown, 2001; Brown and Bal-Price, 2003; Mander *et al.*, 2005; Rousset *et al.*, 2008). Excitotoxicity has also been implicated in the inflammatory, demyelinating disease multiple sclerosis where AMPA receptor antagonists were shown to increase oligodendrocyte survival in a mouse model of experimental autoimmune encephalomyelitis (EAE) (Pitt *et al.*, 2000; Werner *et al.*, 2001). Thus, the significance of excitotoxicity in the pathogenesis of PVL is not dependent on a hypoxic/ischemic origin. This is important, because the pathogenesis of PVL remains unclear and controversial, with recent data favoring the possibility of a two-hit lesion combining both inflammatory and hypoxic/ischemic factors (Rousset *et al.*, 2008). The cellular and molecular mechanisms underlying HI and inflammatory injury, and specifically their role in excitotoxicity, are important for understanding the pathogenesis of PVL.

AMPA RECEPTORS EXPRESSED IN OLIGODENDROCYTES: CULTURE STUDIES

The original studies showing glutamate-evoked currents in cultured oligodendrocytes reported AMPA and kainate receptors to be solely responsible for generating these currents. The presence of functional AMPA glutamate receptors on oligodendrocytes was consistent with mRNA expression of AMPA receptor subunits GluR2, 3, and 4, but not GluR1 (Barres *et al.*, 1990; Borges *et al.*, 1994; Gallo and Russell, 1995; Meucci *et al.*, 1996; Patneau *et al.*, 1994; Puchalski *et al.*, 1994; Sontheimer, 1991; Yoshioka *et al.*, 1995). Similarly, mRNA for subunits GluR6 and 7 and KA-1 and 2, but not GluR5, was found for kainate receptors (Garcia-Barcina and Matute, 1996; Jensen and Chiu, 1993; Matute *et al.*, 1997; Patneau *et al.*, 1994; Yoshioka *et al.*, 1996). To determine whether oligodendrocytes could be injured by excitotoxicity, both oxygen and glucose deprivation (Rivera *et al.*, 2006) and direct application of glutamate agonists have been used as models of HI injury. In culture, pre-oligodendrocytes (O4$^+$O1$^-$MBP$^-$) and immature oligodendrocytes (O4$^+$O1$^+$MBP$^-$) were found to be sensitive to non-NMDA-receptor-mediated excitotoxicity (Matute *et al.*, 1997; McDonald *et al.*, 1998a; Rosenberg *et al.*, 2003; Yoshioka *et al.*, 1995). However, mature oligodendrocytes (O4$^+$O1$^+$MBP$^+$), identified by the MBP marker, were very resistant to excitotoxicity in some studies (Itoh *et al.*, 2002; Rosenberg *et al.*, 2003), but were sensitive to excitotoxicity in another (Leuchtmann *et al.*, 2003; McDonald *et al.*, 1998a, b). The basis for this discrepancy is unclear. The cell culture findings showing increased vulnerability of developing, as opposed to mature, white matter to HI might be due to increased calcium permeability of AMPA receptors on pre-oligodendrocytes. As in the case of NMDA receptors in neurons, non-NMDA-receptor-mediated toxicity is generally accepted to be dependent upon calcium influx into cells. Calcium permeability in AMPA receptors is conferred by the GluR2 subunit. When the GluR2 subunit is edited (Q/R) it is impermeable to calcium, and when it is not edited it is permeable to calcium (Burnashev *et al.*, 1992; Geiger *et al.*, 1995; Hollmann *et al.*, 1991). In oligodendrocyte progenitor cells 95% of GluR2 was found to be edited (Puchalski *et al.*, 1994). In cultures of developing oligodendrocytes intracellular calcium accumulation and electrophysiological responses to kainic acid were enhanced compared with mature oligodendrocytes (Itoh *et al.*, 2002; Rosenberg *et al.*, 2003). This correlates with increased expression of GluR3 and GluR4 receptor subunits compared with GluR2. This receptor-subunit ratio would permit the assembly of GluR2-free, calcium-permeable AMPA receptors. In addition, oxygen and glucose deprivation (OGD) decreased the surface expression of GluR2 on pre-oligodendrocytes causing an increase in calcium permeability compared with untreated pre-oligodendrocytes (Deng *et al.*, 2003).

AMPA RECEPTORS EXPRESSED IN OLIGODENDROCYTES: IN VIVO STUDIES

Consistent with studies in culture, the AMPA receptor antagonist NBQX (6-nitro-7-sulfamoylbenzo(f)quinoxaline-2,3-dione) was protective against cerebral white matter damage in perinatal rats subjected to HI injury at postnatal day seven (P7) (Follett *et al.*, 2000). In rodents the majority of development in the brain occurs postnatally (Dobbing and Sands, 1979). Based on the developmental stages of oligodendrocytes expressed in white matter and the expression of glutamate receptors on these cells, the neonatal rat is considered to be the equivalent of the human fetus at the time of peak vulnerability to PVL (Back *et al.*, 2001, 2002a; Craig *et al.*, 2003; Ferriero, 2006; Follett *et al.*, 2003; Talos *et al.*, 2006). Intracerebral injection of AMPA resulted in a white matter lesion in postnatal day 7 rats with relatively no lesion at postnatal day 11 (P11), demonstrating a developmental change in susceptibility of the perinatal rat cerebral white matter in vivo. The resistance to white matter injury in the P11 rat correlated with increased expression of MBP, again suggesting that the upregulation of calcium-permeable AMPA receptors on developing oligodendrocytes compared with its expression in myelinating oligodendrocytes may contribute to the developmental changes in susceptibility of cerebral white matter to excitotoxicity (Follett et al., 2000). These data have been further corroborated by the developmental expression profile of AMPA receptor subunits in the human and rat forebrain, showing that GluR2-lacking AMPA receptors are highly expressed on developing oligodendrocytes during the time period when cerebral white matter is at greatest risk for injury (Follett et al., 2000; Talos et al., 2006). Recently, evidence has emerged that the NMDA receptor makes a major contribution to ischemic injury in the cerebral white matter.

NMDA RECEPTOR EXPRESSION IN WHITE MATTER

NMDA receptors were assumed to be absent from oligodendrocytes based on previous studies showing the lack of mRNA expression in the optic nerve (Matute et al., 1997) and no NMDA-evoked currents in cultured oligodendrocytes or in brain slices (Barres et al., 1990; Berger et al., 1992; Patneau et al., 1994; Pende et al., 1994). However, during that time period important experiments suggested the contrary. For example, ibotenate (Blaabjerg et al., 2003) injection in P2–P10 rats resulted in both gray and white matter damage that was prevented by an NMDA receptor antagonist but not a metabotropic glutamate receptor antagonist (Gressens et al., 1996; Marret et al., 1995). NMDA receptor antagonists were shown to slow loss of action potentials in rat cerebral white matter (Tekkök and Goldberg, 2001) and were protective to white matter in a rat model of multiple sclerosis (Wallström et al., 1996) and stroke (Schabitz et al., 2000). NMDA-evoked currents were reported in spinal cord oligodendrocytes (Ziak et al., 1998). Almost a decade later, functional NMDA receptors were shown to be expressed in oligodendrocytes and to mediate ischemic injury in the rodent corpus callosum, cerebellar white matter and optic nerve (Karadottir et al., 2005; Micu et al., 2006; Salter and Fern, 2005). These findings demonstrate that the expression of NMDA receptors is mainly found in the oligodendrocyte processes, which may account for the oversight in its earlier detection, while the expression of AMPA receptors is localized to the cell body. In the adult rat optic nerve, NMDA receptors were found to only mediate calcium accumulation in compact myelin, while AMPA receptors were shown to mediate calcium accumulation in oligodendrocyte cell bodies (Micu *et al.*, 2006) providing further insight into how the function of these two receptors is regionally organized on a subcellular level. Similarly, ischemia resulted in loss of developing oligodendrocyte processes, which was blocked by the NMDA receptor antagonist MK801, whereas the AMPA/kainate receptor antagonist NBQX prevented injury to the cell bodies (Salter and Fern, 2005). Expression of NMDA receptors and NMDA-evoked currents was detected at all oligodendrocyte developmental stages identified by the markers for NG2, O4 and MBP (Karadottir *et al.*, 2005). Further exploration of the regional localization and specific subunit expression with regard to the functional differences between AMPA and NMDA receptors is necessary to understand how ischemic injury is mediated in oligodendrocytes (Karadottir and Attwell, 2007).

NMDA receptors are much more sensitive to glutamate than AMPA receptors (Herman and Jahr, 2007; Rosenberg *et al.*, 1992). This fact suggests that, at the receptor level, oligodendrocyte processes would be expected to be more sensitive to excitotoxicity than the cell body. Developing oligodendrocyte processes seek axons, subsequently forming MBP-expressing cells (Back *et al.*, 2002b), each one of which can myelinate internodes of up to 30 different axons. Injury to these oligodendrocyte processes exclusive of oligodendrocyte death may well be expected to produce important changes in myelination affecting multiple axons. While both NMDA and AMPA receptors are ligand-gated ion channels, NMDA receptors are also voltage-dependent and require depolarization to remove the magnesium block and permit an open channel. The magnesium sensitivity of NMDA receptors expressed in oligodendrocytes compared with their expression in neurons varies greatly. The presence of magnesium reduces the current 3- to 5-fold in oligodendrocytes (Karadottir *et al.*, 2005) compared with 20- to 70-fold in neurons. This suggests a variation in receptor subunit composition between these two cell types and may explain why NMDA receptors on oligodendrocytes can generate a significant current even at the cell's resting potential (Karadottir *et al.*, 2005). Expression of NR2C and NR3 subunits has been shown to confer a weak magnesium block on NMDA receptors (Kuner and Schoepfer, 1996; Sasaki *et al.*, 2002). Immunocytochemistry and polymerase chain reaction amplification detected the presence of NR1, NR2A, NR2B, NR2C, NR2D and NR3A on oligodendrocytes, and the relative absence of NR3B, although the receptor subunit composition remains to be elucidated (Karadottir *et al.*, 2005; Micu *et al.*, 2006; Salter and Fern, 2005).

The uncompetitive NMDA receptor antagonist memantine was shown to be protective against the acute loss of myelin basic protein (MBP) in an animal model of PVL (Bakiri *et al.*, 2008; Manning *et al.*, 2008). Interestingly, memantine also prevented the long-term reduction in cerebral mantle thickness observed in this animal model of PVL at postnatal day 21 (Manning *et al.*, 2008). This reduction in cerebral cortical mantle thickness is thought to be representative of the atrophy observed in imaging studies of the cerebral gray matter in human PVL brains (Counsell *et al.*, 2003; Hamrick *et al.*, 2004; Inder *et al.*, 2003; Miller *et al.*, 2003). Memantine is FDA approved for the treatment of Alzheimer's disease, but, as an uncompetitive blocker of the NMDA receptor its effect on the developing brain is unknown. Using NMDA receptors as a therapeutic target in the developing brain is questionable since the clinical use of NMDA receptor channel blockers has been limited by neuronal toxicity (Besancon *et al.*, 2008; Fix *et al.*, 1993; Ikonomidou *et al.*, 1999; Kaindl and Ikonomidou, 2007; Nikizad *et al.*, 2007; Olney *et al.*, 1991). In general, the approach of targeting glutamate receptors for prevention of HI injury in the mature brain has not been successful (Besancon *et al.*, 2008). Perhaps finding a safe drug therapy to block the downstream effects of excessive activation of glutamate receptors will not only attenuate oligodendrocyte death and/or injury, but may also ameliorate the subtle neuronal injury now well recognized as part of the PVL spectrum.

METABOTROPIC GLUTAMATE RECEPTOR EXPRESSION IN WHITE MATTER

Oligodendrocytes also express metabotropic glutamate receptors (D'Antoni *et al.*, 2008). In neurons, metabotropic glutamate receptors consist of eight subtypes (mGluR1–8) and have been classified into three groups based on intracellular signaling properties and physiological activity (Conn and Patel, 1994). Group I metabotropic glutamate receptors include mGluR 1 and mGluR 5, which stimulate phospholipase C leading to the formation of diacylglycerol and inositol triphosphate resulting in activation of protein kinase C (PKC) and the opening of calcium channels, respectively. Group II (mGluR2, 3) and Group III (mGluR 4,6,7, and 8) metabotropic glutamate receptors inhibit the enzyme adenylyl cyclase, preventing the formation of

cyclic adenosine monophosphate (cAMP). In cultured oligodendrocytes, mGluR 1, 2/3, 4 and 5 are expressed in developing oligodendrocytes but are decreased in mature oligodendrocytes (Deng *et al.*,
2004; Luyt *et al.*, 2006). Furthermore, it has been shown that the
group I agonist (*R,S*)-3,5-dihydroxyphenylglycine (DHPG) (Deng *et al.*,
2004; Kelland and Toms, 2001) as well as the broad-spectrum
mGluR agonist (1 *S*,3 *R*)-1-aminocyclopentane-1,3-dicarboxylic acid
(ACPD) (Deng *et al.*, 2004) prevented kainate toxicity in
developing oligodendrocytes. This suggests an important role for
metabotropic glutamate receptors in modulating oligodendrocyte
excitotoxicity. Moreover, in neurons, mGluR agonists have been
shown to be neuroprotective against NMDA-receptor-mediated
excitotoxicity (Ambrosini *et al.*, 1995; Blaabjerg *et al.*, 2003). The
recent finding that NMDA receptors mediate excitotoxicity in developing oligodendrocytes (Karadottir *et al.*, 2005) presents an unex-
plored area for mGluR modulation of NMDA excitotoxicity in
oligodendrocytes.

GLUTAMATE TRANSPORTERS IN WHITE MATTER

Although excitotoxicity may be a fundamental mechanism in the
pathogenesis of PVL, the source of excessive extracellular glutamate
still remains in question. The possible sources of glutamate that
could contribute to the excitotoxic extracellular pool of glutamate
are vesicular release of glutamate from axons (Ziskin *et al.*, 2007) and
astrocytes (Bezzi *et al.*, 1998, 2001; Parpura *et al.*, 1994), or by volume-
sensitive organic osmolyte-anion channels (VSOA) (Kimelberg *et al.*,
1990). The major regulators of extracellular glutamate besides diffusion are glutamate transporters. Glutamate transporters are not ATP
dependent; their uptake capacity is driven primarily by the transmembrane gradients of sodium and potassium. Thus, dissipation of
electrochemical gradients across cell membranes, such as occurs
during HI, will cause reversal of glutamate uptake and release of
glutamate into the extracellular space. Reversal of glutamate transport has been shown to play an important role in HI injury (Deng
et al., 2003; Fern and Möller, 2000; Roettger and Lipton, 1996; Rossi
et al., 2000; Seki *et al.*, 1999). The glutamate transporters GLAST
(EAAT1) and GLT1 (EAAT2) are the predominant glial transporters
and EAAC1 (EAAT3) is the predominant neuronal glutamate transporter (Arriza *et al.*, 1994; Fairman *et al.*, 1995; Pines *et al.*, 1992;
Storck *et al.*, 1992), although recently GLT1 expression was

demonstrated in presynaptic terminals in mouse hippocampus (Chen et al., 2004; Furness et al., 2008). GLT1 is the predominant transporter in the brain. The GLT1 knockout mouse results in a lethal mutation, from which the animals die from intractable seizures several weeks after birth, and have only about 5% of wild-type levels of glutamate uptake activity in cortical synaptosomes (Tanaka et al., 1997). Oligodendrocytes in culture subjected to oxygen-glucose deprivation have been shown to release glutamate by reversal of GLT1, since dihydrokainate, a specific blocker of GLT1, is highly protective (Deng et al., 2003; Fern and Möller, 2000). GLT1 knockout mice are more vulnerable to neuronal loss in the hippocampus and attain higher extracellular glutamate levels in response to a five-minute episode of ischemia than wild-type mice. However, following 20 minutes of ischemia, wild-type mice attain higher glutamate levels than knockout mice (Mitani and Tanaka, 2003). Thus, whether expression of GLT1 in developing human white matter is helpful or harmful may depend on the duration of the ischemic episode.

In the human brain, the glutamate transporter GLT1 is highly expressed in developing oligodendrocytes during the peak window of vulnerability to PVL at a time when calcium-permeable AMPA and NMDA receptors are also present on oligodendrocytes (DeSilva et al., 2007). In mature, MBP-expressing oligodendrocytes, GLT1 is strongly downregulated. Given the previous animal model and cell culture data, these data suggest that during HI injury GLT1 on developing oligodendrocytes in the white matter may play an important role in glutamate release. Additional evidence supporting an important role for GLT1 specifically in oligodendrocytes is the fact that GLT1 was not expressed in astrocytes during early prenatal cerebral white matter development. This is consistent with previous studies showing no astrocytic expression of GLT1 in the developing human CNS (Furuta et al., 2005), human cultured glial progenitors (Maragakis et al., 2004), rat and sheep corpus callosum (Furuta et al., 1997; Northington et al., 1999) and mouse spinal cord (Yamada et al., 1998), until postnatal development. In the adult mammalian brain, it has been assumed that glutamate uptake by GLT1 in astrocytes has a major role in maintaining glutamate homeostasis (Bergles et al., 1999; Danbolt, 2001; Rosenberg et al., 1992; Rosenberg and Aizenman, 1989; Tanaka et al., 1997). The observation that GLT1 is not expressed in astrocytes during cerebral white matter development further suggests that the expression of glutamate transporters specifically in developing oligodendrocytes may play an important role in maintaining glutamate homeostasis. Oligodendrocytes in culture have a similar uptake capacity and affinity for glutamate (DeSilva *et al.*, 2009) compared with astrocytes (Garlin *et al.*, 1995; Schlag *et al.*, 1998; Swanson *et al.*, 1997). Although GLAST, GLT1 and EAAC1 were found to be expressed in oligodendrocytes, interestingly EAAC1, the predominant neuronal glutamate transporter, was responsible for most of the glutamate uptake (DeSilva *et al.*, 2009). The expression profile of GLT1 in cultured oligodendrocytes was different than that in vivo. In culture the expression of GLT1 was high in mature MBP-expressing (MBP$^+$) oligodendrocytes whereas in vivo GLT1 expression was high in developing oligodendrocytes and downregulated in mature MBP-expressing oligodendrocytes (DeSilva *et al.*, 2007, 2009). The culture and in vivo findings suggest a potential role for an axon–oligodendrocyte interaction, missing in the cell culture experiments, that regulates GLT1 expression during myelination. These observations provoke a fundamental question that needs further exploration; namely, what role does glutamatergic signaling play in oligodendrocytes?

GLUTAMATERGIC SIGNALING IN OLIGODENDROCYTE DEVELOPMENT AND MYELINATION

Several lines of evidence suggest that glutamate may be an important signaling factor during oligodendrocyte development and myelination. AMPA and NMDA receptors are known to mediate glutamatergic signaling in neurons, which is precisely regulated by glutamate transporters (Tzingounis and Wadiche, 2007). Glutamate receptors (Karadottir *et al.*, 2005; Micu *et al.*, 2006; Salter and Fern, 2005) and transporters (DeSilva *et al.*, 2009) are expressed throughout the oligodendrocyte lineage implicating a similar function in oligodendrocytes, which have not only been shown to engage in synaptic contacts with axons (Ziskin *et al.*, 2007), but also to express glutamate receptors and transporters (DeSilva *et al.*, 2009). Glutamate and its receptors have been shown to be involved in oligodendrocyte migration, proliferation and differentiation (Gallo *et al.*, 1996; Gudz *et al.*, 2006; Yuan *et al.*, 1998). Vesicular release of glutamate from axons induced AMPA-receptor-mediated currents in postsynaptic oligodendrocyte progenitor cells, demonstrating the functionality of axonal–oligodendrocyte synapses (Ziskin *et al.*, 2007). The predominant expression of NMDA receptors on oligodendrocyte processes, which myelinate axonal internodes, suggests a role for NMDA receptors in glutamatergic axon–oligodendrocyte signaling during myelination (Karadottir *et al.*, 2005). If glutamate signaling is occurring, glutamate homeostasis is critical, and glutamate transporters are the primary mechanism underlying this function. In adult spinal cord, glutamate transporters are expressed on axons and lead to activation of NMDA receptors located in the compact myelin during ischemia, which results in release of glutamate via reversed operation of glutamate transporters (Li *et al.*, 1999). Before myelination occurs in the cerebral white matter, GLT1 expression on developing oligodendrocytes and their processes may be the source of glutamate via reversed transport, causing overactivation of AMPA and NMDA receptors (DeSilva *et al.*, 2007). In contrast, during myelination, release of glutamate from GLT1 located on axons may be the source of the glutamate causing overstimulation of NMDA receptors in the myelinated internode (Li *et al.*, 1999). The studies of Li *et al.* (1999) focus on the dorsal columns of the spinal cord and whether GLT1 expression occurs in cerebral axons in the white matter remains to be seen. However, GLT1 has been shown to be expressed in excitatory axon terminals in the hippocampus (Chen *et al.*, 2004; Furness *et al.*, 2008).

Another important feature of cerebral white matter that may disrupt myelination in the event of energy failure relates to the discovery of synapses between unmyelinated axons and oligodendrocyte progenitor cells that persist in the mature brain (Ziskin *et al.*, 2007). These synapses might be zones of high vulnerability to excitotoxicity due to their dense expression of glutamate receptors. Energy failure that is a consequence of hypoxia/ischemia or inhibition of mitochondrial respiration by nitric oxide could result in reverse transport of GLT1 on oligodendrocytes or on presynaptic terminals. Because vesicular release of glutamate is energy dependent, during energy failure vesicular release of glutamate ceases as ATP levels fall early in the course of ischemia. However, glutamate transporters continue to operate, but in reverse mode, becoming unable to clear recently released synaptic glutamate, and leaking glutamate into the extracellular space (Szatkowski *et al.*, 1990; Zerangue and Kavanaugh, 1996). Recent observations of the depletion of glutamate both from axons and oligodendrocytes in developing rodent white matter subjected to hypoxia/ischemia suggest that both oligodendrocytes and axons are significant sources of the pathological accumulation of glutamate that is produced by this insult (Back *et al.*, 2007).

SUMMARY

Oligodendrocytes have the ability to proliferate after injury (Rivers *et al.*, 2008; Segovia *et al.*, 2008; Zhu *et al.*, 2008) suggesting that a disruption of maturation or an inability to make fully functional contacts with axons during myelination may play an important role in the hypomyelination observed as a result of PVL. In a rat model of perinatal white matter injury, there was an increase in the number of oligodendrocytes as evidenced by staining with Ki67, a marker for cell-cycle proliferation. However, there was an interruption in the progression of oligodendrocyte maturation (Segovia *et al.*, 2008). In human PVL brains, there was no significant difference in Ki67 labeling compared with control, which may reflect the long interval between the insult and the postmortem dissection (Billiards *et al.*, 2008). Recent evidence suggests that during normal physiological conditions, oligodendrocytes can differentiate to form new compact myelin in the adult rat corpus callosum (Rivers *et al.*, 2008). After injury, however, although oligodendrocyte proliferation seems to be maintained, the process of maturation is disrupted (Billiards *et al.*, 2008; Segovia *et al.*, 2008) suggesting that there may be a deficiency in signaling required for differentiation and/or myelination.

The process of myelination is known to involve axon–glial signaling for the selection of axons to be myelinated, the process of myelin ensheathment around axons, formation of the nodes of Ranvier, and regulation of myelin thickness (Franklin and Ffrench-Constant, 2008; Harel and Strittmatter, 2006; Sherman and Brophy, 2005). How injury to the developing cerebral white matter impinges on axon–glial signaling during development has not been studied. Axon–glial signaling may be further complicated by axonal injury (Tekkök and Goldberg, 2001; McCarran and Goldberg, 2007) as evidenced by fractin staining in PVL autopsy brains (Haynes *et al.*, 2008). Whether this axonal injury is in unmyelinated axons that make synaptic contact with oligodendrocyte progenitor cells (Ziskin *et al.*, 2007) or axons in the process of myelination is unclear. While the role of axon–oligodendrocyte synapses in the cerebral white matter is unknown, their existence does suggest a compelling role for glutamatergic signaling during myelination (Bakiri *et al.*, 2009). The regulation of glutamate receptor and transporter expression underlying glutamatergic signaling is likely to be important not only for the pathophysiology of excitotoxicity, but also for cerebral white matter development. Perturbations in this signaling pathway may lie at the root of the deficiency in myelination subsequent to injury of the premature brain.

References

Abelson, J. F., Kwan, K. Y., O'Roak, B. J., *et al.* (2005). Sequence variants in SLITRK1 are associated with Tourette's syndrome. *Science* **310**, 317–320.

Aberg, K., Saetre, P., Lindholm, E., *et al.* (2006). Human QKI, a new candidate gene for schizophrenia involved in myelination. *Am J Med Genet B Neuropsychiatr Genet* **141**, 84–90.

Aboul-Enein, F., Bauer, J., Klein, M., *et al.* (2004). Selective and antigen-dependent effects of myelin degeneration on central nervous system inflammation. *J Neuropathol Exp Neurol* **63**, 1284–1296.

Aboul-Enein, F., Rauschka, H., Kornek, B., *et al.* (2003). Preferential loss of myelin-associated glycoprotein reflects hypoxia-like white matter damage in stroke and inflammatory brain diseases. *J Neuropathol Exp Neurol* **62**, 25–33.

Adams, R. D. and Kubik, C. S. (1952). The morbid anatomy of the demyelinating diseases. *Am J Med* **12**, 510–546.

Adler, C. M., Adams, J., DelBello, M. P., *et al.* (2006). Evidence of white matter pathology in bipolar disorder adolescents experiencing their first episode of mania: a diffusion tensor imaging study. *Am J Psychiatry* **163**, 322–324.

Adrian, E. K., Jr. and Walker, B. E. (1962). Incorporation of thymidine-H3 by cells in normal and injured mouse spinal cord. *J Neuropathol Exp Neurol* **21**, 597–609.

Agrawal, H. C., Randle, C. L., and Agrawal, D. (1982). In vivo acylation of rat brain myelin proteolipid protein. *J Biol Chem.* **257**, 4588–4592.

Aguayo, A. J., Charron, L., and Bray, G. M. (1976). Potential of Schwann cells from unmyelinated nerves to produce myelin: a quantitative ultrastructural and radiographic study. *J Neurocytol* **5**, 565–573.

Ainger, K., Avossa, D., Diana, A. S., Barry, C., Barbarese, E., and Carson, J. H. (1997). Transport and localization elements in myelin basic protein mRNA. *J Cell Biol* **138**, 1077–1087.

Ainger, K., Avossa, D., Morgan, F., *et al.* (1993). Transport and localization of exogenous myelin basic protein mRNA microinjected into oligodendrocytes. *J Cell Biol* **123**, 431–441.

Akiyama, Y., Honmou, O., Kato, T., Uede, T., Hashi, K., and Kocsis, J. D. (2001). Transplantation of clonal neural precursor cells derived from adult human brain establishes functional peripheral myelin in the rat spinal cord. *Exp Neurol* **167**, 27–39.

Akiyama, Y., Radtke, C., Honmou, O., and Kocsis, J. D. (2002a). Remyelination of the spinal cord following intravenous delivery of bone marrow cells. *Glia* **39**, 229–236.

Akiyama, Y., Radtke, C., and Kocsis, J. D. (2002b). Remyelination of the rat spinal cord by transplantation of identified bone marrow stromal cells. *J Neurosci* **22**, 6623–6630.

Aktas, O., Prozorovski, T., and Zipp, F. (2006). Death ligands and autoimmune demyelination. *Neuroscientist* **12**, 305–316.

Alberdi, E., Sanchez-Gomez, M. V., Torre, I., *et al.* (2006). Activation of kainate receptors sensitizes oligodendrocytes to complement attack. *J Neurosci* **26**, 3220–3228.

Albert, M., Antel, J. P., Bruck, W., and Stadelmann, C. (2007). Extensive cortical remyelination in patients with chronic multiple sclerosis. *Brain Pathol* **17**, 129–138.

Alper, G. and Schor, N. F. (2004). Toward the definition of acute disseminated encephalitis of childhood. *Curr Opin Pediatr* **16**, 637–640.

Ambrosini, A., Bresciani, L., Fracchia, S., Brunello, N., and Racagni, G. (1995). Metabotropic glutamate receptors negatively coupled to adenylate cyclase inhibit N-methyl-D-aspartate receptor activity and prevent neurotoxicity in mesencephalic neurons in vitro. *Mol Pharmacol* **47**, 1057–1064.

Ancel, P. Y., Livinec, F., Larroque, B., *et al.* (2006). Cerebral palsy among very preterm children in relation to gestational age and neonatal ultrasound abnormalities: the EPIPAGE cohort study. *Pediatrics* **117**, 828–835.

Andre, P., Castriconi, R., Espeli, M., *et al.* (2004). Comparative analysis of human NK cell activation induced by NKG2D and natural cytotoxicity receptors. *Eur J Immunol* **34**, 961–971.

Anitei, M., Cowan, A. E., Pfeiffer, S. E., and Bansal, R. (2009). Role for Rab3a in oligodendrocyte morphological differentiation. *J Neurosci Res* **87**, 342–352.

Antel, J. P., and Bar-Or, A. (2003). Do myelin-directed antibodies predict multiple sclerosis? *N Engl J Med* **349**, 107–109.

Antel, J. P., McCrea, E., Ladiwala, U., Qin, Y. F., and Becher, B. (1998). Non-MHC-restricted cell-mediated lysis of human oligodendrocytes in vitro: relation with CD56 expression. *J Immunol* **160**, 1606–1611.

Anton, E. S., Hadjiargyrou, M., Patterson, P. H., and Matthew, W. D. (1995). CD9 plays a role in Schwann cell migration in vitro. *J Neurosci* **15**, 584–595.

Antony, J. M., van Marle, G., Opii, W., *et al.* (2004). Human endogenous retrovirus glycoprotein-mediated induction of redox reactants causes oligodendrocyte death and demyelination. *Nat Neurosci* **7**, 1088–1095.

Aquino, J. B., Hjerling-Leffler, J., Koltzenburg, M., Edlund, T., Villar, M. J., and Ernfors, P. (2006). In vitro and in vivo differentiation of boundary cap neural crest stem cells into mature Schwann cells. *Exp Neurol* **198**, 438–449.

Ara, J., Przedborski, S., Naini, A. B., *et al.* (1998). Inactivation of tyrosine hydroxylase by nitration following exposure to peroxynitrite and 1-methyl-4-phenyl-1,2,3,6-tetrahydropyridine (MPTP). *Proc Natl Acad Sci U S A* **95**, 7659–7663.

Araki, T. and Milbrandt, J. (1996). Ninjurin, a novel adhesion molecule, is induced by nerve injury and promotes axonal growth. *Neuron* **17**, 353–361.

Arbuthnott, E. R., Boyd, I. A., and Kalu, K. U. (1980). Ultrastructural dimensions of myelinated peripheral nerve fibres in the cat and their relation to conduction velocity. *J Physiol (Lond)* **308**, 125–157.

Archelos, J. J., Previtali, S. C., and Hartung, H. P. (1999). The role of integrins in immune-mediated diseases of the nervous system. *Trends Neurosci* **22**, 30–38.

Arnett, H. A., Fancy, S. P., Alberta, J. A., *et al.* (2004). bHLH transcription factor Olig1 is required to repair demyelinated lesions in the CNS. *Science* **306**, 2111–2115.

Arquint, M., Roder, J., Chia, L.-S., *et al.* (1987). Molecular cloning and primary structure of myelin-associated glycoproteins. *Proc Natl Acad Sci USA* **84**, 600–604.

Arriza, J. L., Fairman, W. A., Wadiche, J. I., Murdoch, G. H., Kavanaugh, M. P., and Amara, S. G. (1994). Functional comparisons of three glutamate transporter subtypes cloned from human motor cortex. *J Neurosci* **14**, 5559–5569.

Arundine, M. and Tymianski, M. (2004). Molecular mechanisms of glutamate-dependent neurodegeneration in ischemia and traumatic brain injury. *Cell Mol Life Sci* **61**, 657–668.

Atlante, A., Calissano, P., Bobba, A., Giannattasio, S., Marra, E., and Passarella, S. (2001). Glutamate neurotoxicity, oxidative stress and mitochondria. *FEBS Lett* **497**, 1–5.

Azari, M. F., Profyris, C., Karnezis, T., *et al.* (2006). Leukemia inhibitory factor arrests oligodendrocyte death and demyelination in spinal cord injury. *J Neuropathol Exp Neurol* **65**, 914–929.

Babbe, H., Roers, A., Waisman, A., *et al.* (2000). Clonal expansions of CD8(+) T cells dominate the T cell infiltrate in active multiple sclerosis lesions as shown by micromanipulation and single cell polymerase chain reaction. *J Exp Med* **192**, 393–404.

Bachelin, C., Lachapelle, F., Girard, C., *et al.* (2005). Efficient myelin repair in the macaque spinal cord by autologous grafts of Schwann cells. *Brain* **128**, 540–549.

Back, S. A., Craig, A., Kayton, R. J., *et al.* (2007). Hypoxia-ischemia preferentially triggers glutamate depletion from oligodendroglia and axons in perinatal cerebral white matter. *J Cereb Blood Flow Metab* **27**, 334–347.

Back, S. A., Gan, X., Li, Y., Rosenberg, P. A., and Volpe, J. J. (1998). Maturation-dependent vulnerability of oligodendrocytes to oxidative stress-induced death caused by glutathione depletion. *J Neurosci* **18**, 6241–6253.

Back, S. A., Han, B. H., Luo, N. L., *et al.* (2002a). Selective vulnerability of late oligodendrocyte progenitors to hypoxia-ischemia. *J Neurosci* **22**, 455–463.

Back, S. A., Luo, N. L., Borenstein, N. S., Levine, J. M., Volpe, J. J., and Kinney, H. C. (2001). Late oligodendrocyte progenitors coincide with the developmental window of vulnerability for human perinatal white matter injury. *J Neurosci* **21**, 1302–1312.

Back, S. A., Luo, N. L., Borenstein, N. S., Volpe, J. J., and Kinney, H. C. (2002b). Arrested oligodendrocyte lineage progression during human cerebral white matter development: dissociation between the timing of progenitor differentiation and myelinogenesis. *J Neuropathol Exp Neurol* **61**, 197–211.

Back, S. A., Tuohy, T. M., Chen, H., *et al.* (2005). Hyaluronan accumulates in demyelinated lesions and inhibits oligodendrocyte progenitor maturation. *Nat Med* **11**, 966–972.

Badea, T. C., Niculescu, F. I., Soane, L., Shin, M. L., and Rus, H. (1998). Molecular cloning and characterization of RGC-32, a novel gene induced by complement activation in oligodendrocytes. *J Biol Chem* **273**, 26977–26981.

Baechner, D., Liehr, T., Hameister, H., *et al.* (1995). Widespread expression of the peripheral myelin protein-22 gene (PMP22) in neural and non-neural tissues during murine development. *J Neurosci Res* **42**, 733–741.

Baerwald, K. D. and Popko, B. (1998). Developing and mature oligodendrocytes respond differently to the immune cytokine interferon-gamma. *J Neurosci Res* **52**, 230–239.

Bagasra, O., Michaels, F. H., Zheng, Y. M., *et al.* (1995). Activation of the inducible form of nitric oxide synthase in the brains of patients with multiple sclerosis. *Proc Natl Acad Sci USA* **92**, 12041–12045.

Bai, L., Caplan, A., Lennon, D., and Miller, R. H. (2007). Human mesenchymal stem cells signals regulate neural stem cell fate. *Neurochem Res* **32**, 353–362.

Bakiri, Y., Burzomato, V., Frugier, G., Hamilton, N. B., Karadottir, R., and Attwell, D. (2009). Glutamatergic signaling in the brain's white matter. *Neuroscience* **158**, 266–274.

Bakiri, Y., Hamilton, N. B., Karadottir, R., and Attwell, D. (2008). Testing NMDA receptor block as a therapeutic strategy for reducing ischaemic damage to CNS white matter. *Glia* **56**, 233–240.

Bal-Price, A. and Brown, G. C. (2001). Inflammatory neurodegeneration mediated by nitric oxide from activated glia-inhibiting neuronal respiration, causing glutamate release and excitotoxicity. *J Neurosci* **21**, 6480–6491.

Balabanov, R., Strand, K., Goswami, R., *et al.* (2007). Interferon-gamma-oligodendrocyte interactions in the regulation of experimental autoimmune encephalomyelitis. *J Neurosci* **27**, 2013–2024.

Balentine, J. D. (1978a). Pathology of experimental spinal cord trauma. I. The necrotic lesion as a function of vascular injury. *Lab Invest* **39**, 236–253.

Balentine, J. D. (1978b). Pathology of experimental spinal cord trauma. II. Ultrastructure of axons and myelin. *Lab Invest* **39**, 254–266.

Balentine, J. D., and Spector, M. (1977). Calcification of axons in experimental spinal cord trauma. *Ann Neurol* **2**, 520–523.

Balice-Gordon, R. J., Bone, L. J., and Scherer, S. S. (1998). Functional gap junctions in the Schwann cell myelin sheath. *J Cell Biol* **142**, 1095–1104.

Bandtlow, C., Zachleder, T., and Schwab, M. E. (1990). Oligodendrocytes arrest neurite growth by contact inhibition. *J Neurosci* **10**, 3837–3848.

Banker, B. Q., and Larroche, J. C. (1962). Periventricular leukomalacia of infancy. A form of neonatal anoxic encephalopathy. *Arch Neurol* **7**, 386–410.

Bansal, R. and Pfeiffer, S. E. (1992). Novel stage in the oligodendrocyte lineage defined by reactivity of progenitors with R-mAb prior to O1 anti-galactocerebroside. *J Neurosci Res* **32**, 309–316.

Bansal, R. and Pfeiffer, S. E. (1997). FGF-2 converts mature oligodendrocytes to a novel phenotype. *J Neurosci Res* **50**, 215–228.

Baracskay, K. L., Kidd, G. J., Miller, R. H., and Trapp, B. D. (2007). NG2-positive cells generate A2B5-positive oligodendrocyte precursor cells. *Glia* **55**, 1001–1010.

Barbarese, E., Carson, J. H., and Braun, P. E. (1978). Accumulation of the four myelin basic proteins in mouse brain during development. *J Neurochem* **31**, 779–782.

Barbarese, E., Koppel, D. E., Deutscher, M. P., *et al.* (1995). Protein translation components are colocalized in granules in oligodendrocytes. *J Cell Sci* **108**, 2781–2790.

Barkhof, F., Bruck, W., De Groot, C. J., *et al.* (2003). Remyelinated lesions in multiple sclerosis: magnetic resonance image appearance. *Arch Neurol* **60**, 1073–1081.

Barnett, M. H. and Prineas, J. W. (2004). Relapsing and remitting multiple sclerosis: pathology of the newly forming lesion. *Ann Neurol* **55**, 458–468.

Barradas, P. C., Ferraz, A. S., Ferreira, A. A., Daumas, R. P., and Moura, E. G. (2000). 2'3'-Cyclic nucleotide 3'-phosphodiesterase immunohistochemistry shows an impairment on myelin compaction in hypothyroid rats. *Int J Dev Neurosci* **18**, 887–892.

Barres, B. A., Koroshetz, W. J., Swartz, K. J., Chun, L. L. Y., and Corey, D. P. (1990). Ion channel expression by white matter glia: the O2A glial progenitor cell. *Neuron* **4**, 507–524.

Bartel, D. P. (2004). MicroRNAs: genomics, biogenesis, mechanism, and function. *Cell* **116**, 281–297.

Barton, W. A., Liu, B. P., Tzvetkova, D., *et al.* (2003). Structure and axon outgrowth inhibitor binding of the Nogo-66 receptor and related proteins. *EMBO J* **22**, 3291–3302.

Bartsch, S., Montag, D., Schachner, M., and Bartsch, U. (1997). Increased number of unmyelinated axons in optic nerves of adult mice deficient in the myelin-associated glycoprotein (MAG). *Brain Res* **762**, 231–234.

Bartsch, U. (2003). Neural CAMS and their role in the development and organization of myelin sheaths. *Front Biosci* **8**, d477–d490.

Bartsch, U., Bandtlow, C. E., Schnell, L., *et al.* (1995a). Lack of evidence that myelin-associated glycoprotein is a major inhibitor of axonal regeneration in the CNS. *Neuron* **15**, 1375–1381.

Bartsch, U., Kirchhoff, F., and Schachner, M. (1989). Immunohistological localization of the adhesion molecules L1, N-CAM, and MAG in the developing and adult optic nerve of mice. *J Comp Neurol* **284**, 451–462.

Bartsch, U., Montag, D., Bartsch, S., and Schachner, M. (1995b). Multiply myelinated axons in the optic nerve of mice deficient for the myelin-associated glycoprotein. *Glia* **14**, 115–122.

Bartsch, U., Pesheva, P., Raff, M., and Schachner, M. (1993). Expression of janusin (J1-160/180) in the retina and optic nerve of the developing and adult mouse. *Glia* **9**, 57–69.

Bartzokis, G. (2005). Brain myelination in prevalent neuropsychiatric developmental disorders: primary and comorbid addiction. *Adolesc Psychiatry* **29**, 55–96.

Bartzokis, G. (2007). Acetylcholinesterase inhibitors may improve myelin integrity. *Biol Psychiatry* **62**, 294–301.

Bartzokis, G., Lu, P. H., Geschwind, D. H., Edwards, N., Mintz, J., and Cummings, J. L. (2006). Apolipoprotein E genotype and age-related myelin breakdown in healthy individuals: implications for cognitive decline and dementia. *Arch Gen Psychiatry* **63**, 63–72.

Baumann, N. and Pham-Dinh, D. (2001). Biology of oligodendrocyte and myelin in the mammalian central nervous system. *Physiol Rev* **81**, 871–927.

Beattie, M. S. (2004). Inflammation and apoptosis: linked therapeutic targets in spinal cord injury. *Trends Mol Med* **10**, 580–583.

Bechmann, I., Galea, I., and Perry, V. H. (2007). What is the blood-brain barrier (not)? *Trends Immunol* **28**, 5–11.

Becker, T., Anliker, B., Becker, C. G., *et al.* (2000). Tenascin-R inhibits regrowth of optic fibers in vitro and persists in the optic nerve of mice after injury. *Glia* **29**, 330–346.

Behrens, T. E., Johansen-Berg, H., Woolrich, M. W., *et al.* (2003). Non-invasive mapping of connections between human thalamus and cortex using diffusion imaging. *Nat Neurosci* **6**, 750–757.

Belachew, S., Chittajallu, R., Aguirre, A. A., *et al.* (2003). Postnatal NG2 proteoglycan-expressing progenitor cells are intrinsically multipotent and generate functional neurons. *J Cell Biol* **161**, 169–186.

Ben-Hur, T., Einstein, O., Mizrachi-Kol, R., *et al.* (2003). Transplanted multipotential neural precursor cells migrate into the inflamed white matter in response to experimental autoimmune encephalomyelitis. *Glia* **41**, 73–80.

Bengtsson, S. L., Nagy, Z., Skare, S., Forsman, L., Forssberg, H., and Ullen, F. (2005). Extensive piano practicing has regionally specific effects on white matter development. *Nat Neurosci* **8**, 1148–1150.

Benjamins, J. A., Iwata, R., and Hazlett, J. (1978). Kinetics of entry of proteins into the myelin membrane. *J Neurochem* **31**, 1077–1085.

Benjamins, J. A., Nedelkoska, L., and George, E. B. (2003). Protection of mature oligodendrocytes by inhibitors of caspases and calpains. *Neurochem Res* **28**, 143–152.

Bennett, V. and Lambert, S. (1999). Physiological roles of axonal ankyrins in survival of premyelinated axons and localization of voltage-gated sodium channels. *J Neurocytol* **28**, 303–318.

Benninger, Y., Thurnherr, T., Pereira, J. A., *et al.* (2007). Essential and distinct roles for cdc42 and rac1 in the regulation of Schwann cell biology during peripheral nervous system development. *J Cell Biol* **177**, 1051–1061.

Benson, M. D., Romero, M. I., Lush, M. E., Lu, Q. R., Henkemeyer, M., and Parada, L. F. (2005). Ephrin-B3 is a myelin-based inhibitor of neurite outgrowth. *Proc Natl Acad Sci USA* **102**, 10694–10699.

Bentley C. A. and Lee, K. F. (2000). p75 is important for axon growth and Schwann cell migration during development. *J Neurosci* **20**, 7706–7715.

Benveniste, H., Drejer, J., Schousboe, A., and Diemer, N. H. (1984). Elevation of the extracellular concentrations of glutamate and aspartate in rat hippocampus during transient cerebral ischemia monitored by intracerebral microdialysis. *J Neurochem* **43**, 1369–1374.

Bergamaschi, R., Tonietti, S., Franciotta, D., *et al.* (2004). Oligoclonal bands in Devic's neuromyelitis optica and multiple sclerosis: differences in repeated cerebrospinal fluid examinations. *Mult Scler* **10**, 2–4.

Berger, J. R. (2003).Progressive multifocal leukoencephalopathy in acquired immunodeficiency syndrome: explaining the high incidence and disproportionate frequency of the illness relative to other immunosuppressive conditions. *J Neurovirol* **9** Suppl 1, 38–41.

Berger, P., Niemann, A., and Suter, U. (2006). Schwann cells and the pathogenesis of inherited motor and sensory neuropathies (Charcot-Marie-Tooth disease). *Glia* **54**, 243–257.

Berger, T., Rubner, P., Schautzer, F., *et al.* (2003). Antimyelin antibodies as a predictor of clinically definite multiple sclerosis after a first demyelinating event. *N Engl J Med* **349**, 139–145.

Berger, T., Walz, W., Schnitzer, J., and Kettenmann, H. (1992). GABA- and glutamate-activated currents in glial cells of the mouse corpus callosum slice. *J Neurosci Res* **31**, 21–27.

Berghs, S., Aggujaro, D., Dirkx, R., Jr., *et al.* (2000). BetaIV spectrin, a new spectrin localized at axon initial segments and nodes of ranvier in the central and peripheral nervous system. *J Cell Biol* **151**, 985–1002.

Bergles, D. E., Diamond, J. S., and Jahr, C. E. (1999). Clearance of glutamate inside the synapse and beyond. *Curr Opin Neurobiol* **9**, 293–298.

Bergles, D. E., Roberts, J. D., Somogyi, P., and Jahr, C. E. (2000). Glutamatergic synapses on oligodendrocyte precursor cells in the hippocampus. *Nature* **405**, 187–191.

Bergoffen, J., Scherer, S. S., Wang, S., *et al.* (1993). Connexin mutations in X-linked Charcot-Marie-Tooth disease. *Science* **262**, 2039–2042.

Bergsteindottir, K., Brennan, A., Jessen, K. R., and Mirsky, R. (1992). In the presence of dexamethasone, gamma interferon induces rat oligodendrocytes to express major histocompatibility complex class II molecules. *Proc Natl Acad Sci USA* **89**, 9054–9058.

Bernardo, A., Greco, A., Levi, G., and Minghetti, L. (2003). Differential lipid peroxidation, Mn superoxide, and bcl-2 expression contribute to the maturation-dependent vulnerability of oligodendrocytes to oxidative stress. *J Neuropathol Exp Neurol* **62**, 509–519.

Besancon, E., Guo, S., Lok, J., Tymianski, M., and Lo, E. H. (2008). Beyond NMDA and AMPA glutamate receptors: emerging mechanisms for ionic imbalance and cell death in stroke. *Trends Pharmacol Sci* **29**, 268–275.

Bethea, J. R. and Dietrich, W. D. (2002). Targeting the host inflammatory response in traumatic spinal cord injury. *Curr Opin Neurol* **15**, 355–360.

Bezzi, P., Carmignoto, G., Pasti, L., *et al.* (1998). Prostaglandins stimulate calcium-dependent glutamate release in astrocytes. *Nature* **391**, 281–285.

Bezzi, P., Domercq, M., Brambilla, L., *et al.* (2001). CXCR4-activated astrocyte glutamate release via TNFalpha: amplification by microglia triggers neurotoxicity. *Nat Neurosci* **4**, 702–710.

Bhat, M. A., Rios, J. C., Lu, Y., *et al.* (2001). Axon–glia interactions and the domain organization of myelinated axons requires neurexin IV/Caspr/Paranodin. *Neuron* **30**, 369–383.

Billiards, S. S., Haynes, R. L., Folkerth, R. D., *et al.* (2008). Myelin abnormalities without oligodendrocyte loss in periventricular leukomalacia. *Brain Pathol* **18**, 153–163.

Bitsch, A., Kuhlmann, T., da Costa, C., Bunkowski, S., Polak, T., and Brück, W. (2000a). Tumour necrosis factor alpha mRNA expression in early multiple sclerosis lesions: correlation with demyelinating activity and oligodendrocyte pathology. *Glia* **29**, 366–375.

Bitsch, A., Schuchardt, J., Bunkowski, S., Kuhlmann, T., and Bruck, W. (2000b). Acute axonal injury in multiple sclerosis. Correlation with demyelination and inflammation. *Brain* **123**, 1174–1183.

Bixby, J. L., Lilien, J., and Reichardt, L. F. (1988). Identification of the major proteins that promote neuronal process outgrowth on Schwann cells in vitro. *J Cell Biol* **107**, 353–361.

Bizzozero, O. A., McGarry, J. F., and Lees, M. B. (1986). Acylation of rat brain myelin proteolipid protein with different fatty acids. *J Neurochem* **47**, 772–778.

Bjartmar, C. and Trapp, B. D. (2001). Axonal and neuronal degeneration in multiple sclerosis: mechanisms and functional consequences. *Curr Opin Neurol* **14**, 271–278.

Blaabjerg, M., Fang, L., Zimmer, J., and Baskys, A. (2003). Neuroprotection against NMDA excitotoxicity by group I metabotropic glutamate receptors is associated with reduction of NMDA stimulated currents. *Exp Neurol* **183**, 573–580.

Black, J. A., Kocsis, J. D., and Waxman, S. G. (1990). Ion channel organization of the myelinated fiber. *Trends Neurosci* **13**, 48–54.

Black, J. A., Waxman, S. G., and Smith, K. J. (2006). Remyelination of dorsal column axons by endogenous Schwann cells restores the normal pattern of Nav1.6 and Kv1.2 at nodes of Ranvier. *Brain* **129**, 1319–1329.

Blakemore, W. F. (1969). Schmidt–Lantermann incisures in the central nervous system. *J Ultrastruct Res* **29**, 496–498.

Blakemore, W. F. (1974). Pattern of remyelination in the CNS. *Nature* **249**, 577–578.

Blakemore, W. F. (1977). Remyelination of CNS axons by Schwann cells transplanted from the sciatic nerve. *Nature* **266**, 68–69.

Blakemore, W. F. (1981). Observations on myelination and remyelination in the central nervous system. In *Development in the Nervous System*, D. R. Garrod and J. D. Feldman, eds. (Cambridge University Press), pp. 289–308.

Blakemore, W. F. and Keirstead, H. S. (1999). The origin of the remyelinating cells in the central nervous system. *J Neuroimmunol* **98**, 69–76.

Blaschuk, K. L., Frost, E. E., and Ffrench-Constant, C. (2000). The regulation of proliferation and differentiation in oligodendrocyte progenitor cells by alphaV integrins. *Development* **127**, 1961–1969.

Blau, H. M. (2002). A twist of fate. *Nature* **419**, 437.

Blight, A. R. (1983). Cellular morphology of chronic spinal cord injury in the cat: analysis of myelinated axons by line-sampling. *Neuroscience* **10**, 521–543.

Bo, L., Mork, S., Kong, P. A., Nyland, H., Pardo, C. A., and Trapp, B. D. (1994). Detection of MHC class II-antigens on macrophages and microglia, but not on astrocytes and endothelia in active multiple sclerosis lesions. *J Neuroimmunol* **51**, 135–146.

Bo, L., Quarles, R. H., Fujita, N., Bartoszewicz, Z., Sato, S., and Trapp, B. D. (1995). Endocytic depletion of L-MAG from CNS myelin in quaking mice. *J Cell Biol* **131**, 1811–1820.

Boggs, J. M. (2006). Myelin basic protein: a multifunctional protein. *Cell Mol Life Sci* **63**, 1945–1961.

Bogler, O., Wren, D., Barnett, S. C., Land, H., and Noble, M. (1990). Cooperation between two growth factors promotes extended self-renewal and inhibits differentiation of oligodendrocyte-type-2 astrocyte (O-2A) progenitor cells. *Proc Natl Acad Sci USA* **87**, 6368–6372.

Boison, D. and Stoffel, W. (1994). Disruption of the compacted myelin sheath of axons of the central nervous system in proteolipid protein-deficient mice. *Proc Natl Acad Sci USA* **91**, 11709–11713.

Borges, K., Ohlemeyer, C., Trotter, J., and Kettenmann, H. (1994). AMPA/kainate receptor activation in murine oligodendrocyte precursor cells leads to activation of a cation conductance, calcium influx and blockade of delayed rectifying K+ channels. *Neuroscience* **63**, 135–149.

Bosio, A., Bussow, H., Adam, J., and Stoffel, W. (1998). Galactosphingolipids and axono-glial interaction in myelin of the central nervous system. *Cell Tissue Res* **292**, 199–210.

Bouvier-Labit, C., Liprandi, A., Monti, G., Pellissier, J. F., and Figarella-Branger, D. (2002). CD44H is expressed by cells of the oligodendrocyte lineage and by oligodendrogliomas in humans. *J Neurooncol* **60**, 127–134.

Boyle, M. E., Berglund, E. O., Murai, K. K., Weber, L., Peles, E., and Ranscht, B. (2001). Contactin orchestrates assembly of the septate-like junctions at the paranode in myelinated peripheral nerve. *Neuron* **30**, 385–397.

Brady, S. T., Witt, A. S., Kirkpatrick, L. L., *et al.* (1999). Formation of compact myelin is required for maturation of the axonal cytoskeleton. *J Neurosci* **19**, 7278–7288.

Braude, P., Minger, S. L., and Warwick, R. M. (2005). Stem cell therapy: hope or hype? *BMJ* **330**, 1159–1160.

Braun, P. E., Sandillon, F., Edwards, A., Matthieu, J.-M., and Privat, A. (1988). Immunocytochemical localization by electron microscopy of 2′,3′-cyclic nucleotide 3′-phosphodiesterase in developing oligodendrocytes of normal and mutant brain. *J Neurosci* **8**, 3057–3066.

Bre, M.-H., Kreis, T. E., and Karsenti, E. (1987). Control of microtubule nucleation and stability in Madin-Darby canine kidney cells: the occurrence of noncentrosomal, stable detyrosinated microtubules. *J Cell Biol* **105**, 1283–1296.

Bregman, B. S., Kunkel-Bagden, E., Schnell, L., Dai, H. N., Gao, D., and Schwab, M. E. (1995). Recovery from spinal cord injury mediated by antibodies to neurite growth inhibitors. *Nature* **378**, 498–501.

Brenner, T., Brocke, S., Szafer, F., *et al.* (1997). Inhibition of nitric oxide synthase for treatment of experimental autoimmune encephalomyelitis. *J Immunol* **158**, 2940–2946.

Brierley, C. M., Crang, A. J., Iwashita, Y., *et al.* (2001). Remyelination of demyelinated CNS axons by transplanted human Schwann cells: the deleterious effect of contaminating fibroblasts. *Cell Transplant* **10**, 305–315.

Brinkmann, B. G., Agarwal, A., Sereda, M. W., *et al.* (2008). Neuregulin-1/ErbB signaling serves distinct functions in myelination of the peripheral and central nervous system. *Neuron* **59**, 581–595.

Brophy, P. J. (2001). Axoglial junctions: separate the channels or scramble the message. *Curr Biol* **11**, R555–R557.

Brosamle, C., Huber, A. B., Fiedler, M., Skerra, A., and Schwab, M. E. (2000). Regeneration of lesioned corticospinal tract fibers in the adult rat induced by a recombinant, humanized IN-1 antibody fragment. *J Neurosci* **20**, 8061–8068.

Brosnan, C. F., Bornstein, M. B., and Bloom, B. R. (1981). The effects of macrophage depletion on the clinical and pathologic expression of experimental allergic encephalomyelitis. *J Immunol* **126**, 614–620.

Brown, G. C. and Bal-Price, A. (2003). Inflammatory neurodegeneration mediated by nitric oxide, glutamate, and mitochondria. *Mol Neurobiol* **27**, 325–355.

Brownell, B. and Hughes, J. T. (1962). The distribution of plaques in the cerebrum in multiple sclerosis. *J Neurol Neurosurg Psychiatry* **25**, 315–320.

Brück, W., Schmied, M., Suchanek, G., *et al.* (1994). Oligodendrocytes in the early course of multiple sclerosis. *Ann Neurol* **35**, 65–73.

Brunner, C., Lassmann, H., Waehneldt, T. V., Matthieu, J. M., and Linington, C. (1989). Differential ultrastructural localization of myelin basic protein, myelin/oligodendroglial glycoprotein, and 2′,3′-cyclic nucleotide 3′-phosphodiesterase in the CNS of adult rats. *J Neurochem* **52**, 296–304.

Brushart, T. M. E. (1990). Preferential motor reinnervation: a sequential double-labeling study. *Restor Neurol Neurosci* 281–287.

Brushart, T. M. E. (1993). Motor axons preferentially reinnervate motor pathways. *J Neurosci* **13**, 2730–2738.

Brustle, O., Jones, K. N., Learish, R. D., *et al.* (1999). Embryonic stem cell-derived glial precursors: a source of myelinating transplants. *Science* **285**, 754–756.

Bruzzone, R., White, T. W., Scherer, S. S., Fischbeck, K. H., and Paul, D. L. (1994). Null mutations of connexin32 in patients with X-linked Charcot-Marie-Tooth disease. *Neuron* **13**, 1253–1260.

Bsibsi, M., Ravid, R., Gveric, D., and van Noort, J. M. (2002). Broad expression of Toll-like receptors in the human central nervous system. *J Neuropathol Exp Neurol* **61**, 1013–1021.

Buffo, A., Zagrebelsky, M., Huber, A. B., *et al.* (2000). Application of neutralizing antibodies against NI-35/250 myelin-associated neurite growth inhibitory proteins to the adult rat cerebellum induces sprouting of uninjured Purkinje cell axons. *J Neurosci* **20**, 2275–2286.

Bunge, M. B. and Pearse, D. D. (2003). Transplantation strategies to promote repair of the injured spinal cord. *J Rehabil Res Dev* **40**, 55–62.

Bunge, M. B. Bunge, R. P., and Ris, H. (1961). Ultrastructural study of remyelination in an experimental lesion in adult cat spinal cord. *J Biophys Biochem Cytol* **10**, 67–94.

Bunge, R. P., Bunge, M. B., and Ris, H. (1960). Electron microscopic study of demyelination in an experimentally induced lesion in adult cat spinal cord. *J Biophys Biochem Cytol* **7**, 685–696.

Buntinx, M., Moreels, M., Vandenabeele, F., *et al.* (2004). Cytokine-induced cell death in human oligodendroglial cell lines: I. Synergistic effects of IFN-gamma and TNF-alpha on apoptosis. *J Neurosci Res* **76**, 834–845.

Burgmaier, G., Schönrock, M. L., Kuhlmann, T., Richter-Landsberg, C., and Brück, W. (2000). Association of increased bcl-2 expression with rescue from TNF-α induced cell death in the oligodendrocyte cell line OLN-93. *J Neurochem* **75**, 2270–2276.

Burke, R. E. (2007). Sir Charles Sherrington's the integrative action of the nervous system: a centenary appreciation. *Brain* **130**, 887–894.

Burnashev, N., Monyer, H., Seeburg, P. H., and Sakmann, B. (1992). Divalent ion permeability of AMPA receptor channels is dominated by the edited form of a single subunit. *Neuron* **8**, 189–198.

Burns, J., Rosenzweig, A., Zweiman, B., and Lisak, R. (1983). Isolation of myelin basic protein-reactive T-cell lines from normal human blood. *Cell Immunol* **81**, 435–440.

Burt, R. K., Loh, Y., Pearce, W., *et al.* (2008). Clinical applications of blood-derived and marrow-derived stem cells for nonmalignant diseases. *J Am Med Assoc* **299**, 925–936.

Bushati, N. and Cohen, S. M. (2007). microRNA functions. *Annu Rev Cell Dev Biol* **23**, 175–205.

Butt, A. M., Duncan, A., Hornby, M. F., *et al.* (1999). Cells expressing the NG2 antigen contact nodes of Ranvier in adult CNS white matter. *Glia* **26**, 84–91.

Butt, A. M., Hamilton, N., Hubbard, P., Pugh, M., and Ibrahim, M. (2005). Synantocytes: the fifth element. *J Anat* **207**, 695–706.

Butt, A. M., Kiff, J., Hubbard, P., and Berry, M. (2002). Synantocytes: new functions for novel NG2 expressing glia. *J Neurocytol* **31**, 551–565.

Butzkueven, H., Emery, B., Cipriani, T., Marriott, M. P., and Kilpatrick, T. J. (2006). Endogenous leukemia inhibitory factor production limits autoimmune demyelination and oligodendrocyte loss. *Glia* **53**, 696–703.

Byravan, S., Foster, L. M., Phan, T., Verity, A. N., and Campagnoni, A. T. (1994). Murine oligodendroglial cells express nerve growth factor. *Proc Natl Acad Sci USA* **91**, 8812–8816.

Cai, D., Qiu, J., Cao, Z., McAtee, M., Bregman, B. S., and Filbin, M. T. (2001). Neuronal cyclic AMP controls the developmental loss in ability of axons to regenerate. *J Neurosci* **21**, 4731–4739.

Cai, J., Qi, Y., Hu, X., *et al.* (2005). Generation of oligodendrocyte precursor cells from mouse dorsal spinal cord independent of Nkx6 regulation and Shh signaling. *Neuron* **45**, 41–53.

Cai, Z., Pan, Z. L., Pang, Y., Evans, O. B., and Rhodes, P. G. (2000). Cytokine induction in fetal rat brains and brain injury in neonatal rats after maternal lipopolysaccharide administration. *Pediatr Res* **47**, 64–72.

Caldwell, J. H., Schaller, K. L., Lasher, R. S., Peles, E., and Levinson, S. R. (2000). Sodium channel Na(v)1.6 is localized at nodes of Ranvier, dendrites, and synapses. *Proc Natl Acad Sci USA* **97**, 5616–5620.

Cameron-Curry, P. and Le Douarin, N. M. (1995). Oligodendrocyte precursors originate from both the dorsal and the ventral parts of the spinal cord. *Neuron* **15**, 1299–1310.

Campagnoni, A. T., Pribyl, T. M., Campagnoni, C. W., *et al.* (1993). Structure and developmental regulation of Golli-mbp, a 105 kilobase gene that encompasses the myelin basic protein gene and is expressed in cells in the oligodendrocytes lineage in the brain. *J Biol Chem* **268**, 4930–4938.

Cannella, B. and Raine, C. S. (2004). Multiple sclerosis: cytokine receptors on oligodendrocytes predict innate regulation. *Ann. Neurol.* **55**, 46–57.

Cannella, B., Gaupp, S., Omari, K. M., and Raine, C. S. (2007). Multiple sclerosis: death receptor expression and oligodendrocyte apoptosis in established lesions. *J Neuroimmunol* **188**, 128–137.

Cao, Q., Zhang, Y. P., Iannotti, C., *et al.* (2005). Functional and electrophysiological changes after graded traumatic spinal cord injury in adult rat. *Exp Neurol* **191** Suppl 1, S3–S16.

Carbonetto, S., Evans, D., and Cochard, P. (1987). Nerve fiber growth in culture on tissue substrata from central and peripheral nervous systems. *J Neurosci* **7**, 610–620.

Carenini, S., Montag, D., Cremer, H., Schachner, M., and Martini, R. (1997). Absence of the myelin-associated glycoprotein (MAG) and the neural cell adhesion molecule (N-CAM) interferes with the maintenance, but not with the formation of peripheral myelin. *Cell Tissue Res* **287**, 3–9.

Carnegie, P. R., Dunkley, P. R., Kemp, B. E., and Murray, A. W. (1974). Phosphorylation of selected serine and threonine residues in myelin basic protein by endogenous and exogenous protein kinases. *Nature* **249**, 147–150.

Caroni, P. and Schwab, M. E. (1988a). Antibody against myelin-associated inhibitor of neurite growth neutralizes nonpermissive substrate properties of CNS white matter. *Neuron* **1**, 85–96.

Caroni, P. and Schwab, M. E. (1988b). Two membrane protein fractions from rat central myelin with inhibitory properties for neurite growth and fibroblast spreading. *J Cell Biol* **106**, 1281–1288.

Carroll, S. L., Miller, M. L., Frohnert, P. W., Kim, S. S., and Corbett, J. A. (1997). Expression of neuregulins and their putative receptors, ErbB2 and ErbB3, is induced during Wallerian degeneration. *J Neurosci* **17**, 1642–1659.

Carroll, W. M. and Jennings, A. R. (1994). Early recruitment of oligodendrocyte precursors in CNS demyelination. *Brain* **117**, 563–578.

Carroll, W. M., Jennings, A. R., and Ironside, L. J. (1998). Identification of the adult resting progenitor cell by autoradiographic tracking of oligodendrocyte precursors in experimental CNS demyelination. *Brain* **121** (Pt 2), 293–302.

Carson, J. H., Cui, H., and Barbarese, E. (2001). The balance of power in RNA trafficking. *Curr Opin Neurobiol* **11**, 558–563.

Carson, J. H., Gao, Y., Tatavarty, V., *et al.* (2008). Multiplexed RNA trafficking in oligodendrocytes and neurons. *Biochim Biophys Acta* **1779**, 453–458.

Carson, J. H., Worboys, K., Ainger, K., and Barbarese, E. (1997). Translocation of myelin basic protein mRNA in oligodendrocytes requires microtubules and kinesin. *Cell Motil Cytoskeleton* **38**, 318–328.

Carson, M. J., Behringer, R. R., Brinster, R. L., and McMorris, F. A. (1993). Insulin-like growth factor I increases brain growth and central nervous system myelination in transgenic mice. *Neuron* **10**, 729–740.

Casha, S., Yu, W. R., and Fehlings, M. G. (2001). Oligodendroglial apoptosis occurs along degenerating axons and is associated with FAS and p75 expression following spinal cord injury in the rat. *Neuroscience* **103**, 203–218.

Cassiani-Ingoni, R., Greenstone, H. L., Donati, D., *et al.* (2005). CD46 on glial cells can function as a receptor for viral glycoprotein-mediated cell-cell fusion. *Glia* **52**, 252–258.

Chan, J. A., Krichevsky, A. M., and Kosik, K. S. (2005). MicroRNA-21 is an anti-apoptotic factor in human glioblastoma cells. *Cancer Res* **65**, 6029–6033.

Chan, J. R., Watkins, T. A., Cosgaya, J. M., *et al.* (2004). NGF controls axonal receptivity to myelination by Schwann cells or oligodendrocytes. *Neuron* **43**, 183–191.

Chang, A., Nishiyama, A., Peterson, J., Prineas, J., and Trapp, B. D. (2000). NG2-positive oligodendrocyte progenitor cells in adult human brain and multiple sclerosis lesions. *J Neurosci* **20**, 6404–6412.

Chang, A., Tourtellotte, W. W., Rudick, R., and Trapp, B. D. (2002). Premyelinating oligodendrocytes in chronic lesions of multiple sclerosis. *New Engl J Med* **346**, 165–173.

Charcot, J. (1868). Histologie de la sclérose en plaque. *Gaz Hop Civ Mil Empire Ottoman* **41**, 554–566.

Charcot, J M. (1877). Lecture VI. Disseminated sclerosis. Pathological anatomy. In *Lectures on The Diseases of the Nervous System*, Trans. George Sigerson. (London: The New Sydenham Society), pp. 157–181.

Charles, P., Hernandez, M. P., Stankoff, B., *et al.* (2000). Negative regulation of central nervous system myelination by polysialylated-neural cell adhesion molecule. *Proc Natl Acad Sci USA* **97**, 7585–7590.

Charles, P., Reynolds, R., Seilhean, D., *et al.* (2002a). Re-expression of PSA-NCAM by demyelinated axons: an inhibitor of remyelination in multiple sclerosis? *Brain* **125**, 1972–1979.

Charles, P., Tait, S., Faivre-Sarrailh, C., *et al.* (2002b). Neurofascin is a glial receptor for the paranodin/Caspr-contactin axonal complex at the axoglial junction. *Curr Biol* **12**, 217–220.

Charo, I. F. and Ransohoff, R. M. (2006). The many roles of chemokines and chemokine receptors in inflammation. *N Engl J Med* **354**, 610–621.

Chaudhry, N. and Filbin, M. T. (2007). Myelin-associated inhibitory signaling and strategies to overcome inhibition. *J Cereb Blood Flow Metab* **27**, 1096–1107.

Chaudhuri, A. (2006). Lessons for clinical trials from natalizumab in multiple sclerosis. *BMJ* **332**, 416–419.

Chaudhuri, A. and Behan, P. O. (2005). Multiple sclerosis: looking beyond auto-immunity. *J R Soc Med* **98**, 303–306.

Chen, J. T., Kuhlmann, T., Jansen, G. H., *et al.* (2007a). Voxel-based analysis of the evolution of magnetization transfer ratio to quantify remyelination and demyelination with histopathological validation in a multiple sclerosis lesion. *Neuroimage* **36**, 1152–1158.

Chen, K. and Rajewsky, N. (2006). Natural selection on human microRNA binding sites inferred from SNP data. *Nat Genet* **38**, 1452–1456.

Chen, M. S., Huber, A. B., van der Haar, M. E., *et al.* (2000). Nogo-A is a myelin-associated neurite outgrowth inhibitor and an antigen for monoclonal antibody IN-1. *Nature* **403**, 434–439.

Chen, Q., Long, Y., Yuan, X., *et al.* (2005). Protective effects of bone marrow stromal cell transplantation in injured rodent brain: synthesis of neurotrophic factors. *J Neurosci Res* **80**, 611–619.

Chen, W., Mahadomrongkul, V., Berger, U. V., *et al.* (2004). The glutamate transporter GLT1a is expressed in excitatory axon terminals of mature hippocampal neurons. *J Neurosci* **24**, 1136–1148.

Chen, Z. L., Yu, W. M., and Strickland, S. (2007b). Peripheral regeneration. *Annu Rev Neurosci* **30**, 209–233.

Cheong, K. H., Zacchetti, D., Schneeberger, E. E., and Simons, K. (1999). VIP17/MAL, a lipid raft-associated protein, is involved in apical transport in MDCK cells. *Proc Natl Acad Sci USA* **96**, 6241–6248.

Chew, L. J., King, W. C., Kennedy, A., and Gallo, V. (2005). Interferon-gamma inhibits cell cycle exit in differentiating oligodendrocyte progenitor cells. *Glia* **52**, 127–143.

Chitnis, T., Imitola, J., Wang, Y., *et al.* (2007). Elevated neuronal expression of CD200 protects Wlds mice from inflammation-mediated neurodegeneration. *Am J Pathol* **170**, 1695–1712.

Chivatakarn, O., Kaneko, S., He, Z., Tessier-Lavigne, M., and Giger, R. J. (2007). The Nogo-66 receptor NgR1 is required only for the acute growth cone-collapsing but not the chronic growth-inhibitory actions of myelin inhibitors. *J Neurosci* **27**, 7117–7124.

Choi, D. W. (1988). Glutamate neurotoxicity and diseases of the nervous system. *Neuron* **1**, 623–634.

Choi, J., Opalenik, S. R., Wu, W. C., Thompson, J. A., and Forman, H. J. (2000). Modulation of glutathione synthetic enzymes by acidic fibroblast growth factor. *Arch Biochem Biophys* **375**, 201–209.

Chopp, M., Zhang, X. H., Li, Y., *et al.* (2000). Spinal cord injury in rat: treatment with bone marrow stromal cell transplantation. *NeuroReport* **11**, 3001–3005.

Chow, E., Mottahedeh, J., Prins, M., Ridder, W., Nusinowitz, S., and Bronstein, J. M. (2005). Disrupted compaction of CNS myelin in an OSP/Claudin-11 and PLP/DM20 double knockout mouse. *Mol Cell Neurosci* **29**, 405–413.

Chun, S. J., Rasband, M. N., Sidman, R. L., Habib, A. A., and Vartanian, T. (2003). Integrin-linked kinase is required for laminin-2-induced oligodendrocyte cell spreading and CNS myelination. *J Cell Biol* **163**, 397–408.

Ciutat, D., Caldero, J., Oppenheim, R. W., and Esquerda, J. E. (1996). Schwann cell apoptosis during normal development and after axonal degeneration induced by neurotoxins in the chick embryo. *J Neurosci* **16**, 3979–3990.

Cleveland, D. W. (1987). The multitubulin hypothesis revisited: what have we learned? *J. Cell Biol* **104**, 381–383.

Cogle, C. R., Yachnis, A. T., Laywell, E. D., *et al.* (2004). Bone marrow transdifferentiation in brain after transplantation: a retrospective study. *Lancet* **363**, 1432–1437.

Cohen, N. R., Taylor, J. S., Scott, L. B., Guillery, R. W., Soriano, P., and Furley, A. J. (1998). Errors in corticospinal axon guidance in mice lacking the neural cell adhesion molecule L1. *Curr Biol* **8**, 26–33.

Colello, R. J., Pott, U., and Schwab, M. E. (1994). The role of oligodendrocytes and myelin on axon maturation in the developing rat retinofugal pathway. *J Neurosci* **14**, 2594–2605.

Coleman M. P. and Perry, V. H. (2002). Axon pathology in neurological disease: a neglected therapeutic target. *Trends Neurosci* **25**, 532–537.

Coles, A., Wing, M. G., Molyneux, P., Paolillo, A., Davie, C. A., and Hale, G. (1999). Monoclonal antibody treatment exposes three mechanisms underlying the clinical course of multiple sclerosis. *Ann Neurol* **46**, 304.

Colman, D. R., Kreibich, G., Frey, A. B., and Sabatini, D. D. (1982). Synthesis and incorporation of myelin polypeptide into CNS myelin. *J Cell Biol* **95**, 598–608.

Coman, I., Aigrot, M. S., Seilhean, D., *et al.* (2006). Nodal, paranodal and juxtaparanodal axonal proteins during demyelination and remyelination in multiple sclerosis. *Brain* **129**, 3186–3195.

Coman, I., Barbin, G., Charles, P., Zalc, B., and Lubetzki, C. (2005). Axonal signals in central nervous system myelination, demyelination and remyelination. *J Neurol Sci* **233**, 67–71.

Compston, D. A. S. (1996). Remyelination of the central nervous system. *Mult Scler* **1**, 388–392.

Compston, D. A. S., Morgan, B. P., Campbell, A. K., *et al.* (1989). Immunocytochemical localization of the terminal complement complex in multiple sclerosis. *Neuropathol Appl Neurobiol* **15**, 307–316.

Conde, J. R. and Streit, W. J. (2006). Microglia in the aging brain. *J Neuropathol Exp Neurol* **65**, 199–203.

Confavreux, C., Vukusic, S., Moreau, T., and Adeleine, P. (2000). Relapses and progression of disability in multiple sclerosis. *N Engl J Med* **343**, 1430–1438.

Conn, J. P. and Patel, J. (1994). *The Metabotropic Glutamate Receptors*. (Totowa, NJ: Humana Press).

Connor, J. R. and Menzies, S. L. (1996). Relationship of iron to oligodendrocytes and myelination. *Glia* **17**, 83–93.

Corfas, G., Velardez, M. O., Ko, C. P., Ratner, N., and Peles, E. (2004). Mechanisms and roles of axon-Schwann cell interactions. *J Neurosci* **24**, 9250–9260.

Cornbrooks, C. J., Carey, D. J., McDonald, J. A., Timpl, R., and Bunge, R. P. (1983). In vivo and in vitro observations on laminin production by Schwann cells. *Proc Natl Acad Sci USA* **80**, 3850–3854.

Counsell, S. J., Allsop, J. M., Harrison, M. C., *et al.* (2003). Diffusion-weighted imaging of the brain in preterm infants with focal and diffuse white matter abnormality. *Pediatrics* **112**, 1–7.

Craig, A., Ling Luo, N., Beardsley, D. J., *et al.* (2003). Quantitative analysis of perinatal rodent oligodendrocyte lineage progression and its correlation with human. *Exp Neurol* **181**, 231–240.

Craner, M. J., Lo, A. C., Black, J. A., and Waxman, S. G. (2003). Abnormal sodium channel distribution in optic nerve axons in a model of inflammatory demyelination. *Brain* **126**, 1552–1561.

Craner, M. J., Newcombe, J., Black, J. A., Hartle, C., Cuzner, M. L., and Waxman, S. G. (2004). Molecular changes in neurons in multiple sclerosis: altered axonal expression of Nav1.2 and Nav1.6 sodium channels and Na$^+$/Ca^{2+} exchanger. *Proc Natl Acad Sci USA* **101**, 8168–8173.

Crespo, D., Asher, R. A., Lin, R., Rhodes, K. E., and Fawcett, J. W. (2007). How does chondroitinase promote functional recovery in the damaged CNS? *Exp Neurol* **206**, 159–171.

Cross, A. H., Manning, P. T., Stern, M. K., and Misko, T. P. (1997). Evidence for the production of peroxynitrite in inflammatory CNS demyelination. *J Neuroimmunol* **80**, 121–130.

Cross, A. H., Trotter, J. L., and Lyons, J.-A. (2001). B cells and antibodies in CNS demyelinating disease. *J Neuroimmunol* **112**, 1–14.

Cross, D., Farias, G., Dominguez, J., Avila, J., and Maccioni, R. B. (1994). Carboxyl terminal sequences of beta-tubulin involved in the interaction of HMW-MAPs. Studies using site-specific antibodies. *Mol Cell Biochem* **132**, 81–90.

Crow, J. P., Ye, Y. Z., Strong, M., Kirk, M., Barnes, S., and Beckman, J. S. (1997). Superoxide dismutase catalyzes nitration of tyrosines by peroxynitrite in the rod and head domains of neurofilament-L. *J Neurochem* **69**, 1945–1953.

Crowe, M. J., Bresnahan, J. C., Shuman, S. L., Masters, J. N., and Beattie, M. S. (1997). Apoptosis and delayed degeneration after spinal cord injury in rats and monkeys. *Nat Med* **3**, 73–76.

Cudrici, C., Niculescu, F., Jensen, T., *et al.* (2006). C5b-9 terminal complex protects oligodendrocytes from apoptotic cell death by inhibiting caspase-8 processing and up-regulating FLIP. *J Immunol* **176**, 3173–3180.

Cummings, B. J., Uchida, N., Tamaki, S. J., *et al.* (2005). Human neural stem cells differentiate and promote locomotor recovery in spinal cord-injured mice. *Proc Natl Acad Sci USA* **102**, 14069–14074.

Cuzner, M. L., Loughlin, A. J., Mosley, K., and Woodroofe, M. N. (1994). The role of microglia macrophages in the processes of inflammatory demyelination and remyelination. *Neuropathol Appl Neurobiol* **20**, 200–201.

D'Antoni, S., Berretta, A., Bonaccorso, C. M., *et al.* (2008). Metabotropic glutamate receptors in glial cells. *Neurochem Res* **33**, 2436–2443.

da Cunha A., Jefferson, J. A., Jackson, R. W., and Vitkovic, L. (1993). Glial cell-specific mechanisms of TGF-beta 1 induction by IL-1 in cerebral cortex. *J. Neuroimmunol.* **42**, 71–85.

Dahme, M., Bartsch, U., Martini, R., Anliker, B., Schachner, M., and Mantei, N. (1997). Disruption of the mouse L1 gene leads to malformations of the nervous system. *Nat Genet* **17**, 346–349.

Dai, X., Lercher, L. D., Clinton, P. M., *et al.* (2003). The trophic role of oligodendrocytes in the basal forebrain. *J Neurosci* **23**, 5846–5853.

Dalitz, P., Harding, R., Rees, S. M., and Cock, M. L. (2003). Prolonged reductions in placental blood flow and cerebral oxygen delivery in preterm fetal sheep exposed to endotoxin: possible factors in white matter injury after acute infection. *J Soc Gynecol Investig* **10**, 283–290.

Dammann, O. and Leviton, A. (2000). Role of the fetus in perinatal infection and neonatal brain damage. *Curr Opin Pediatr* **12**, 99–104.

Dammann, O., Kuban, K. C., and Leviton, A. (2002). Perinatal infection, fetal inflammatory response, white matter damage, and cognitive limitations in children born preterm. *Men Retard Dev Dis* **8**, 46–50.

Danbolt, N. C. (2001). Glutamate uptake. *Prog Neurobiol* **65**, 1–105.

Dashiell, S. M., Tanner, S. L., Pant, H. C., and Quarles, R. H. (2002). Myelin-associated glycoprotein modulates expression and phosphorylation of neuronal cytoskeletal elements and their associated kinases. *J Neurochem* **81**, 1263–1272.

David, S. and Aguayo, A. J. (1981). Axonal elongation into peripheral nervous system "bridges" after central nervous system injury in adult rats. *Science* **214**, 931–933.

David, S., Braun, P. E., Jackson, D. L., Kottis, V., and McKerracher, L. (1995). Laminin overrides the inhibitory effects of peripheral nervous system and central nervous system myelin-derived inhibitors of neurite growth. *J Neurosci Res* **42**, 594–602.

Davis, A. D., Weatherby, T. M., Hartline, D. K., and Lenz, P. H. (1999). Myelin-like sheaths in copepod axons. *Nature* **398**, 571.

Davis, J. Q., Lambert, S., and Bennett, V. (1996). Molecular composition of the node of Ranvier: identification of ankyrin-binding cell adhesion molecules neurofascin (mucin+/third FNIII domain–) and NrCAM at nodal axon segments. *J Cell Biol* **135**(5), 1355–1367.

Dawson, J. W. (1916). The histology of disseminated sclerosis. *Edinb Med J* **17**, 229–410.

Dawson, M. R., Levine, J. M., and Reynolds, R. (2000). NG2-expressing cells in the central nervous system: are they oligodendroglial progenitors? *J Neurosci Res* **61**, 471–479.

Dawson, M. R., Polito, A., Levine, J. M., and Reynolds, R. (2003). NG2-expressing glial progenitor cells: an abundant and widespread population of cycling cells in the adult rat CNS. *Mol Cell Neurosci* **24**, 476–488.

de Vries, H. and Hoekstra, D. (2000). On the biogenesis of the myelin sheath: cognate polarized trafficking pathways in oligodendrocytes. *Glycoconj J* **17**, 181–190.

de Waegh, S. M., Lee, V. M., and Brady, S. T. (1992). Local modulation of neurofilament phosphorylation, axonal caliber, and slow axonal transport by myelinating Schwann cells. *Cell* **68**, 451–463.

Decker, L., Avellana-Adalid, V., Nait-Oumesmar, B., Durbec, P., and Baron-Van Evercooren, A. (2000). Oligodendrocyte precursor migration and differentiation: combined effects of PSA residues, growth factors, and substrates. *Mol Cell Neurosci* **16**, 422–439.

Delarasse, C., Daubas, P., Mars, L. T., *et al.* (2003). Myelin/oligodendrocyte glycoprotein-deficient (MOG-deficient) mice reveal lack of immune tolerance to MOG in wild-type mice. *J Clin Invest* **112**, 544–553.

Deloire-Grassin, M. S., Brochet, B., Quesson, B., *et al.* (2000). In vivo evaluation of remyelination in rat brain by magnetization transfer imaging. *J Neurol Sci* **178**, 10–16.

Demerens, C., Stankoff, B., Logak, M., *et al.* (1996). Induction of myelination in the central nervous system by electrical activity. *Proc Natl Acad Sci USA* **93**, 9887–9892.

Deng, W., Rosenberg, P. A., Volpe, J. J., and Jensen, F. E. (2003). Calcium-permeable AMPA/kainate receptors mediate toxicity and preconditioning by oxygen-glucose deprivation in oligodendrocyte precursors. *Proc Natl Acad Sci USA* **100**, 6801–6806.

Deng, W., Wang, H., Rosenberg, P. A., Volpe, J. J., and Jensen, F. E. (2004). Role of metabotropic glutamate receptors in oligodendrocyte excitotoxicity and oxidative stress. *Proc Natl Acad Sci USA* **101**, 7751–7756.

Denisenko-Nehrbass, N., Oguievetskaia, K., Goutebroze, L., *et al.* (2003). Protein 4.1B associates with both Caspr/paranodin and Caspr2 at paranodes and juxtaparanodes of myelinated fibres. *Eur J Neurosci* **17**, 411–416.

Dermietzel, R., Traub, O., Hwang, T. K., *et al.* (1989). Differential expression of three gap junction proteins in developing and mature brain tissues. *Proc Natl Acad Sci USA* **86**, 10148–10152.

DeSilva, T. M., Kabakov, A. Y., Goldhoff, P. E., Volpe, J. J., and Rosenberg, P. A. (2009). Regulation of glutamate transport in developing rat oligodendrocytes. *J Neurosci* **29**, 7898–7908.

DeSilva, T. M., Kinney, H. C., Borenstein, N. S., *et al.* (2007). The glutamate transporter EAAT2 is transiently expressed in developing human cerebral white matter. *J Comp Neurol* **501**, 879–890.

Devaux, J. J. and Scherer, S. S. (2005). Altered ion channels in an animal model of Charcot-Marie-Tooth disease type IA. *J Neurosci* **25**, 1470–1480.

Dhaunchak, A. S. and Nave, K. A. (2007). A common mechanism of PLP/DM20 misfolding causes cysteine-mediated endoplasmic reticulum retention in oligodendrocytes and Pelizaeus-Merzbacher disease. *Proc Natl Acad Sci USA* **104**, 17813–17818.

Diers-Fenger, M., Kirchhoff, F., Kettenmann, H., Levine, J. M., and Trotter, J. (2001). AN2/NG2 protein-expressing glial progenitor cells in the murine CNS: isolation, differentiation, and association with radial glia. *Glia* **34**, 213–228.

Dimos, J. T., Rodolfa, K. T., Niakan, K. K., et al. (2008). Induced pluripotent stem cells generated from patients with ALS can be differentiated into motor neurons. *Science* **321**, 1218–1221.

Dimou, L., Schnell, L., Montani, L., *et al.* (2006). Nogo-A-deficient mice reveal strain-dependent differences in axonal regeneration. *J Neurosci* **26**, 5591–5603.

Dingledine, R., Borges, K., Bowie, D., and Traynelis, S. F. (1999). The glutamate receptor ion channels. *Pharmacol Rev* **51**, 7–61.

Disanza, A., Steffen, A., Hertzog, M., Frittoli, E., Rottner, K., and Scita, G. (2005). Actin polymerization machinery: the finish line of signaling networks, the starting point of cellular movement. *Cell Mol Life Sci* **62**, 955–970.

Dobbing, J. and Sands, J. (1979). Comparative aspects of the brain growth spurt. *Early Hum Dev* **3**, 79–83.

Dolei, A. and Perron, H. (2009). The multiple sclerosis-associated retrovirus and its HERV-W endogenous family: a biological interface between virology, genetics, and immunology in human physiology and disease. *J Neurovirol* **15**, 4–13.

Domeniconi, M., Cao, Z., Spencer, T., *et al.* (2002). Myelin-associated glycoprotein interacts with the Nogo66 receptor to inhibit neurite outgrowth. *Neuron* **35**, 283–290.

Domercq, M., Sanchez-Gomez, M. V., Sherwin, C., Etxebarria, E., Fern, R., and Matute, C. (2007). System xc- and glutamate transporter inhibition mediates microglial toxicity to oligodendrocytes. *J Immunol* **178**, 6549–6556.

Dong, Z., Brennan, A., Liu, N., *et al.* (1995). Neu differentiation factor is a neuron-glia signal and regulates survival, proliferation, and maturation of rat Schwann cell precursors. *Neuron* **15**, 585–596.

Dorr, J., Bechmann, I., Waiczies, S., *et al.* (2002). Lack of tumor necrosis factor-related apoptosis-inducing ligand but presence of its receptors in the human brain. *J Neurosci* **22**, RC209–RC211.

Dowling, P., Husar, W., Menonna, J., Donnenfeld, H., Cook, S., and Sidhu, M. (1997). Cell death and birth in multiple sclerosis brain. *J Neurol Sci* **149**, 1–11.

D'Souza, S. D., Bonetti, B., Balasingam, V., Cashman, N. R., Barker, P. A., Troutt, A. B., Raine, C. S., and Antel, J P. *et al.* (1996). Multiple sclerosis: Fas signaling in oligodendrocyte cell death. *J Exp Med* **184**, 2361–2370.

Dubois-Dalcq, M., Behar, T., Hudson, L., and Lazzarini, R. A. (1986). Emergence of three myelin proteins in oligodendrocytes cultured without neurons. *J Cell Biol* **102**, 384–392.

Duce, J. A., Hollander, W., Jaffe, R., and Abraham, C. R. (2006). Activation of early components of complement targets myelin and oligodendrocytes in the aged rhesus monkey brain. *Neurobiol Aging* **27**, 633–644.

Ducker, T. B., Salcman, M., Perot, P. L., Jr., and Ballantine, D. (1978). Experimental spinal cord trauma. I. Correlation of blood flow, tissue oxygen and neurologic status in the dog. *Surg Neurol* **10**, 60–63.

Dugas, J. C., Tai, Y. C., Speed, T. P., Ngai, J., and Barres, B. A. (2006). Functional genomic analysis of oligodendrocyte differentiation. *J Neurosci* **26**, 10967–10983.

Duncan, I. D., Griffiths, I. R., and Munz, M. (1983). "Shaking pups": a disorder of central myelination in the spaniel dog. III. Quantitative aspects of glia and myelin in the spinal cord and optic nerve. *Neuropathol Appl Neurobiol* **9**, 355–368.

Duncan, I. D., Hammang, J. P., and Trapp, B. D. (1988). Abnormal compact myelin in the myelin-deficient rat: absence of proteolipid protein correlates with a defect in the intraperiod line. *Proc Natl Acad Sci USA* **84**, 6287–6291.

Duncan, J. R., Cock, M. L., Scheerlinck, J. P., *et al.* (2002). White matter injury after repeated endotoxin exposure in the preterm ovine fetus. *Pediatr Res* **52**, 941–949.

Dupree, J. L., Coetzee, T., Blight, A., Suzuki, K., and Popko, B. (1998). Myelin galactolipids are essential for proper node of Ranvier formation in the CNS. *J Neurosci* **18**, 1642–1649.

Dupree, J. L., Girault, J. A., and Popko, B. (1999). Axo-glial interactions regulate the localization of axonal paranodal proteins. *J Cell Biol* **147**, 1145–1152.

Dyer, C. A. and Benjamins, J. A. (1989). Organization of oligodendroglial membrane sheets. I. Association of myelin basic protein and 2′,3′-cyclic nucleotide 3′-phosphohydrolase with cytoskeleton. *J Neurosci Res* **24**, 201–211.

Dzhashiashvili, Y., Zhang, Y., Galinska, J., Lam, I., Grumet, M., and Salzer, J. L. (2007). Nodes of Ranvier and axon initial segments are ankyrin

G-dependent domains that assemble by distinct mechanisms. *J Cell Biol* **177**, 857–870.

Dziembowska, M., Tham, T. N., Lau, P., Vitry, S., Lazarini, F., and Dubois-Dalcq, M. (2005). A role for CXCR4 signaling in survival and migration of neural and oligodendrocyte precursors. *Glia* **50**, 258–269.

Eash, S., Tavares, R., Stopa, E. G., Robbins, S. H., Brossay, L., and Atwood, W. J. (2004). Differential distribution of the JC virus receptor-type sialic acid in normal human tissues. *Am J Pathol* **164**, 419–428.

Eberhardt, K. A., Irintchev, A., Al-Majed, A. A., *et al.* (2006). BDNF/TrkB signaling regulates HNK-1 carbohydrate expression in regenerating motor nerves and promotes functional recovery after peripheral nerve repair. *Exp Neurol* **198**, 500–510.

Edgar, J. M., McLaughlin, M., Yool, D., *et al.* (2004). Oligodendroglial modulation of fast axonal transport in a mouse model of hereditary spastic paraplegia. *J Cell Biol* **166**, 121–131.

Einheber, S., Zanazzi, G., Ching, W., *et al.* (1997). The axonal membrane protein Caspr, a homologue of neurexin IV, is a component of the septate-like paranodal junctions that assemble during myelination. *J Cell Biol* **139**, 1495–1506.

Einstein, O., Fainstein, N., Vaknin, I., *et al.* (2007). Neural precursors attenuate autoimmune encephalomyelitis by peripheral immunosuppression. *Ann Neurol* **61**, 209–218.

Einstein, O., Grigoriadis, N., Mizrachi-Kol, R., *et al.* (2006). Transplanted neural precursor cells reduce brain inflammation to attenuate chronic experimental autoimmune encephalomyelitis. *Exp Neurol* **198**, 275–284.

Eltayeb, S., Berg, A. L., Lassmann, H., *et al.* (2007). Temporal expression and cellular origin of CC chemokine receptors CCR1, CCR2 and CCR5 in the central nervous system: insight into mechanisms of MOG-induced EAE. *J Neuroinflammation* **4**, 14.

Engelhardt, B. (2008). The blood–central nervous system barriers actively control immune cell entry into the central nervous system. *Curr Pharm Des* **14**, 1555–1565.

Eshed, Y., Feinberg, K., Carey, D. J., and Peles, E. (2007). Secreted gliomedin is a perinodal matrix component of peripheral nerves. *J Cell Biol* **177**, 551–562.

Eshed, Y., Feinberg, K., Poliak, S., *et al.* (2005). Gliomedin mediates Schwann cell–axon interaction and the molecular assembly of the nodes of Ranvier. *Neuron* **47**, 215–229.

Esper, R. M., Pankonin, M. S., and Loeb, J. A. (2006). Neuregulins: versatile growth and differentiation factors in nervous system development and human disease. *Brain Res Rev* **51**, 161–175.

Fairman, W. A., Vandenberg, R. J., Arriza, J. L., Kavanaugh, M. P., and Amara, S. G. (1995). An excitatory amino-acid transporter with properties of a ligand-gated chloride channel. *Nature* **375**, 599–603.

Falls, D. L. (2003). Neuregulins: functions, forms, and signaling strategies. *Exp Cell Res* **284**, 14–30.

Fancy, S. P., Zhao, C., and Franklin, R. J. (2004). Increased expression of Nkx2.2 and Olig2 identifies reactive oligodendrocyte progenitor cells responding to demyelination in the adult CNS. *Mol Cell Neurosci* **27**, 247–254.

Fannon, A. M., Sherman, D. L., Ilyina-Gragerova, G., Brophy, P. J., Friedrich, V. L., Jr., and Colman, D. R. (1995). Novel E-cadherin-mediated adhesion in peripheral nerve: Schwann cell architecture is stabilized by autotypic adherens junctions. *J Cell Biol* **129**, 189–202.

Farh, K. K., Grimson, A., Jan, C., *et al.* (2005). The widespread impact of mammalian MicroRNAs on mRNA repression and evolution. *Science* **310**, 1817–1821.

Fehlings, M. G. and Nashmi, R. (1995). Assessment of axonal dysfunction in an in vitro model of acute compressive injury to adult rat spinal cord axons. *Brain Res* **677**, 291–299.

Fehlings, M. G. and Tator, C. H. (1995). The relationships among the severity of spinal cord injury, residual neurological function, axon counts, and counts of retrogradely labeled neurons after experimental spinal cord injury. *Exp Neurol* **132**, 220–228.

Feldman, M. L., and Peters, A. (1998). Ballooning of myelin sheaths in normally aged macaques. *J Neurocytol* **27**, 605–614.

Feltri, M. L., Graus Porta, D., Previtali, S. C., *et al.* (2002). Conditional disruption of beta 1 integrin in Schwann cells impedes interactions with axons. *J Cell Biol* **156**, 199–209.

Ferguson, B., Matyszak, M. K., Esiri, M. M., and Perry, V. H. (1997). Axonal damage in acute multiple sclerosis lesions. *Brain* **120**, 393–399.

Fern, R. and Möller, T. (2000). Rapid ischemic cell death in immature oligodendrocytes: a fatal glutamate release feedback loop. *J Neurosci* **20**, 34–42.

Fernandez-Valle, C., Bunge, R. P., and Bunge, M. B. (1995). Schwann cells degrade myelin and proliferate in the absence of macrophages: evidence from in vitro studies of Wallerian degeneration. *J Neurocytol* **24**, 667–679.

Ferriero, D. M. (2006). Can we define the pathogenesis of human periventricular white-matter injury using animal models? *J Child Neurol* **21**, 580–581.

Fewou, S. N., Ramakrishnan, H., Bussow, H., Gieselmann, V., and Eckhardt, M. (2007). Down-regulation of polysialic acid is required for efficient myelin formation. *J Biol Chem* **282**, 16700–16711.

Ffrench-Constant, C., and Raff, M. C. (1986). Proliferating bipotential glial progenitor cells in adult rat optic nerve. *Nature* **319**, 499–502.

Fields, R. D. (2005). Myelination: an overlooked mechanism of synaptic plasticity? *Neuroscientist* **11**, 528–531.

Fields, R. D. (2008a). Oligodendrocytes changing the rules: action potentials in glia and oligodendrocytes controlling action potentials. *Neuroscientist* **14**, 540–543.

Fields, R. D. (2008b). White matter in learning, cognition and psychiatric disorders. *Trends Neurosci* **31**, 361–370.

Fields, R. D. (2008c). White matter matters. *Sci Am* **298**, 42–49.

Fields, R. D. and Burnstock, G. (2006). Purinergic signalling in neuron-glia interactions. *Nat Rev Neurosci* **7**, 423–436.

Filbin, M. T. (2003). Myelin-associated inhibitors of axonal regeneration in the adult mammalian CNS. *Nat Rev Neurosci* **4**, 703–713.

Filippi, M. and Rocca, M. A. (2005). MRI evidence for multiple sclerosis as a diffuse disease of the central nervous system. *J Neurol* **252** Suppl 5, v16–v24.

Fischer, D., He, Z., and Benowitz, L. I. (2004). Counteracting the Nogo receptor enhances optic nerve regeneration if retinal ganglion cells are in an active growth state. *J Neurosci* **24**, 1646–1651.

Fischer, I., Konola, J., and Cochary, E. (1990). Microtubule associated protein (MAP1B) is present in cultured oligodendrocytes and co-localizes with tubulin. *J Neurosci Res* **27**, 112–124.

Fix, A. S., Horn, J. W., Wightman, K. A., *et al.* (1993). Neuronal vacuolization and necrosis induced by the noncompetitive *N*-methyl-D-aspartate (NMDA) antagonist MK(+)801 (dizocilpine maleate): a light and electron microscopic evaluation of the rat retrosplenial cortex. *Exp Neurol* **123**, 204–215.

Flores, A. I., Narayanan, S. P., Morse, E. N., *et al.* (2008). Constitutively active Akt induces enhanced myelination in the CNS. *J Neurosci* **28**, 7174–7183.

Fogarty, M., Richardson, W. D., and Kessaris, N. (2005). A subset of oligodendrocytes generated from radial glia in the dorsal spinal cord. *Development* **132**, 1951–1959.

Folkerth, R. D. and Kinney, H. C. (2008). Disorders of the perinatal period. In *Greenfield's Neuropathology* (London: Hodder Arnold), pp. 241–315.

Follett, P. L., Rosenberg, P. A., Volpe, J. J., and Jensen, F. E. (2000). NBQX attenuates excitotoxic injury in developing white matter. *J Neurosci* **20**, 9235–9241.

Follett, P. L., Talos, D. M., Volpe, J. J., and Jensen, F. E. (2003). AMPA receptor subunit expression in human white matter during window of susceptibility to periventricular leukomalacia. *Ann Neurol* **54**(S3), S103.

Foote, A. K. and Blakemore, W. F. (2005). Inflammation stimulates remyelination in areas of chronic demyelination. *Brain* **128**, 528–539.

Fortin, D., Rom, E., Sun, H., Yayon, A., and Bansal, R. (2005). Distinct fibroblast growth factor (FGF)/FGF receptor signaling pairs initiate diverse cellular responses in the oligodendrocyte lineage. *J Neurosci* **25**, 7470–7479.

Fournier, A. E., GrandPre, T., and Strittmatter, S. M. (2001). Identification of a receptor mediating Nogo-66 inhibition of axonal regeneration. *Nature* **409**, 341–346.

Fournier, A. E., Takizawa, B. T., and Strittmatter, S. M. (2003). Rho kinase inhibition enhances axonal regeneration in the injured CNS. *J Neurosci* **23**, 1416–1423.

Fox, E. J. (2004). Mechanism of action of mitoxantrone. *Neurology* **63**, S15–S18.

Franco, P. G., Silvestroff, L., Soto, E. F., and Pasquini, J. M. (2008). Thyroid hormones promote differentiation of oligodendrocyte progenitor cells and improve remyelination after cuprizone-induced demyelination. *Exp Neurol* **212**, 458–467.

Frank, M. (2000). MAL, a proteolipid in glycosphingolipid enriched domains: functional implications in myelin and beyond. *Prog Neurobiol* **60**, 531–544.

Franklin, R. J. (2002). Why does remyelination fail in multiple sclerosis? *Nat Rev Neurosci* **3**, 705–714.

Franklin, R. J. and Barnett, S. C. (2004). Olfactory ensheathing cells. In *Myelin Biology and Disorders*, R. A. Lazzarini, ed. (New York: Elsevier), pp. 371–384.

Franklin, R. J. and Ffrench-Constant, C. (2008). Remyelination in the CNS: from biology to therapy. *Nat Rev Neurosci* **9**, 839–855.

Freedman, M. S., Buu, N. N., Ruijs, T. C., Williams, K., and Antel, J. P. (1992). Differential expression of heat shock proteins by human glial cells. *J Neuroimmunol* **41**, 231–238.

Freedman, M. S., Ruijs, T. C., Selin, L. K., and Antel, J. P. (1991). Peripheral blood gamma-delta T cells lyse fresh human brain-derived oligodendrocytes. *Ann Neurol* **30**, 794–800.

Friede, R. L. (1972). Control of myelin formation by axon caliber (with a model of the control mechanism). *J Comp Neurol* **144**, 233–252.

Frost, E. E., Zhou, Z., Krasnesky, K., and Armstrong, R. C. (2009). Initiation of oligodendrocyte progenitor cell migration by a PDGF-A activated extracellular regulated kinase (ERK) signaling pathway. *Neurochem Res* **34**, 169–181.

Fruttiger, M., Montag, D., Schachner, M., and Martini, R. (1995). Crucial role for the myelin-associated glycoprotein in the maintenance of axon-myelin integrity. *Eur J Neurosci* **7**, 511–515.

Fry, E. J., Ho, C., and David, S. (2007). A role for Nogo receptor in macrophage clearance from injured peripheral nerve. *Neuron* **53**, 649–662.

Fukushima, N., Furuta, D., Hidaka, Y., Moriyama, R., and Tsujiuchi, T. (2009). Post-translational modifications of tubulin in the nervous system. *J Neurochem* **109**, 683–693.

Furley, A. J., Morton, S. B., Manalo, D., Karagogeos, D., Dodd, J., and Jessell, T. M. (1990). The axonal glycoprotein TAG-1 is an immunoglobulin superfamily member with neurite outgrowth-promoting activity. *Cell* **61**, 157–170.

Furness, D. N., Dehnes, Y., Akhtar, A. Q., *et al.* (2008). A quantitative assessment of glutamate uptake into hippocampal synaptic terminals and astrocytes: new insights into a neuronal role for excitatory amino acid transporter 2 (EAAT2). *Neuroscience* **157**, 80–94.

Furuta, A., Rothstein, J. D., and Martin, L. J. (1997). Glutamate transporter protein subtypes are expressed differentially during rat CNS development. *J Neurosci* **17**, 8363–8375.

Furuta, A., Takashima, S., Yokoo, H., Rothstein, J. D., Wada, K., and Iwaki, T. (2005). Expression of glutamate transporter subtypes during normal human corticogenesis and type II lissencephaly. *Brain Res Dev Brain Res* **155**, 155–164.

Gage, F. H. (2000). Mammalian neural stem cells. *Science* **287**, 1433–1438.

Galiano, M. R., Bosc, C., Schweitzer, A., Andrieux, A., Job, D., and Hallak, M. E. (2004). Astrocytes and oligodendrocytes express different STOP protein isoforms. *J Neurosci Res* **78**, 329–337.

Gallo, V. and Russell, J. T. (1995). Excitatory amino acid receptors in glia: different subtypes for distinct functions. *J. Neurosci. Res.* **42**, 1–8.

Gallo, V., Mangin, J. M., Kukley, M., and Dietrich, D. (2008). Synapses on NG2-expressing progenitors in the brain: multiple functions? *J Physiol (Lond)* **586**, 3767–3781.

Gallo, V., Zhou, J. M., McBain, C. J., Wright, P., Knutson, P. L., and Armstrong, R. C. (1996). Oligodendrocyte progenitor cell proliferation and lineage progression are regulated by glutamate receptor-mediated K$^+$ channel block. *J Neurosci* **16**, 2659–2670.

Gao, L. and Miller, R. H. (2006). Specification of optic nerve oligodendrocyte precursors by retinal ganglion cell axons. *J Neurosci* **29**, 7619–7628.

Gao, X., Gillig, T. A., Ye, P., D'Ercole, A. J., Matsushima, G. K., and Popko, B. (2000). Interferon-gamma protects against cuprizone-induced demyelination. *Mol Cell Neurosci* **16**, 338–349.

Garbern, J. Y. (2007). Pelizaeus–Merzbacher disease: genetic and cellular pathogenesis. *Cell Mol Life Sci* **64**, 50–65.

Garbern, J. Y., Cambi, F., Tang, X. M., *et al.* (1997). Proteolipid protein is necessary in peripheral as well as central myelin. *Neuron* **19**, 205–218.

Garbern, J. Y., Yool, D. A., Moore, G. J., *et al.* (2002). Patients lacking the major CNS myelin protein, proteolipid protein 1, develop length-dependent axonal degeneration in the absence of demyelination and inflammation. *Brain* **125**, 551–561.

Garcia, R., Aguiar, J., Alberti, E., de la Cuetara, K., and Pavon, N. (2004). Bone marrow stromal cells produce nerve growth factor and glial cell line-derived neurotrophic factors. *Biochem Biophys Res Commun* **316**, 753–754.

Garcia-Barcina, J. M. and Matute, C. (1996). Expression of kainate-selective glutamate receptor subunits in glial cells of the adult bovine white matter. *Eur J Neurosci* **8**, 2379–2387.

Gard, A. L., Williams, W. C., and Burrell, M. R. (1995). Oligodendroblasts distinguished from O-2A glial progenitors by surface phenotype (O4+GalC–) and response to cytokines using signal transducer LIFR beta. *Dev Biol* **167**, 596–608.

Garlin, A. B., Sinor, A. D., Sinor, J. D., Jee, S. H., Grinspan, J. B., and Robinson, M. B. (1995). Pharmacology of sodium-dependent high-affinity L-[^{3}H]glutamate transport in glial cultures. *J Neurochem* **64**, 2572–2580.

Garratt, A. N., Britsch, S., and Birchmeier, C. (2000). Neuregulin, a factor with many functions in the life of a Schwann cell. *Bioessays* **22**, 987–996.

Gasque, P. and Morgan, B. P. (1996). Complement regulatory protein expression by a human oligodendrocyte cell line: cytokine regulation and comparison with astrocytes. *Immunology* **89**, 338–347.

Gasque, P., Singhrao, S. K., Neal, J. W., Gotze, O., and Morgan, B. P. (1997). Expression of the receptor for complement C5a (CD88) is up-regulated on reactive astrocytes, microglia, and endothelial cells in the inflamed human central nervous system. *Am J Pathol* **150**, 31–41.

Gatzinsky, K. P., Persson, G. H., and Berthold, C. H. (1997). Removal of retrogradely transported material from rat lumbosacral alpha-motor axons by paranodal axon–Schwann cell networks. *Glia* **20**, 115–126.

Gay, C. T., Hardies, L. J., Rauch, R. A., *et al.* (1997). Magnetic resonance imaging demonstrates incomplete myelination in 18q- syndrome: evidence for myelin basic protein haploinsufficiency. *Am J Med Genet* **74**, 422–431.

Ge, W. P., Zhou, W., Luo, Q., Jan, L. Y., and Jan, Y. N. (2009). Dividing glial cells maintain differentiated properties including complex morphology and functional synapses. *Proc Natl Acad Sci USA* **106**, 328–333.

Geiger, J. R., Melcher, T., Koh, D. S., *et al.* (1995). Relative abundance of subunit mRNAs determines gating and Ca^{2+} permeability of AMPA receptors in principal neurons and interneurons in rat CNS. *Neuron* **15**, 193–204.

Geiger, K., Howes, E., Gallina, M., Huang, X. J., Travis, G. H., and Sarvetnick, N. (1994). Transgenic mice expressing IFN-gamma in the retina develop inflammation of the eye and photoreceptor loss. *Invest Ophthalmol Vis Sci* **35**, 2667–2681.

Genain, C. P., Cannella, B., Hauser, S. L., and Raine, C. S. (1999). Identification of autoantibodies associated with myelin damage in multiple sclerosis. *Nature Med* **5**, 170–175.

Genain, C. P., Nguyen, M. H., Letvin, N. L., *et al.* (1995). Antibody facilitation of multiple sclerosis-like lesions in a nonhuman primate. *J Clin Invest* **96**, 2966–2974.

Gencic, S. and Hudson, L. D. (1990). Conservative amino acid substitution in the myelin proteolipid protein of jimpymsd mice. *J Neurosci* **10**, 117–124.

Genoud, S., Lappe-Siefke, C., Goebbels, S., *et al.* (2002). Notch1 control of oligodendrocyte differentiation in the spinal cord. *J Cell Biol* **158**, 709–718.

Gensert, J. M. and Goldman, J. E. (1997). Endogenous progenitors remyelinate demyelinated axons in the adult CNS. *Neuron* **19**, 197–203.

George, E. B., Glass, J. D., and Griffin, J. W. (1995). Axotomy-induced axonal degeneration is mediated by calcium influx through ion-specific channels. *J Neurosci* **15**, 6445–6452.

Gerdoni, E., Gallo, B., Casazza, S., *et al.* (2007). Mesenchymal stem cells effectively modulate pathogenic immune response in experimental autoimmune encephalomyelitis. *Ann Neurol* **61**, 219–227.

Ghabriel, M. N. and Allt, G. (1981). Incisures of Schmidt–Lanterman. *Prog Neurobiol* **17**, 25–58.

Ghandour, M. S. and Skoff, R. P. (1991). Double-labeling in situ hybridization analysis of mRNAs for carbonic anhydrase II and myelin basic protein: expression in developing cultured glial cells. *Glia* **4**, 1–10.

Ghatak, N. R., Hirano, A., Doron, Y., and Zimmerman, H. M. (1973). Remyelination in multiple sclerosis with peripheral type myelin. *Arch Neurol* **29**, 262–267.

Giese, K. P., Martini, R., Lemke, G., Soriano, P., and Schachner, M. (1992). Mouse P0 gene disruption leads to hypomyelination, abnormal expression of recognition molecules, and degeneration of myelin and axons. *Cell* **71**, 565–576.

Gill, A. S. and Binder, D. K. (2007). Wilder Penfield, Pio del Hortega, and the discovery of oligodendroglia. *Neurosurgey* **60**, 940–948.

Gilles, F. H., Leviton, A., and Kerr, C. S. (1976). Endotoxin leucoencephalopathy in the telencephalon of the newborn kitten. *J Neurol Sci* **27**, 183–191.

Gillespie, C. S., Trapp, B. D., Colman, D. R., and Brophy, P. J. (1990). Distribution of myelin basic protein and P2 mRNA's in rabbit spinal cord oligodendrocytes. *J Neurochem* **54**, 1556–1561.

Gilmour, D. T., Maischein, H. M., and Nusslein-Volhard, C. (2002). Migration and function of a glial subtype in the vertebrate peripheral nervous system. *Neuron* **34**, 577–588.

Giovannoni, G. and Hartung, H. P. (1996). The immunopathogenesis of multiple sclerosis and Guillain–Barre syndrome. *Curr Opin Neurol* **9**, 165–177.

Giraldez, A. J., Mishima, Y., Rihel, J., et al. (2006). Zebrafish MiR-430 promotes deadenylation and clearance of maternal mRNAs. *Science* **312**, 75–79.

Giulian, D., Young, D. G., Woodward, J., Brown, D. C., and Lachman, L. B. (1988). Interleukin-1 is an astroglial growth factor in the developing brain. *J Neurosci* **8**, 709–714.

Giuliani, F., Goodyer, C. G., Antel, J. P., and Yong, V. W. (2003). Vulnerability of human neurons to T cell-mediated cytotoxicity. *J Immunol* **171**, 368–379.

Gledhill, R. F. and McDonald, W. I. (1977). Morphological characteristics of central demyelination and remyelination: a single-fiber study. *Ann Neurol* **1**, 552–560.

Gledhill, R. F. Harrison, B. M., and McDonald, W. I. (1973a). Demyelination and remyelination after acute spinal cord compression. *Exp Neurol* **38**, 472–487.

Gledhill, R. F., Harrison, B. M., and McDonald, W. I. (1973b). Pattern of remyelination in the CNS. *Nature* **244**, 443–444.

Gocht, A. (1992). The subcellular localization of the carbohydrate epitope 3-fucosyl-*N*-acetyllactosamine is different in normal and reactive astrocytes. *Acta Anat (Basel)* **145**, 434–441.

Goddard, D. R., Berry, M., and Butt, A. M. (1999). In vivo actions of fibroblast growth factor-2 and insulin-like growth factor-I on oligodendrocyte development and myelination in the central nervous system. *J Neurosci Res* **57**, 74–85.

Goldberg, J. L., Vargas, M. E., Wang, J. T., et al. (2004). An oligodendrocyte lineage-specific semaphorin, Sema5A, inhibits axon growth by retinal ganglion cells. *J Neurosci* **24**, 4989–4999.

Goldman, J. E., Geier, S. S., and Hirano, M. (1986). Differentiation of astrocytes and oligodendrocytes from germinal matrix cells in primary culture. *J Neurosci* **6**, 52–60.

Goldstein, L. S. and Yang, Z. (2000). Microtubule-based transport systems in neurons: the roles of kinesins and dyneins. *Annu Rev Neurosci* **23**, 39–71.

Gollan, L., Sabanay, H., Poliak, S., Berglund, E. O., Ranscht, B., and Peles, E. (2002). Retention of a cell adhesion complex at the paranodal junction requires the cytoplasmic region of Caspr. *J Cell Biol* **157**, 1247–1256.

Gomes, W. A., Mehler, M. F., and Kessler, J. A. (2003). Transgenic overexpression of BMP4 increases astroglial and decreases oligodendroglial lineage commitment. *Dev Biol* **255**, 164–177.

Gorath, M., Stahnke, T., Mronga, T., Goldbaum, O., and Richter-Landsberg, C. (2001). Developmental changes of tau protein and mRNA in cultured rat brain oligodendrocytes. *Glia* **36**, 89–101.

Gordon, D., Kidd, G. J., and Smith, R. (2008a). Antisense suppression of tau in cultured rat oligodendrocytes inhibits process formation. *J Neurosci Res* **86**, 2591–2601.

Gordon, D., Pavlovska, G., Glover, C. P., Uney, J. B., Wraith, D., and Scolding, N. J. (2008b). Human mesenchymal stem cells abrogate experimental allergic encephalomyelitis after intraperitoneal injection, and with sparse CNS infiltration. *Neurosci Lett* **448**, 71–73.

Gorman, M. P., Golomb, M. R., Walsh, L. E., *et al.* (2007). Steroid-responsive neurologic relapses in a child with a proteolipid protein-1 mutation. *Neurology* **68**, 1305–1307.

Gould, R. M., Byrd, A. L., and Barbarese, E. (1995). The number of Schmidt–Lanterman incisures is more than doubled in shiverer PNS myelin sheaths. *J Neurocytol* **24**, 85–98.

Gould, R. M., Freund, C. M., Palmer, F., and Feinstein, D. L. (2000). Messenger RNAs located in myelin sheath assembly sites. *J Neurochem* **75**, 1834–1844.

Gow, A. and Lazzarini, R. A. (1996). A cellular mechanism governing the severity of Pelizaeus–Merzbacher disease. *Nat Genet* **13**, 422–428.

Gow, A., Friedrich, V. L., Jr., and Lazzarini, R. A. (1994). Many naturally occurring mutations of myelin proteolipid protein impair its intracellular transport. *J Neursci Res* **37**, 574–583.

Gow, A., Southwood, C. M., and Lazzarini, R. A. (1998). Disrupted proteolipid protein trafficking results in oligodendrocyte apoptosis in an animal model of Pelizaeus–Merzbacher disease. *J Cell Biol* **140**, 925–934.

Gow, A., Southwood, C. M., Li, J. S., *et al.* (1999). CNS myelin and Sertoli cell tight junction strands are absent in Osp/claudin-11 null mice. *Cell* **99**, 649–659.

GrandPre, T., Li, S., and Strittmatter, S. M. (2002). Nogo-66 receptor antagonist peptide promotes axonal regeneration. *Nature* **417**, 547–551.

GrandPre, T., Nakamura, F., Vartanian, T., and Strittmatter, S. M. (2000). Identification of the Nogo inhibitor of axon regeneration as a Reticulon protein. *Nature* **403**, 439–444.

Graumann, U., Reynolds, R., Steck, A. J., and Schaeren-Wiemers, N. (2003). Molecular changes in normal appearing white matter in multiple sclerosis are characteristic of neuroprotective mechanisms against hypoxic insult. *Brain Pathol* **13**, 554–573.

Gregori, N., Proschel, C., Noble, M., and Mayer-Proschel, M. (2002). The tripotential glial-restricted precursor (GRP) cell and glial development in the spinal cord: generation of bipotential oligodendrocyte-type-2 astrocyte progenitor cells and dorsal-ventral differences in GRP cell function. *J Neurosci* **22**, 248–256.

Grenier, Y., Ruijs, T. C., Robitaille, Y., Olivier, A., and Antel, J. P. (1989). Immunohistochemical studies of adult human glial cells. *J Neuroimmunol* **21**, 103–115.

Gressens, P., Marret, S., and Evrard, P. (1996). Developmental spectrum of the excitotoxic cascade induced by ibotenate: a model of hypoxic insults in fetuses and neonates. *Neuropathol Appl Neurobiol* **22**, 498–502.

Griffiths, I. and McCulloch, M. C. (1983). Nerve fibres in spinal cord impact injuries. Part 1. Changes in the myelin sheath during the initial 5 weeks. *J Neurol Sci* **58**, 335–349.

Griffiths, I., Klugmann, M., Anderson, T., Thomson, C., Vouyiouklis, D., and Nave, K. A. (1998a). Current concepts of PLP and its role in the nervous system. *Microsc Res Tech* **41**, 344–358.

Griffiths, I., Klugmann, M., Anderson, T., *et al.* (1998b). Axonal swellings and degeneration in mice lacking the major proteolipid of myelin. *Science* **280**, 1610–1613.

Grinspan, J. B., Stern, J. L., Franceschini, B., and Pleasure, D. (1993). Trophic effects of basic fibroblast growth factor (bFGF) on differentiated oligodendroglia: a mechanism for regeneration of the oligodendroglial lineage. *J Neurosci Res* **36**, 672–680.

Griot-Wenk, M., Griot, C., Pfister, H., and Vandevelde, M. (1991). Antibody-dependent cellular cytotoxicity in antimyelin antibody-induced oligodendrocyte damage in vitro. *J Neuroimmunol* **33**, 145–155.

Groom, A. J., Smith, T., and Turski, L. (2003). Multiple sclerosis and glutamate. *Ann N Y Acad Sci* **993**, 229–275.

Grossman, S. D., Rosenberg, L. J., and Wrathall, J. R. (2001). Temporal-spatial pattern of acute neuronal and glial loss after spinal cord contusion. *Exp Neurol* **168**, 273–282.

Grove, M., Komiyama, N. H., Nave, K. A., Grant, S. G., Sherman, D. L., and Brophy, P. J. (2007). FAK is required for axonal sorting by Schwann cells. *J Cell Biol* **176**, 277–282.

Groves, A. K., Barnett, S. C., Franklin, R. J. M., *et al.* (1993). Repair of demyelinated lesions by transplantation of purified O-2A progenitor cells. *Nature* **362**, 453–455.

Grumet, M., Mauro, V., Burgoon, M. P., Edelman, G. M., and Cunningham, B. A. (1991). Structure of a new nervous system glycoprotein, Nr-CAM, and its relationship to subgroups of neural cell adhesion molecules. *J Cell Biol* **113** (6), 1399–1412.

Gudz, T. I., Komuro, H., and Macklin, W. B. (2006). Glutamate stimulates oligodendrocyte progenitor migration mediated via an alphav integrin/myelin proteolipid protein complex. *J Neurosci* **26**, 2458–2466.

Guertin, A. D., Zhang, D. P., Mak, K. S., Alberta, J. A., and Kim, H. A. (2005). Microanatomy of axon/glial signaling during Wallerian degeneration. *J Neurosci* **25**, 3478–3487.

Guidotti, G. (1972). Membrane proteins. *Annu Rev Biochem* **41**, 731–752.

Hafler, D. A., Compston, A., Sawcer, S., *et al.* (2007). Risk alleles for multiple sclerosis identified by a genomewide study. *N Engl J Med* **357**, 851–862.

Hagberg, H. (1992). Hypoxic-ischemic damage in the neonatal brain: excitatory amino acids. *Dev Pharmacol Ther* **18**, 139–144.

Haines, J. D., Fragoso, G., Hossain, S., Mushynski, W. E., and Almazan, G. (2008). p38 mitogen-activated protein kinase regulates myelination. *J Mol Neurosci* **35**, 23–33.

Hakak, Y., Walker, J. R., Li, C., *et al.* (2001). Genome-wide expression analysis reveals dysregulation of myelination-related genes in chronic schizophrenia. *Proc Natl Acad Sci USA* **98**, 4746–4751.

Halfpenny, C. A. and Scolding, N. J. (2003). Immune-modifying agents do not impair the survival, migration or proliferation of oligodendrocyte progenitors (CG-4) in vitro. *J. Neuroimmunol.* **139**, 9–16.

Halfpenny, C., Benn, T., and Scolding, N. J. (2002). Cell transplantation, myelin repair and multiple sclerosis. *Lancet Neurol* **1**, 31–40.

Hall, A. K. and Miller, R. (2004). Emerging roles for bone morphogenetic proteins in central nervous system glial biology. *J Neurosci Res* **76**, 1–8.

Hall, S. (2005). The response to injury in the peripheral nervous system. *J Bone Joint Surg Br* **87**, 1309–1319.

Hall, S. M. and Gregson, N. A. (1974). The effects of mitomycin C on remyelination in the peripheral nervous system. *Nature* **252**, 303–305.

Hamamoto, Y., Ogata, T., Morino, T., Hino, M., and Yamamoto, H. (2007). Real-time direct measurement of spinal cord blood flow at the site of compression: relationship between blood flow recovery and motor deficiency in spinal cord injury. *Spine* **32**, 1955–1962.

Hamanoue, M., Yoshioka, A., Ohashi, T., Eto, Y., and Takamatsu, K. (2004). NF-kappaB prevents TNF-alpha-induced apoptosis in an oligodendrocyte cell line. *Neurochem Res* **29**, 1571–1576.

Hamrick, S. E., Miller, S. P., Leonard, C., *et al.* (2004). Trends in severe brain injury and neurodevelopmental outcome in premature newborn infants: the role of cystic periventricular leukomalacia. *J Pediatr* **145**, 593–599.

Haney, C. A., Sahenk, Z., Li, C., Lemmon, V. P., Roder, J., and Trapp, B. D. (1999). Heterophilic binding of L1 on unmyelinated sensory axons mediates Schwann cell adhesion and is required for axonal survival. *J Cell Biol* **146**, 1173–1184.

Hansen, T., Olsen, L., Lindow, M., *et al.* (2007). Brain expressed microRNAs implicated in schizophrenia etiology. *PLoS ONE* **2**, e873.

Hansen-Pupp, I., Harling, S., Berg, A. C., Cilio, C., Hellstrom-Westas, L., and Ley, D. (2005). Circulating interferon-gamma and white matter brain damage in preterm infants. *Pediatr Res* **58**, 946–952.

Harada, A., Oguchi, K., Okabe, S., *et al.* (1994). Altered microtubule organization in small-calibre axons of mice lacking tau protein. *Nature* **369**, 488–491.

Harauz, G., Ishiyama, N., Hill, C. M., Bates, I. R., Libich, D. S., and Fares, C. (2004). Myelin basic protein-diverse conformational states of an intrinsically unstructured protein and its roles in myelin assembly and multiple sclerosis. *Micron* **35**, 503–542.

Harel, N. Y. and Strittmatter, S. M. (2006). Can regenerating axons recapitulate developmental guidance during recovery from spinal cord injury? *Nat Rev Neurosci* **7**, 603–616.

Harrison, B. M. and McDonald, W. I. (1977). Remyelination after transient experimental compression of the spinal cord. *Ann Neurol* **1**, 542–551.

Harrison, B. M., Gledhill, R. F., and McDonald, W. J. (1975). Remyelination after transient compression of the spinal cord. *Proc Aust Assoc Neurol* **12**, 117–122.

Harsan, L. A., Steibel, J., Zaremba, A., *et al.* (2008). Recovery from chronic demyelination by thyroid hormone therapy: myelinogenesis induction and assessment by diffusion tensor magnetic resonance imaging. *J Neurosci* **28**, 14189–14201.

Hart, I. K., Richardson, W. D., Heldin, C. H., Westermark, B., and Raff, M. C. (1989). PDGF receptors on cells of the oligodendrocyte-type-2 astrocyte (O-2A) cell lineage. *Development* **105**, 595–603.

Hartline, D. K. and Colman, D. R. (2007). Rapid conduction and the evolution of giant axons and myelinated fibers. *Curr Biol* **17**, R29–R35.

Hartung, H. P. (2009). New cases of progressive multifocal leukoencephalopathy after treatment with natalizumab. *Lancet Neurol* **8**, 28–31.

Hartung, H. P., Gonsette, R., Konig, N., *et al.* (2002). Mitoxantrone in progressive multiple sclerosis: a placebo-controlled, double-blind, randomised, multicentre trial. *Lancet* **360**, 2018–2025.

Hasegawa, M. (2006). Biochemistry and molecular biology of tauopathies. *Neuropathology* **26**, 484–490.

Hata, K., Fujitani, M., Yasuda, Y., *et al.* (2006). RGMa inhibition promotes axonal growth and recovery after spinal cord injury. *J Cell Biol* **173**, 47–58.

Hatano, Y., Miura, I., Horiuchi, T., *et al.* (1997). Cerebellar myeloblastoma formation in CD7-positive, neural cell adhesion molecule (CD56)-positive acute myelogenous leukemia (M1). *Ann Hematol* **75**, 125–128.

Hauser, S. L., Waubant, E., Arnold, D. L., *et al.* (2008). B-cell depletion with rituximab in relapsing-remitting multiple sclerosis. *N Engl J Med.* **358**, 676–688.

Hayes, G. M., Woodroofe, M. N., and Cuzner, M. L. (1987). Microglia are the major cell type expressing MHC class II in human white matter. *J Neurol Sci* **80**, 25–37.

Haynes, R. L., Billiards, S. S., Borenstein, N. S., Volpe, J. J. and Kinney, H. C. (2008). Diffuse axonal injury in periventricular leukomalacia as determined by apoptotic marker fractin. *Pediatr Res* **63**, 656–661.

Haynes, R. L., Borenstein, N. S., DeSilva, T. M., *et al.* (2005). Axonal development in the cerebral white matter of the human fetus and infant. *J Comp Neurol* **484**, 156–167.

He, X. L., Bazan, J. F., McDermott, G., *et al.* (2003). Structure of the Nogo receptor ectodomain: a recognition module implicated in myelin inhibition. *Neuron* **38**, 177–185.

Hedtjarn, M., Mallard, C., Arvidsson, P., and Hagberg, H. (2005). White matter injury in the immature brain: role of interleukin-18. *Neurosci Lett* **373**, 16–20.

Heese, K., Hock, C., and Otten, U. (1998). Inflammatory signals induce neurotrophin expression in human microglial cells. *J Neurochem* **70**, 699–707.

Heick, A. and Skriver, E. (2000). *Chlamydia pneumoniae*-associated ADEM. *Eur J Neurol* **7**, 435–438.

Heine, S., Ebnet, J., Maysami, S., and Stangel, M. (2006). Effects of interferon-beta on oligodendroglial cells. *J Neuroimmunol* **177**, 173–180.

Hemmer, B., Nessler, S., Zhou, D., Kieseier, B., and Hartung, H. P. (2006). Immunopathogenesis and immunotherapy of multiple sclerosis. *Nat Clin Pract Neurol* **2**, 201–211.

Henneke, M., Combes, P., Diekmann, S., *et al.* (2008). GJA12 mutations are a rare cause of Pelizaeus-Merzbacher-like disease. *Neurology* **70**, 744–745.

Henson, J. W. (1994). Regulation of the glial-specific JC virus early promoter by the transcription factor Sp1. *J Biol Chem* **269**, 1046–1050.

Herman, M. A. and Jahr, C. E. (2007). Extracellular glutamate concentration in hippocampal slice. *J Neurosci* **27**, 9736–9741.

Heumann, R., Korsching, S., Bandtlow, C., and Thoenen, H. (1987). Changes of nerve growth factor synthesis in nonneuronal cells in response to sciatic nerve transection. *J Cell Biol* **104**, 1623–1631.

Hildebrand, C., Remahl, S., Persson, H., and Bjartmar, C. (1993). Myelinated nerve fibres in the CNS. *Prog Neurobiol* **40**, 319–384.

Hilliard, B., Wilmen, A., Seidel, C., Liu, T.-S. T., Göke, R., and Chen, Y. (2001). Roles of TNF-related apoptosis-inducing ligand in experimental autoimmune encephalomyelitis. *J Immunol* **166**, 1314–1319.

Hirayama, M., Yokochi, T., Shimokata, K., Iida, M., and Fujiki, N. (1986). Induction of human leukocyte antigen-A, B, C and -DR on cultured human oligodendrocytes and astrocytes by human gamma-interferon. *Neurosci Lett* **72**, 369–374.

Hisahara, S., Araki, T., Sugiyama, F., *et al.* (2000). Targeted expression of baculovirus p35 caspase inhibitor in oligodendrocytes protects mice against autoimmune-mediated demyelination. *EMBO J* **19**, 341–348.

Hobart, J., Kalkers, N., Barkhof, F., Uitdehaag, B., Polman, C., and Thompson, A. (2004). Outcome measures for multiple sclerosis clinical trials: relative measurement precision of the Expanded Disability Status Scale and Multiple Sclerosis Functional Composite. *Mult Scler* **10**, 41–46.

Hobart, J., Lamping, D., Fitzpatrick, R., Riazi, A., and Thompson, A. (2001). The Multiple Sclerosis Impact Scale (MSIS-29): a new patient-based outcome measure. *Brain* **124**, 962–973.

Hoek, K. S., Kidd, G. J., Carson, J. H., and Smith, R. (1998). hnRNP A2 selectively binds the cytoplasmic transport sequence of myelin basic protein mRNA. *Biochemistry* **37**, 7021–7029.

Hoftberger, R., Aboul-Enein, F., Brueck, W., *et al.* (2004). Expression of major histocompatibility complex class I molecules on the different cell types in multiple sclerosis lesions. *Brain Pathol* **14**, 43–50.

Hoke, A. (2006). Mechanisms of disease: what factors limit the success of peripheral nerve regeneration in humans? *Nat Clin Pract Neurol* **2**, 448–454.

Hoke, A., Redett, R., Hameed, H., *et al.* (2006). Schwann cells express motor and sensory phenotypes that regulate axon regeneration. *J Neurosci* **26**, 9646–9655.

Hollmann, M., Hartley, M., and Heinemann, S. (1991). Ca^{2+} permeability of KA-AMPA-gated glutamate receptor channels depends on subunit composition. *Science* **252**, 851–853.

Holmes, G. (1907). On the relation between loss of function and structural change in focal lesions of the central nervous system, with special reference to secondary degeneration. *Brain* **29**, 514–523.

Holz, A., Schaeren-Wiemers, N., Schaefer, C., Pott, U., Colello, R. J., and Schwab, M. E. (1996). Molecular and developmental characterization of novel cDNAs of the myelin-associated/oligodendrocytic basic protein. *J Neurosci* **16**, 467–477.

Honke, K., Hirahara, Y., Dupree, J., *et al.* (2002). Paranodal junction formation and spermatogenesis require sulfoglycolipids. *Proc Natl Acad Sci USA* **99**, 4227–4232.

Hooper, D. C., Spitsin, S., Kean, R. B., *et al.* (1998). Uric acid, a natural scavenger of peroxynitrite, in experimental allergic encephalomyelitis and multiple sclerosis. *Proc Natl Acad Sci USA* **95**, 675–680.

Horky, L. L., Galimi, F., Gage, F. H., and Horner, P. J. (2006). Fate of endogenous stem/progenitor cells following spinal cord injury. *J Comp Neurol* **498**, 525–538.

Horner, P. J., Power, A. E., Kempermann, G., *et al.* (2000). Proliferation and differentiation of progenitor cells throughout the intact adult rat spinal cord. *J Neurosci* **20**, 2218–2228.

Horner, P. J., Thallmair, M., and Gage, F. H. (2002). Defining the NG2-expressing cell of the adult CNS. *J Neurocytol* **31**, 469–480.

Hortega, P. D. R. (1928). Tercera aportacion al cenocimiento morfologico e interpretacion funcional de la oligodendroglia. *Mem Real Soc Esp Hist Nat* **14**, 40–122.

van Horssen, J., Schreibelt, G., Bo, L., *et al.* (2006). NAD(P)H:quinone oxidoreductase 1 expression in multiple sclerosis lesions. *Free Radic Biol Med* **41**, 311–317.

Hovelmeyer, N., Hao, Z., Kranidioti, K., *et al.* (2005). Apoptosis of oligodendrocytes via Fas and TNF-R1 is a key event in the induction of experimental autoimmune encephalomyelitis. *J Immunol* **175**, 5875–5884.

Howe, C. L., Bieber, A. J., Warrington, A. E., Pease, L. R., and Rodriguez, M. (2004). Antiapoptotic signaling by a remyelination-promoting human antimyelin antibody. *Neurobiol Dis* **15**, 120–131.

Hsieh, S.-T., Kidd, G. J., Crawford, T. O., *et al.* (1994). Regional modulation of neurofilament organization by myelination in normal axons. *J Neurosci* **14**, 6392–6401.

Hu, Q. D., Ang, B. T., Karsak, M., *et al.* (2003). F3/contactin acts as a functional ligand for Notch during oligodendrocyte maturation. *Cell* **115**, 163–175.

Hu, X., Hicks, C. W., He, W., *et al.* (2006). Bace1 modulates myelination in the central and peripheral nervous system. *Nat Neurosci* **9**, 1520–1525.

Huang, J. K., Phillips, G. R., Roth, A. D., *et al.* (2005). Glial membranes at the node of Ranvier prevent neurite outgrowth. *Science* **310**, 1813–1817.

Huangfu, D., Maehr, R., Guo, W., *et al.* (2008). Induction of pluripotent stem cells by defined factors is greatly improved by small-molecule compounds. *Nat Biotechnol* **26**, 795–797.

Huber, A. B., Weinmann, O., Brosamle, C., Oertle, T., and Schwab, M. E. (2002). Patterns of Nogo mRNA and protein expression in the developing and adult rat and after CNS lesions. *J Neurosci* **22**, 3553–3567.

Hudson, L. D. (2003). Pelizaeus–Merzbacher disease and spastic paraplegia type 2: two faces of myelin loss from mutations in the same gene. *J Child Neurol* **18**, 616–624.

Hudson, L. D., Garbern, J. Y., and Kamholz, J. A. (2004). Pelizaeus–Merzbacher disease. In *Myelin Biology and Disorders*, R. A. Lazzarini, ed. (Amsterdam: Elsevier Academic Press), pp. 867–885.

Huitinga, I., Van Rooijen, N., De Groot, C. J., Uitdehaag, B. M., and Dijkstra, C. D. (1990). Suppression of experimental allergic encephalomyelitis in Lewis rats after elimination of macrophages. *J Exp Med* **172**, 1025–1033.

Hulsebosch, C. E. (2002). Recent advances in pathophysiology and treatment of spinal cord injury. *Adv Physiol Educ* **26**, 238–255.

Hulshof, S., Montagne, L., De Groot, C. J., and Van Der Valk, P. (2002). Cellular localization and expression patterns of interleukin-10, interleukin-4, and their receptors in multiple sclerosis lesions. *Glia* **38**, 24–35.

Husain, J. and Juurlink, B. H. (1995). Oligodendroglial precursor cell susceptibility to hypoxia is related to poor ability to cope with reactive oxygen species. *Brain Res* **698**, 86–94.

Huseby, E. S., Liggitt, D., Brabb, T., Schnabel, B., Ohlen, C., and Goverman, J. (2001). A pathogenic role for myelin-specific CD8(+) T cells in a model for multiple sclerosis. *J Exp Med* **194**, 669–676.

Ide, C., Tohyama, K., Yokota, R., Nitatori, T., and Onodera, S. (1983). Schwann cell basal lamina and nerve regeneration. *Brain Res* **288**, 61–75.

Iglesias, A., Bauer, J., Litzenburger, T., Schubart, A., and Linington, C. (2001). T- and B-cell responses to myelin oligodendrocyte glycoprotein in experimental autoimmune encephalomyelitis and multiple sclerosis. *Glia* **36**, 220–234.

Ikonomidou, C., Bosch, F., Miksa, M., *et al.* (1999). Blockade of NMDA receptors and apoptotic neurodegeneration in the developing brain. *Science* **283**, 70–74.

Inder, T. E., Anderson, N. J., Spencer, C., Wells, S., and Volpe, J. J. (2003). White matter injury in the premature infant: a comparison between serial cranial sonographic and MR findings at term. *AJNR Am J Neuroradiol* **24**, 805–809.

Inouye, H., Ganser, A. L., and Kirschner, D. A. (1985). Shiverer and normal peripheral myelin compared: basic protein localization, membrane interactions, and lipid composition. *J Neurochem* **45**, 1911–1922.

Irvine, K. A. and Blakemore, W. F. (2008). Remyelination protects axons from demyelination-associated axon degeneration. *Brain* **131**, 1464–1477.

Ishibashi, T., Dakin, K. A., Stevens, B., *et al.* (2006). Astrocytes promote myelination in response to electrical impulses. *Neuron* **49**, 823–832.

Ishibashi, T., Ding, L., Ikenaka, K., *et al.* (2004). Tetraspanin protein CD9 is a novel paranodal component regulating paranodal junctional formation. *J Neurosci* **24**, 96–102.

Itoh, T., Beesley, J., Itoh, A., *et al.* (2002). AMPA glutamate receptor-mediated calcium signaling is transiently enhanced during development of oligodendrocytes. *J Neurochem* **81**, 390–402.

Itoyama, Y., Ohnishi, A., Tateishi, J., Kuroiwa, Y., and Webster, H. D. (1985). Spinal cord multiple sclerosis lesions in Japanese patients: Schwann cell remyelination occurs in areas that lack glial fibrillary acidic protein (GFAP). *Acta Neuropathol Berl* **65**, 217–223.

Itoyama, Y., Sternberger, N. H., Webster, H. D., Quarles, R. H., Cohen, S. R., and Richardson, E. P., Jr. (1980). Immunocytochemical observations on the distribution of myelin associated glycoprotein and myelin basic protein in multiple sclerosis lesions. *Ann Neurol* **7**, 167–177.

Itoyama, Y., Webster, H. D., Richardson, E. P., Jr., and Trapp, B. D. (1983). Schwann cell remyelination of demyelinated axons in spinal cord multiple sclerosis lesions. *Ann Neurol* **14**, 339–346.

Jack, C., Antel, J. P., Bruck, W., and Kuhlmann, T. (2007). Contrasting potential of nitric oxide and peroxynitrite to mediate oligodendrocyte injury in multiple sclerosis. *Glia* **55**, 926–934.

Jacobs, J. M., Cavanagh, J. B., and Chen, F. C. K. (1972). Spinal subarachnoid injection of colchicine in rats. *J Neurol Sci* **17**, 461–480.

Jacobsen, M., Schweer, D., Ziegler, A., *et al.* (2000). A point mutation in PTPRC is associated with the development of multiple sclerosis. *Nat Genet* **26**, 495–499.

Jacobson, M. (1978). *Developmental Neurobiology* (New York: Plenum.)

Jahng, A. W., Maricic, I., Pedersen, B., *et al.* (2001). Activation of natural killer T cells potentiates or prevents experimental autoimmune encephalomyelitis. *J Exp Med* **194**, 1789–1799.

Jeffery, N. D. and Blakemore, W. F. (1997). Locomotor deficits induced by experimental spinal cord demyelination are abolished by spontaneous remyelination. *Brain* **120**, 27–37.

Jensen, A. M. and Chiu, S. Y. (1993). Expression of glutamate receptor genes in white matter: developing and adult rat optic nerve. *J Neurosci* **13**, 1664–1675.

Jessell, T. M. (2000). Neuronal specification in the spinal cord: inductive signals and transcriptional codes. *Nature Rev Genet* **1**, 20–29.

Jessen, K. R. and Mirsky, R. (2005a). The origin and development of glial cells in peripheral nerves. *Nat Rev Neurosci* **6**, 671–682.

Jessen, K. R. and Mirsky, R. (2005b). The Schwann cell lineage. In *Neuroglia*, H. Kettenmann and B. R. Ransom, eds. (New York: Oxford University Press), pp. 85–100.

Ji, B., Case, L. C., Liu, K., *et al.* (2008). Assessment of functional recovery and axonal sprouting in oligodendrocyte-myelin glycoprotein (OMgp) null mice after spinal cord injury. *Mol Cell Neurosci* **39**, 258–267.

Johansson, C. B., Youssef, S., Koleckar, K., *et al.* (2008). Extensive fusion of haematopoietic cells with Purkinje neurons in response to chronic inflammation. *Nat Cell Biol* **10**, 575–583.

John, G. R., Shankar, S. L., Shafit-Zagardo, B., *et al.* (2002). Multiple sclerosis: re-expression of a developmental pathway that restricts oligodendrocyte maturation. *Nat Med* **8**, 1115–1121.

Johns, T. G. and Bernard, C. C. (1997). Binding of complement component Clq to myelin oligodendrocyte glycoprotein: a novel mechanism for regulating CNS inflammation. *Mol Immunol* **34**, 33–38.

Johns, T. G. and Bernard, C. C. (1999). The structure and function of myelin oligodendrocyte glycoprotein. *J Neurochem* **72**, 1–9.

Johnson, P. W., Abramow-Newerly, W., Seilheimer, B., *et al.* (1989). Recombinant myelin-associated glycoprotein confers neural adhesion and neurite out-growth function. *Neuron* **3**, 377–385.

Joseph, N. M., Mukouyama, Y. S., Mosher, J. T., *et al.* (2004). Neural crest stem cells undergo multilineage differentiation in developing peripheral nerves to generate endoneurial fibroblasts in addition to Schwann cells. *Development* **131**, 5599–5612.

Jurewicz, A., Biddison, W. E., and Antel, J. P. (1998). MHC-Class I-restricted lysis of human oligodendrocytes by myelin basic protein peptide-specific CD8 T lymphocytes. *J Immunol* **160**, 3056–3059.

Jurewicz, A., Matysiak, M., Andrzejak, S., and Selmaj, K. (2006). TRAIL-induced cell death of human adult oligodendrocytes is mediated by JNK pathway. *Glia* **15**, 158–166.

Jurewicz, A., Matysiak, M., Tybor, K., Kilianek, L., Raine, C. S., and Selmaj, K. (2005). Tumor necrosis factor-induced death of adult human oligoden-drocytes is mediated by apoptosis inducing factor. *Brain* **128**, 2675–2688.

Jurewicz, A., Matysiak, M., Tybor, K., and Selmaj, K. (2003). TNF-induced death of adult human oligodendrocytes is mediated by c-jun NH(2)-terminal kinase-3. *Brain* **126**, 1358–1370.

Juurlink, B. J. H. (1997). Response of glial cells to ischemia: roles of reactive oxygen species and glutathione. *Neurosci Biobehav Rev* **21**, 151–166.

Juurlink, B. J. H., Thorburne, S. K., and Hertz, L. (1998). Peroxide-scavenging deficit underlies oligodendrocyte susceptibility to oxidative stress. *Glia* **22**, 371–378.

Kachar, B., Behar, T., and Dubois-Dalcq, M. (1986). Cell shape and motility of oligodendrocytes cultured without neurons. *Cell Tissue Res* **244**, 27–38.

Kadi, L., Selvaraju, R., de Lys, P., Proudfoot, A. E., Wells, T. N., and Boschert, U. (2006). Differential effects of chemokines on oligodendrocyte precursor proliferation and myelin formation in vitro. *J Neuroimmunol* **174**, 133–146.

Kagawa, T., Ikenaka, K., Inoue, Y., *et al.* (1994). Glial cell degeneration and hypomyelination caused by overexpression of myelin proteolipid protein gene. *Neuron* **13**, 427–442.

Kagawa, T., Mekada, E., Shishido, Y., and Ikenaka, K. (1997). Immune system-related CD9 is expressed in mouse central nervous system myelin at a very late stage of myelination. *J Neurosci Res* **50**, 312–320.

Kaindl, A. M. and Ikonomidou, C. (2007). Glutamate antagonists are neurotoxins for the developing brain. *Neurotox Res* **11**, 203–218.

Kakulas, B. A. (1999). A review of the neuropathology of human spinal cord injury with emphasis on special features. *J Spinal Cord Med* **22**, 119–124.

Kamasawa, N., Sik, A., Morita, M., *et al.* (2005). Connexin-47 and connexin-32 in gap junctions of oligodendrocyte somata, myelin sheaths, paranodal loops and Schmidt–Lanterman incisures: implications for ionic homeostasis and potassium siphoning. *Neuroscience* **136**, 65–86.

Kanwar, J. R., Kanwar, R. K., and Krissansen, G. W. (2004). Simultaneous neuro-protection and blockade of inflammation reverses autoimmune encephalo-myelitis. *Brain* **127**, 1313–1331.

Kaplan, M. R., Cho, M. H., Ullian, E. M., Isom, L. L., Levinson, S. R., and Barres, B. A. (2001). Differential control of clustering of the sodium channels Na(v)1.2 and Na(v)1.6 at developing CNS nodes of Ranvier. *Neuron* **30**, 105–119.

Kaplan, M. R., Meyer-Franke, A., Lambert, S., *et al.* (1997). Induction of sodium channel clustering by oligodendrocytes. *Nature* **386**, 724–728.

Kapsimali, M., Kloosterman, W. P., de Bruijn, E., Rosa, F., Plasterk, R. H., and Wilson, S. W. (2007). MicroRNAs show a wide diversity of expression profiles in the developing and mature central nervous system. *Genome Biol* **8**, R173.

Karadottir, R. and Attwell, D. (2007). Neurotransmitter receptors in the life and death of oligodendrocytes. *Neuroscience* **145**, 1426–1438.

Karadottir, R., Cavelier, P., Bergersen, L. H., and Attwell, D. (2005). NMDA receptors are expressed in oligodendrocytes and activated in ischaemia. *Nature* **438**, 1162–1166.

Karadottir, R., Hamilton, N. B., Bakiri, Y., and Attwell, D. (2008). Spiking and nonspiking classes of oligodendrocyte precursor glia in CNS white matter. *Nat Neurosci* **11**, 450–456.

Karimi-Abdolrezaee, S., Eftekharpour, E., and Fehlings, M. G. (2004). Temporal and spatial patterns of Kv1.1 and Kv1.2 protein and gene expression in spinal cord white matter after acute and chronic spinal cord injury in rats: implications for axonal pathophysiology after neurotrauma. *Eur J Neurosci* **19**, 577–589.

Karimi-Abdolrezaee, S., Eftekharpour, E., Wang, J., Morshead, C. M., and Fehlings, M. G. (2006). Delayed transplantation of adult neural precursor cells promotes remyelination and functional neurological recovery after spinal cord injury. *J Neurosci* **26**, 3377–3389.

Karoutzou, G., Emrich, H. M., and Dietrich, D. E. (2008). The myelin-pathogenesis puzzle in schizophrenia: a literature review. *Mol Psychiatry* **13**, 245–260.

Kassis, I., Grigoriadis, N., Gowda-Kurkalli, B., et al. (2008). Neuroprotection and immunomodulation with mesenchymal stem cells in chronic experimental autoimmune encephalomyelitis. *Arch Neurol* **65**, 753–761.

Kassmann, C. M., Lappe-Siefke, C., Baes, M., et al. (2007). Axonal loss and neuro-inflammation caused by peroxisome-deficient oligodendrocytes. *Nat Genet* **39**, 969–976.

Kato, T., Kakiuchi, C., and Iwamoto, K. (2007). Comprehensive gene expression analysis in bipolar disorder. *Can J Psychiatry* **52**, 763–771.

Keirstead, H. S., Hasan, S. J., Muir, G. D., and Steeves, J. D. (1992). Suppression of the onset of myelination extends the permissive period for the functional repair of embryonic spinal cord. *Proc Natl Acad Sci USA* **89**, 11664–11668.

Keirstead, H. S., Nistor, G., Bernal, G., et al. (2005). Human embryonic stem cell-derived oligodendrocyte progenitor cell transplants remyelinate and restore locomotion after spinal cord injury. *J Neurosci* **25**, 4694–4705.

Kelland, E. E. and Toms, N. J. (2001). Group I metabotropic glutamate receptors limit AMPA receptor-mediated oligodendrocyte progenitor cell death. *Eur J Pharmacol* **424**, R3–R4.

Kelm, S., Pelz, A., Schauer, R., et al. (1994). Sialoadhesin, myelin-associated glycoprotein and CD22 define a new family of sialic acid-dependent adhesion molecules of the immunoglobulin superfamily. *Curr Biol* **4**, 965–972.

Kerlero de Rosbo, N., Hoffman, M., Mendel, I., et al. (1997). Predominance of the autoimmune response to myelin oligodendrocyte glycoprotein in multiple sclerosis: reactivity to the extracellular domain of MOG is directed against three main regions. *Eur J Immunol* **27**, 3059–3069.

Kerlero de Rosbo, N., Milo, R., Lees, M. B., Burger, D., Bernard, C. C., and Ben Nun, A. (1993). Reactivity to myelin antigens in multiple sclerosis. Peripheral blood lymphocytes respond predominantly to myelin oligodendrocyte glycoprotein. *J Clin Invest* **92**, 2602–2608.

Kerschensteiner, M., Gallmeier, E., Behrens, L., et al. (1999). Activated human T cells, B cells, and monocytes produce brain-derived neurotrophic factor in vitro and in inflammatory brain lesions: a neuroprotective role of inflammation? *J Exp Med* **189**, 865–870.

Kerschensteiner, M., Meinl, E., and Hohlfeld, R. (2009). Neuro-immune crosstalk in CNS diseases. *Neuroscience* **158**, 1122–1132.

Kessaris, N., Fogarty, M., Iannarelli, P., Grist, M., Wegner, M., and Richardson, W. D. (2006). Competing waves of oligodendrocytes in the forebrain and postnatal elimination of an embryonic lineage. *Nat Neurosci* **9**, 173–179.

Kessaris, N., Pringle, N., and Richardson, W. D. (2008). Specification of CNS glia from neural stem cells in the embryonic neuroepithelium. *Philos Trans R Soc Lond B Biol Sci* **363**, 71–85.

Kettenmann, H. and Ransom, B. R. (2005). The concept of neuroglia: a historical perspective. In *Neuroglia*, H. Kettenmann and B. R. Ransom, eds. (New York: Oxford University Press), pp. 1–16.

Kettenmann, H. and Verkhratsky, A. (2008). Neuroglia: the 150 years after. *Trends Neurosci* **31**, 653–659.

Kidd, G. J., Andrews, S. B., and Trapp, B. D. (1996). Axons regulate the distribution of Schwann cell microtubules. *J Neurosci* **16**, 946–954.

Kidd, G. J., Hauer, P. E., and Trapp, B. D. (1990). Axons modulate myelin protein messenger RNA levels during central nervous system myelination in vivo. *J Neurosci Res* **26**, 409–418.

Kidd, G. J., Yadav, V. K., Huang, P., *et al.* (2006). A dual tyrosine-leucine motif mediates myelin protein P0 targeting in MDCK cells. *Glia* **54**, 135–145.

Kierstead, H. S. and Blakemore, W. F. (1997). Identification of post-mitotic oligodendrocytes incapable of remyelination within the demyelinated adult spinal cord. *J Neuropathol Exp Neurol* **56**, 1191–1201.

Kim, H. J., DiBernardo, A. B., Sloane, J. A., *et al.* (2006). WAVE1 is required for oligodendrocyte morphogenesis and normal CNS myelination. *J Neurosci* **26**, 5849–5859.

Kim, J. E., Krichevsky, A., Grad, Y., *et al.* (2004a). Identification of many microRNAs that copurify with polyribosomes in mammalian neurons. *Proc Natl Acad Sci USA* **101**, 360–365.

Kim, J. E., Li, S., GrandPre, T., Qiu, D., and Strittmatter, S. M. (2003). Axon regeneration in young adult mice lacking Nogo-A/B. *Neuron* **38**, 187–199.

Kim, J. E., Liu, B. P., Park, J. H., and Strittmatter, S. M. (2004b). Nogo-66 receptor prevents raphespinal and rubrospinal axon regeneration and limits functional recovery from spinal cord injury. *Neuron* **44**, 439–451.

Kim, S. U., Moretto, G., and Shin, D. H. (1985). Expression of Ia antigens on the surface of human oligodendrocytes and astrocytes in culture. *J Neuroimmunol* **10**, 141–149.

Kim, Y. J., Park, H. J., Lee, G., *et al.* (2009). Neuroprotective effects of human mesenchymal stem cells on dopaminergic neurons through anti-inflammatory action. *Glia* **57**, 13–23.

Kimelberg, H. K., Goderie, S. K., Higman, S., Pang, S., and Waniewski, R. A. (1990). Swelling-induced release of glutamate, aspartate, and taurine from astrocyte cultures. *J Neurosci* **10**, 1583–1591.

Kimura, H., Weisz, A., Kurashima, Y., *et al.* (2000). Hypoxia response element of the human vascular endothelial growth factor gene mediates transcriptional regulation by nitric oxide: control of hypoxia-inducible factor-1 activity by nitric oxide. *Blood* **95**, 189–197.

Kimura, M., Sato, M., Akatsuka, A., *et al.* (1989). Restoration of myelin formation by a single type of myelin basic protein in transgenic shiverer mice. *Proc Natl Acad Sci USA* **86**, 5661–5665.

Kinney, H. C. and Volpe, J. J. (2009). Perinatal panencephalopathy in premature infants: is it due to hypoxia-ischemia? In *Brain Hypoxia and Ischemia*, (Totowa, NJ: Humana Press).

Kinney, H. C., Brody, B. A., Kloman, A. S., and Gilles, F. H. (1988). Sequence of central nervous system myelination in human infancy. *J Neuropathol Exp Neurol* **47**, 217–234.

Kinney, H. C., Panigrahy, A., Newburger, J. W., Jonas, R. A., and Sleeper, L. A. (2005). Hypoxic-ischemic brain injury in infants with congenital heart disease dying after cardiac surgery. *Acta Neuropathol* **110**, 563–578.

Kirby, B. B., Takada, N., Latimer, A. J., *et al.* (2006). In vivo time-lapse imaging shows dynamic oligodendrocyte progenitor behavior during zebrafish development. *Nat Neurosci* **9**, 1506–1511.

Kirkpatrick, L. L., Witt, A. S., Payne, H. R., Shine, H. D., and Brady, S. T. (2001). Changes in microtubule stability and density in myelin-deficient shiverer mouse CNS axons. *J Neurosci* **21**, 2288–2297.

Kirschner, D. A. and Ganser, A. L. (1980). Compact myelin exists in the absence of basic protein in the shiverer mutant mouse. *Nature* **283**, 207–210.

Kitada, M. and Rowitch, D. H. (2006). Transcription factor co-expression patterns indicate heterogeneity of oligodendroglial subpopulations in adult spinal cord. *Glia* **54**, 35–46.

Kleopa, K. A., Orthmann, J. L., Enriquez, A., Paul, D. L., and Scherer, S. S. (2004). Unique distributions of the gap junction proteins connexin29, connexin32, and connexin47 in oligodendrocytes. *Glia* **47**, 346–357.

Klugmann, M., Schwab, M. H., Puhlhofer, A., *et al.* (1997). Assembly of CNS myelin in the absence of proteolipid protein. *Neuron* **18**, 59–70.

Koch, T., Brugger, T., Bach, A., Gennarini, G., and Trotter, J. (1997). Expression of the immunoglobulin superfamily cell adhesion molecule F3 by oligodendrocyte-lineage cells. *Glia* **19**, 199–212.

Kocsis, J. D. and Waxman, S. G. (2007). Schwann cells and their precursors for repair of central nervous system myelin. *Brain* **130**, 1978–1980.

Kohama, I., Lankford, K. L., Preiningerova, J., White, F. A., Vollmer, T. L., and Kocsis, J. D. (2001). Transplantation of cryopreserved adult human Schwann cells enhances axonal conduction in demyelinated spinal cord. *J Neurosci* **21**, 944–950.

Kondo, T. and Raff, M. (2000). Oligodendrocyte precursor cells reprogrammed to become multipotential CNS stem cells [see comments]. *Science* **289**, 1754–1757.

Korbling, M. and Estrov, Z. (2003). Adult stem cells for tissue repair. *N Engl J Med* **349**, 570–582.

Kordeli, E., Davis, J. D., Trapp, B. D., and Bennett, V. (1990). An isoform of ankyrin is localized at nodes of Ranvier in myelinated axons of central and peripheral nerves. *J Cell Biol* **110**, 1341–1352.

Kordeli, E., Lambert, S., and Bennett, V. (1995). AnkyrinG. A new ankyrin gene with neural-specific isoforms localized at the axonal initial segment and node of Ranvier. *J Biol Chem* **270**, 2352–2359.

Kornek, B., Storch, M. K., Weissert, R., *et al.* (2000). Multiple sclerosis and chronic autoimmune encephalomyelitis: a comparative quantitative study of axonal injury in active, inactive, and remyelinated lesions. *Am J Pathol* **157**, 267–276.

Koticha, D., Maurel, P., Zanazzi, G., *et al.* (2006). Neurofascin interactions play a critical role in clustering sodium channels, ankyrin G and beta IV spectrin at peripheral nodes of Ranvier. *Dev Biol* **293**, 1–12.

Kotter, M. R., Li, W. W., Zhao, C., and Franklin, R. J. (2006). Myelin impairs CNS remyelination by inhibiting oligodendrocyte precursor cell differentiation. *J Neurosci* **26**, 328–332.

Kotter, M. R., Setzu, A., Sim, F. J., Van Rooijen, N., and Franklin, R. J. (2001). Macrophage depletion impairs oligodendrocyte remyelination following lysolecithin-induced demyelination. *Glia* **35**, 204–212.

Kottis, V., Thibault, P., Mikol, D., *et al.* (2002). Oligodendrocyte-myelin glycoprotein (OMgp) is an inhibitor of neurite outgrowth. *J Neurochem* **82**, 1566–1569.

Kramer, E. M., Schardt, A., and Nave, K. A. (2001). Membrane traffic in myelinating oligodendrocytes. *Microsc Res Tech* **52**, 656–671.

Krammer, P. H. (1999). CD95(APO-1/Fas)-mediated apoptosis: live and let die. *Adv Immunol* **71**, 163–210.

Krause, G., Winkler, L., Mueller, S. L., Haseloff, R. F., Piontek, J., and Blasig, I. E. (2008). Structure and function of claudins. *Biochim Biophys Acta* **1778**, 631–645.

Kress, G. J., Dineley, K. E., and Reynolds, I. J. (2002). The relationship between intracellular free iron and cell injury in cultured neurons, astrocytes, and oligodendrocytes. *J Neurosci* **22**, 5848–5855.

Krichevsky, A. M., King, K. S., Donahue, C. P., Khrapko, K., and Kosik, K. S. (2003). A microRNA array reveals extensive regulation of microRNAs during brain development. *RNA* **9**, 1274–1281.

Kroepfl, J. F. and Gardinier, M. V. (2001). Mutually exclusive apicobasolateral sorting of two oligodendroglial membrane proteins, proteolipid protein and myelin/oligodendrocyte glycoprotein, in Madin-Darby canine kidney cells. *J Neurosci Res* **66**, 1140–1148.

Kroepfl, J. F., Viise, L. R., Charron, A. J., Linington, C., and Gardinier, M. V. (1996). Investigation of myelin/oligodendrocyte glycoprotein membrane topology. *J Neurochem* **67**, 2219–2222.

Kuhlmann, T., Lucchinetti, C., Zettl, U. K., Bitsch, A., Lassmann, H., and Brück, W. (1999). Bcl-2-expressing oligodendrocytes in multiple sclerosis lesions. *Glia* **28**, 34–39.

Kuhlmann, T., Miron, V., Cuo, Q., Wegner, C., Antel, J., and Bruck, W. (2008). Differentiation block of oligodendroglial progenitor cells as a cause for remyelination failure in chronic multiple sclerosis. *Brain* **131**, 1749–1758.

Kuhlmann, T., Wendling, U., Nolte, C., *et al.* (2002). Differential regulation of myelin phagocytosis by macrophages/microglia: involvement of target myelin, Fc receptors and activation by intravenous immunoglobulins. *J Neurosci Res* **67**, 185–190.

Kukley, M., Capetillo-Zarate, E., and Dietrich, D. (2007). Vesicular glutamate release from axons in white matter. *Nat Neurosci* **10**, 311–320.

Kukley, M., Kiladze, M., Tognatta, R., *et al.* (2008). Glial cells are born with synapses. *FASEB J* **22**, 2957–2969.

Kuner, T. and Schoepfer, R. (1996). Multiple structural elements determine subunit specificity of Mg^{2+} block in NMDA receptor channels. *J Neurosci* **16**, 3549–3558.

Kutzelnigg, A., Lucchinetti, C. F., Stadelmann, C., *et al.* (2005). Cortical demyelination and diffuse white matter injury in multiple sclerosis. *Brain* **128**, 2705–2712.

Kwiatkowski, D. J. (1999). Functions of gelsolin: motility, signaling, apoptosis, cancer. *Curr Opin Cell Biol* **11**, 103–108.

Kwiecien, J. M., O'Connor, L. T., Goetz, B. D., Delaney, K. H., Fletch, A. L., and Duncan, I. D. (1998). Morphological and morphometric studies of the dysmyelinating mutant, the Long Evans shaker rat. *J Neurocytol* **27**, 581–591.

Kwon, B. K., Oxland, T. R., and Tetzlaff, W. (2002). Animal models used in spinal cord regeneration research. *Spine (Phila Pa 1976)* **27**, 1504–1510.

Laabs, T., Carulli, D., Geller, H. M., and Fawcett, J. W. (2005). Chondroitin sulfate proteoglycans in neural development and regeneration. *Curr Opin Neurobiol* **15**, 116–120.

Labauge, P., Fogli, A., Niel, F., Rodriguez, D., and Boespflug-Tanguy, O. (2007). [CACH/VWM syndrome and leucodystrophies related to EIF2B mutations.] *Rev Neurol (Paris)* **163**, 793–799.

Lacas-Gervais, S., Guo, J., Strenzke, N., *et al.* (2004). BetaIVSigma1 spectrin stabilizes the nodes of Ranvier and axon initial segments. *J Cell Biol* **166**, 983–990.

Lachance, C., Arbour, N., Cashman, N. R., and Talbot, P. J. (1998). Involvement of aminopeptidase N (CD13) in infection of human neural cells by human coronavirus 229E. *J Virol* **72**, 6511–6519.

Lagos-Quintana, M., Rauhut, R., Yalcin, A., Meyer, J., Lendeckel, W., and Tuschl, T. (2002). Identification of tissue-specific microRNAs from mouse. *Curr Biol* **12**, 735–739.

Lampasona, V., Franciotta, D., Furlan, R., *et al.* (2004). Similar low frequency of anti-MOG IgG and IgM in MS patients and healthy subjects. *Neurology* **62**, 2092–2094.

Langford, L. A., Porter, S., and Bunge, R. P. (1988). Immortalized rat Schwann cells produce tumours in vivo. *J Neurocytol* **17**, 521–529.

Lappe-Siefke, C., Goebbels, S., Gravel, M., *et al.* (2003). Disruption of Cnp1 uncouples oligodendroglial functions in axonal support and myelination. *Nat Genet* **33**, 366–374.

Lasiene, J., Matsui, A., Sawa, Y., Wong, F., and Horner, P. J. (2009). Age-related myelin dynamics revealed by increased oligodendrogenesis and short internodes. *Aging Cell* **8**, 201–213.

Lassmann, H. (1983). *Comparative Neuropathology of Chronic Experimental Allergic Encephalomyelitis and Multiple Sclerosis* (Berlin: Springer-Verlag).

Lassmann, H. (2003). Axonal injury in multiple sclerosis. *J Neurol Neurosurg Psychiatry* **74**, 695–697.

Lassmann, H., Brück, W., Lucchinetti, C., and Rodriguez, M. (1997). Remyelination in multiple sclerosis. *Mult Scler* **3**, 133–136.

Lavdas, A., Franceschini, I., Dubois-Dalcq, M., and Matsas, R. (2006). Schwann cells genetically engineered to express PSA show enhanced migratory potential without impairment of their myelinating ability in vitro. *Glia* **53**, 868–878.

Lavdas, A. A., Papastefanaki, F., Thomaidou, D., and Matsas, R. (2008). Schwann cell transplantation for CNS repair. *Curr Med Chem* **15**, 151–160.

Le Douarin, N. M. and Smith, J. (1988). Development of the peripheral nervous system from the neural crest. *Annu Rev Cell Biol* **4**, 375–404.

Lee, J., Gravel, M., Zhang, R., Thibault, P., and Braun, P. E. (2005). Process outgrowth in oligodendrocytes is mediated by CNP, a novel microtubule assembly myelin protein. *J Cell Biol* **170**, 661–673.

Lee, K. K., de Repentigny, Y., Saulnier, R., Rippstein, P., Macklin, W. B., and Kothary, R. (2006). Dominant-negative beta1 integrin mice have region-specific myelin defects accompanied by alterations in MAPK activity. *Glia* **53**, 836–844.

Lee, R. C., Feinbaum, R. L., and Ambros, V. (1993). The *C. elegans* heterochronic gene lin-4 encodes small RNAs with antisense complementarity to lin-14. *Cell* **75**, 843–854.

Lee, S. C. and Raine, C. S. (1989). Multiple sclerosis: oligodendrocytes in active lesions do not express class II major histocompatibility complex molecules. *J Neuroimmunol* **25**, 261–266.

Lee, X., Yang, Z., Shao, Z., *et al.* (2007). NGF regulates the expression of axonal LINGO-1 to inhibit oligodendrocyte differentiation and myelination. *J Neurosci* **27**, 220–225.

Leegwater, P. A., Vermeulen, G., Konst, A. A., *et al.* (2001). Subunits of the translation initiation factor eIF2B are mutant in leukoencephalopathy with vanishing white matter. *Nat Genet* **29**, 383–388.

Lees, M. B. (1998). A history of proteolipids: a personal memoir. *Neurochem Res* **23**, 261–271.

Legrand, C., Ferraz, C., Clavel, M. C., and Rabie, A. (1986). Immunocytochemical localisation of gelsolin in oligodendroglia of the developing rabbit central nervous system. *Brain Res* **395**, 231–235.

Lemke, G. (1986). Molecular biology of the major myelin genes. *Trends Neurosci* **96**, 266–270.

Lena, J. Y., Legrand, C., Faivre-Sarrailh, C., Sarlieve, L. L., Ferraz, C., and Rabie, A. (1994). High gelsolin content of developing oligodendrocytes. *Int J Dev Neurosci* **12**, 375–386.

Lennon, V. A., Wingerchuk, D. M., Kryzer, T. J., *et al.* (2004). A serum autoantibody marker of neuromyelitis optica: distinction from multiple sclerosis. *Lancet* **364**, 2106–2112.

Leocani, L., Rovaris, M., Boneschi, F. M., *et al.* (2006). Multimodal evoked potentials to assess the evolution of multiple sclerosis: a longitudinal study. *J Neurol Neurosurg Psychiatry* **77**, 1030–1035.

Lepore, A. C. and Fischer, I. (2005). Lineage-restricted neural precursors survive, migrate, and differentiate following transplantation into the injured adult spinal cord. *Exp Neurol* **194**, 230–242.

Leuchtmann, E. A., Ratner, A. E., Vijitruth, R., Qu, Y., and McDonald, J. W. (2003). AMPA receptors are the major mediators of excitotoxic death in mature oligodendrocytes. *Neurobiol Dis* **14**, 336–348.

Levi, A. D. O. and Bunge, R. P. (1994). Studies of myelin formation after transplantation of human Schwann cells into the severe combined immunodeficient mouse. *Exp Neurol* **130**, 41–52.

Levine, J. M. and Reynolds, R. (1999). Activation and proliferation of endogenous oligodendrocyte precursor cells during ethidium bromide-induced demyelination. *Exp Neurol* **160**, 333–347.

Levine, J. M., Reynolds, R., and Fawcett, J. W. (2001). The oligodendrocyte precursor cell in health and disease. *Trends Neurosci* **24**, 39–47.

Levine, J. M., Stincone, F., and Lee, Y. S. (1993). Development and differentiation of glial precursor cells in the rat cerebellum. *Glia* **7**, 307–321.

Leviton, A. and Gilles, F. H. (1973). An epidemiologic study of perinatal telencephalic leucoencephalopathy in an autopsy population. *J Neurol Sci* **18**, 53–66.

Li, C., Tropak, M. B., Gerlai, R., *et al.* (1994). Myelination in the absence of myelin-associated glycoprotein. *Nature* **369**, 747–750.

Li, G. L., Brodin, G., Farooque, M., *et al.* (1996). Apoptosis and expression of Bcl-2 after compression trauma to rat spinal cord. *J Neuropathol Exp Neurol* **55**, 280–289.

Li, J., Baud, O., Vartanian, T., Volpe, J. J., and Rosenberg, P. A. (2005). Peroxynitrite generated by inducible nitric oxide synthetase and NADPH oxidase mediates microglia toxicity to oligodendrocytes. *Proc Natl Acad Sci USA* **102**, 9936–9941.

Li, J., Hertzberg, E. L., and Nagy, J. I. (1997). Connexin32 in oligodendrocytes and association with myelinated fibers in mouse and rat brain. *J Comp Neurol* **379**, 571–591.

Li, M., Shibata, A., Li, C., *et al.* (1996). Myelin-associated glycoprotein inhibits neurite/axon growth and causes growth cone collapse. *J Neurosci Res* **46**, 404–414.

Li, S., Kim, J. E., Budel, S., Hampton, T. G., and Strittmatter, S. M. (2005). Transgenic inhibition of Nogo-66 receptor function allows axonal sprouting and improved locomotion after spinal injury. *Mol Cell Neurosci* **29**, 26–39.

Li, S., Liu, B. P., Budel, S., *et al.* (2004). Blockade of Nogo-66, myelin-associated glycoprotein, and oligodendrocyte myelin glycoprotein by soluble Nogo-66 receptor promotes axonal sprouting and recovery after spinal injury. *J Neurosci* **24**, 10511–10520.

Li, S. and Strittmatter, S. M. (2003). Delayed systemic Nogo-66 receptor antagonist promotes recovery from spinal cord injury. *J Neurosci* **23**, 4219–4227.

Li, S., Mealing, G. A., Morley, P., and Stys, P. K. (1999). Novel injury mechanism in anoxia and trauma of spinal cord white matter: glutamate release via reverse Na$^+$-dependent glutamate transport. *J Neurosci* **19**, RC16.

Li, W., Maeda, Y., Ming, X., *et al.* (2002). Apoptotic death following Fas activation in human oligodendrocyte hybrid cultures. *J Neurosci Res* **69**, 189–196.

Li, Y., Chen, J., Chen, X. G., *et al.* (2002). Human marrow stromal cell therapy for stroke in rat: neurotrophins and functional recovery. *Neurology* **59**, 514–523.

Li, Y., Chen, J., Wang, L., Lu, M., and Chopp, M. (2001a). Treatment of stroke in rat with intracarotid administration of marrow stromal cells. *Neurology* **56**, 1666–1672.

Li, Y., Chen, J., Wang, L., Zhang, L., Lu, M., and Chopp, M. (2001b). Intracerebral transplantation of bone marrow stromal cells in a 1-methyl-4-phenyl-1,2,3,6-tetrahydropyridine mouse model of Parkinson's disease. *Neurosci Lett* **316**, 67–70.

Li, Y., Chen, J., Zhang, C. L., *et al.* (2005). Gliosis and brain remodeling after treatment of stroke in rats with marrow stromal cells. *Glia* **49**, 407–417.

Li, Y., Field, P. M., and Raisman, G. (1997). Repair of adult rat corticospinal tract by transplants of olfactory ensheathing cells. *Science* **277**, 2000–2002.

Liebscher, T., Schnell, L., Schnell, D., *et al.* (2005). Nogo-A antibody improves regeneration and locomotion of spinal cord-injured rats. *Ann Neurol* **58**, 706–719.

Lin, S. C. and Bergles, D. E. (2004). Synaptic signaling between neurons and glia. *Glia* **47**, 290–298.

Lin, W., Bailey, S. L., Ho, H., *et al.* (2007). The integrated stress response prevents demyelination by protecting oligodendrocytes against immune-mediated damage. *J Clin Invest* **117**, 448–456.

Lin, W., Kemper, A., Dupree, J. L., Harding, H. P., Ron, D., and Popko, B. (2006). Interferon-gamma inhibits central nervous system remyelination through a process modulated by endoplasmic reticulum stress. *Brain* **129**, 1306–1318.

Linington, C., Bradl, M., Lassmann, H., Brunner, C., and Vass, K. (1988). Augmentation of demyelination in rat acute allergic encephalomyelitis by circulating mouse monoclonal antibodies directed against a myelin/oligodendrocyte glycoprotein. *Am J Pathol* **130**, 443–454.

Linington, C., Engelhardt, B., Kapocs, G., and Lassmann, H. (1992). Induction of persistently demyelinated lesions in the rat following the repeated adoptive transfer of encephalitogenic T cells and demyelinating antibody. *J Neuroimmunol* **40**, 219–224.

Linington, C., Lassmann, H., Morgan, B. P., and Compston, D. A. S. (1989). Immunohistochemical localization of terminal complement component C9 in experimental allergic encephalomyelitis. *Acta Neuropathol* **79**, 78–85.

Linnington, C., Webb, M., and Woodhams, P. L. (1984). A novel myelin-associated glycoprotein defined by a mouse monoclonal antibody. *J Neuroimmunol* **6**, 387–396.

Lipton, S. A. (1986). Blockade of electrical-activity promotes the death of mammalian retinal ganglion-cells in culture. *Proc Natl Acad Sci USA* **83**, 9774–9778.

Lipton, S. A. and Rosenberg, P. A. (1994). Mechanisms of disease: excitatory amino acids as a final common pathway for neurologic disorders. *N Engl J Med* **330**, 613–622.

Liu, B. P., Cafferty, W. B., Budel, S. O., and Strittmatter, S. M. (2006a). Extracellular regulators of axonal growth in the adult central nervous system. *Philos Trans R Soc Lond B Biol Sci* **361**, 1593–1610.

Liu, B. P., Fournier, A., GrandPre, T., and Strittmatter, S. M. (2002). Myelin-associated glycoprotein as a functional ligand for the Nogo-66 receptor. *Science* **297**, 1190–1193.

Liu, D., Liu, J., Sun, D., Alcock, N. W., and Wen, J. (2003). Spinal cord injury increases iron levels: catalytic production of hydroxyl radicals. *Free Radic Biol Med* **34**, 64–71.

Liu, D., Liu, J., and Wen, J. (1999). Elevation of hydrogen peroxide after spinal cord injury detected by using the Fenton reaction. *Free Radic Biol Med* **27**, 478–482.

Liu, J., Marino, M. W., Wong, G., *et al.* (1998). TNF is a potent anti-inflammatory cytokine in autoimmune-mediated demyelination. *Nat Med* **4**, 78–83.

Liu, J. S., Zhao, M. L., Brosnan, C. F., and Lee, S. C. (2001). Expression of inducible nitric oxide synthase and nitrotyrosine in multiple sclerosis lesions. *Am J Pathol* **158**, 2057–2066.

Liu, X. Z., Xu, X. M., Hu, R., *et al.* (1997). Neuronal and glial apoptosis after traumatic spinal cord injury. *J Neurosci* **17**, 5395–5406.

Liu, Y., Hao, W., Letiembre, M., *et al.* (2006b). Suppression of microglial inflammatory activity by myelin phagocytosis: role of p47-PHOX-mediated generation of reactive oxygen species. *J Neurosci* **26**, 12904–12913.

Lobsiger, C. S., Schweitzer, B., Taylor, V., and Suter, U. (2000). Platelet-derived growth factor-BB supports the survival of cultured rat Schwann cell precursors in synergy with neurotrophin-3. *Glia* **30**, 290–300.

Loeliger, M., Watson, C. S., Reynolds, J. D., *et al.* (2003). Extracellular glutamate levels and neuropathology in cerebral white matter following repeated umbilical cord occlusion in the near term fetal sheep. *Neuroscience* **116**, 705–714.

Loevner, L. A., Shapiro, R. M., Grossman, R. I., Overhauser, J., and Kamholz, J. (1996). White matter changes associated with deletions of the long arm of chromosome 18 (18q- syndrome): a dysmyelinating disorder? *AJNR Am J Neuroradiol* **17**, 1843–1848.

Lohse, D. C., Senter, H. J., Kauer, J. S., and Wohns, R. (1980). Spinal cord blood flow in experimental transient traumatic paraplegia. *J Neurosurg* **52**, 335–345.

Lopez-Munoz, F., Boya, J., and Alamo, C. (2006). Neuron theory, the cornerstone of neuroscience, on the centenary of the Nobel Prize award to Santiago Ramón y Cajal. *Brain Res Bull* **70**, 391–405.

LoPresti, P., Szuchet, S., Papasozomenos, S. C., Zinkowski, R. P., and Binder, L. I. (1995). Functional implications for the microtubule-associated protein tau: localization in oligodendrocytes. *Proc Natl Acad Sci USA* **92**, 10369–10373.

Love, S. (2006). Demyelinating diseases. *J Clin Pathol* **59**, 1151–1159.

Low, K., Culbertson, M., Bradke, F., Tessier-Lavigne, M., and Tuszynski, M. H. (2008). Netrin-1 is a novel myelin-associated inhibitor to axon growth. *J Neurosci* **28**, 1099–1108.

Low, S. H., Roche, P. A., Anderson, H. A., *et al.* (1998). Targeting of SNAP-23 and SNAP-25 in polarized epithelial cells. *J Biol Chem* **273**, 3422–3430.

Lu, Q. R., Sun, T., Zhu, Z., *et al.* (2002). Common developmental requirement for Olig function indicates a motor neuron/oligodendrocyte connection. *Cell* **109**, 75–86.

Lu, Q. R., Yuk, D., Alberta, J. A., *et al.* (2000). Sonic hedgehog – regulated oligodendrocyte lineage genes encoding bHLH proteins in the mammalian central nervous system. *Neuron* **25**, 317–329.

Lucchinetti, C., Brück, W., Parisi, J., Scheithauer, B., Rodriguez, M., and Lassmann, H. (1999). A quantitative analysis of oligodendrocytes in multiple sclerosis lesions. A study of 113 cases. *Brain* **122**, 2279–2295.

Lucchinetti, C., Brück, W., Parisi, J., Scheithauer, B., Rodriguez, M., and Lassmann, H. (2000). Heterogeneity of multiple sclerosis lesions: implications for the pathogenesis of demyelination. *Ann Neurol* **47**, 707–717.

Lucchinetti, C. F., Brück, W., Rodriguez, M., and Lassmann, H. (1996). Distinct patterns of multiple sclerosis pathology indicates heterogeneity in pathogenesis. *Brain Pathol* **6**, 259–274.

Lucchinetti, C. F., Mandler, R. N., McGavern, D., *et al.* (2002). A role for humoral mechanisms in the pathogenesis of Devic's neuromyelitis optica. *Brain* **125**, 1450–1461.

Luduena, R. F. (1998). Multiple forms of tubulin: different gene products and covalent modifications. *Int Rev Cytol* **178**, 207–275.

Ludwin, S. K. (1980). Chronic demyelination inhibits remyelination of the central nervous system. *Lab Invest* **43**, 382–387.

Ludwin, S. K. (1988). Remyelination in the central nervous system and the peripheral nervous system. *Adv Neurol* **47**, 215–254.

Ludwin, S. K. and Maitland, M. (1984). Long-term remyelination fails to reconstitute normal thickness of central myelin sheaths. *J Neurol Sci* **64**, 193–198.

Luetjens, C. M., Bui, N. T., Sengpiel, B., *et al.* (2000). Delayed mitochondrial dysfunction in excitotoxic neuron death: cytochrome c release and a secondary increase in superoxide production. *J Neurosci* **20**, 5715–5723.

Lumsden, C. E. (1951). Fundamental problems in the pathology of multiple sclerosis and allied demyelinating diseases. *Br Med J* 1035–1043.

Lunn, E. R., Scourfield, J., Keynes, R. J., and Stern, C. D. (1987). The neural tube origin of ventral root sheath cells in the chick embryo. *Development* **101**, 247–254.

Lunn, K. F., Baas, P. W., and Duncan, I. D. (1997). Microtubule organization and stability in the oligodendrocyte. *J Neurosci* **17**, 4921–4932.

Luyt, K., Slade, T. P., Dorward, J. J., *et al.* (2007). Developing oligodendrocytes express functional GABA(B) receptors that stimulate cell proliferation and migration. *J Neurochem* **100**, 822–840.

Luyt, K., Varadi, A., Durant, C. F., and Molnar, E. (2006). Oligodendroglial metabotropic glutamate receptors are developmentally regulated and involved in the prevention of apoptosis. *J Neurochem* **99**, 641–656.

Luyt, K., Varadi, A., Halfpenny, C. A., Scolding, N. J., and Molnar, E. (2004). Metabotropic glutamate receptors are expressed in adult human glial progenitor cells. *Biochem Biophys Res Commun* **319**, 120–129.

Luzi, P., Zaka, M., Rao, H. Z., Curtis, M., Rafi, M. A., and Wenger, D. A. (2004). Generation of transgenic mice expressing insulin-like growth factor-1 under the control of the myelin basic protein promoter: increased myelination and potential for studies on the effects of increased IGF-1 on experimentally and genetically induced demyelination. *Neurochem Res* **29**, 881–889.

Macklin, W. B., Campagnoni, C. W., Deininger, P. L., and Gardinier, M. V. (1987a). Structure and expression of the mouse myelin proteolipid gene. *J Neurosci Res* **18**, 383–394.

Macklin, W. B., Gardinier, M. V., King, K. D., and Kampf, K. (1987b). An AG-GG transition at a splice site in the myelin PLP gene in jimpy mice results in the removal of an exon. *FEBS Lett* **223**, 417–421.

Madison, D. L., Krueger, W. H., Cheng, D., Trapp, B. D., and Pfeiffer, S. E. (1999). SNARE complex proteins, including the cognate pair VAMP-2 and syntaxin-4, are expressed in cultured oligodendrocytes. *J Neurochem* **72**, 988–998.

Madison, D. L., Krueger, W. H., Kim, T., and Pfeiffer, S. E. (1996). Differential expression of rab3 isoforms in oligodendrocytes and astrocytes. *J Neurosci Res* **45**, 258–268.

Maeda, Y., Solanky, M., Menonna, J., Chapin, J., Li, W., and Dowling, P. (2001). Platelet-derived growth factor-alpha receptor-positive oligodendroglia are frequent in multiple sclerosis lesions. *Ann Neurol* **49**, 776–785.

Maggipinto, M., Rabiner, C., Kidd, G. J., Hawkins, A. J., Smith, R., and Barbarese, E. (2004). Increased expression of the MBP mRNA binding protein HnRNP A2 during oligodendrocyte differentiation. *J Neurosci Res* **75**, 614–623.

Magner, L. N. (2002). Problems in generation: preformation and epigenesis. In *A History of the Life Sciences* (Chicago, IL: CRC Press), pp. 152–204.

Maier, O., van der Heide, T., Johnson, R., de Vries, H., Baron, W., and Hoekstra, D. (2006). The function of neurofascin155 in oligodendrocytes is regulated by metalloprotease-mediated cleavage and ectodomain shedding. *Exp Cell Res* **312**, 500–511.

Makeyev, E. V., Zhang, J., Carrasco, M. A., and Maniatis, T. (2007). The MicroRNA miR-124 promotes neuronal differentiation by triggering brain-specific alternative pre-mRNA splicing. *Mol Cell* **27**, 435–448.

Maletkovic, J., Schiffmann, R., Gorospe, J. R., *et al.* (2008). Genetic and clinical heterogeneity in eIF2B-related disorder. *J Child Neurol* **23**, 205–215.

Mallard, C., Welin, A. K., Peebles, D., Hagberg, H., and Kjellmer, I. (2003). White matter injury following systemic endotoxemia or asphyxia in the fetal sheep. *Neurochem Res* **28**, 215–223.

Mander, P., Borutaite, V., Moncada, S., and Brown, G. C. (2005). Nitric oxide from inflammatory-activated glia synergizes with hypoxia to induce neuronal death. *J Neurosci Res* **79**, 208–215.

Manitt, C., Wang, D., Kennedy, T. E., and Howland, D. R. (2006). Positioned to inhibit: netrin-1 and netrin receptor expression after spinal cord injury. *J Neurosci Res* **84**, 1808–1820.

Mann, S. A., Versmold, B., Marx, R., *et al.* (2008). Corticosteroids reverse cytokine-induced block of survival and differentiation of oligodendrocyte progenitor cells from rats. *J Neuroinflammation* **5**, 39.

Manning, S. M., Talos, D. M., Zhou, C., *et al.* (2008). NMDA receptor blockade with memantine attenuates white matter injury in a rat model of periventricular leukomalacia. *J Neurosci* **28**, 6670–6678.

Maragakis, N. J., Dietrich, J., Wong, V., *et al.* (2004). Glutamate transporter expression and function in human glial progenitors. *Glia* **45**, 133–143.

Marcus, J., Dupree, J. L., and Popko, B. (2000). Effects of galactolipid elimination on oligodendrocyte development and myelination. *Glia* **30**, 319–328.

Markham, J. A. and Greenough, W. T. (2004). Experience-driven brain plasticity: beyond the synapse. *Neuron Glia Biol* **1**, 351–363.

Maro, G. S., Vermeren, M., Voiculescu, O., *et al.* (2004). Neural crest boundary cap cells constitute a source of neuronal and glial cells of the PNS. *Nat Neurosci* **7**, 930–938.

Marret, S., Mukendi, R., Gadisseux, J. F., Gressens, P., and Evrard, P. (1995). Effect of ibotenate on brain development: an excitotoxic mouse model of microgyria and post-hypoxic-like lesions. *J Neuropathol Exp Neurol* **54**, 358–370.

Marriott, M. P., Emery, B., Cate, H. S., *et al.* (2008). Leukemia inhibitory factor signaling modulates both central nervous system demyelination and myelin repair. *Glia* **56**, 686–698.

Martin, R., McFarland, H. F., and McFarlin, D. E. (1992). Immunological aspects of demyelinating diseases. *Annu Rev Immunol* **10**, 153–187.

Martini, R. (1994). Expression and functional roles of neural cell surface molecules and extracellular matrix components during development and regeneration of peripheral nerves. *J Neurocytol* **23**, 1–28.

Martini, R. (2005). Schwann cells and myelin. In *Neuroglia*, B. R. Ransom and H. Kettenmann, eds. (Oxford: Oxford University Press), pp. 48–59.

Martini, R. and Schachner, M. (1986). Immunoelectron microscopic localization of neural cell adhesion molecules (L1, N-CAM, and MAG) and their shared carbohydrate epitope and myelin basic protein in developing sciatic nerve. *J Cell Biol* **103**, 2439–2448.

Martini, R. and Schachner, M. (1988). Immunoelectron microscopic localization of neural cell adhesion molecules (L1, N-CAM, and myelin-associated glycoprotein) in regenerating adult mouse sciatic nerve. *J Cell Biol* **106**, 1735–1746.

Martini, R. and Schachner, M. (1991). Complex expression pattern of tenascin during innervation of the posterior limb buds of the developing chicken. *J Neurosci Res* **28**, 261–279.

Martini, R., Fischer, S., Lopez-Vales, R., and David, S. (2008). Interactions between Schwann cells and macrophages in injury and inherited demyelinating disease. *Glia* **56**, 1566–1577.

Martini, R., Mohajeri, M. H., Kasper, S., Giese, K. P., and Schachner, M. (1995). Mice doubly deficient in the genes for P0 and myelin basic protein show that both proteins contribute to the formation of the major dense line in peripheral nerve myelin. *J Neurosci* **15**, 4488–4495.

Martini, R., Schachner, M., and Brushart, T. M. (1994). The L2/HNK-1 carbohydrate is preferentially expressed by previously motor axon-associated Schwann cells in reinnervated peripheral nerves. *J Neurosci* **14**, 7180–7191.

Martini, R., Schachner, M., and Faissner, A. (1990). Enhanced expression of the extracellular matrix molecule J1/tenascin in the regenerating adult mouse sciatic nerve. *J Neurocytol* **19**, 601–616.

Martini, R., Xin, Y., Schmitz, B., and Schachner, M. (1992). The L2/HNK-1 carbohydrate epitope is involved in the preferential outgrowth of motor neurons on ventral roots and motor nerves. *Eur J Neurosci* **4**, 628–639.

Martino, G. and Hartung, H. P. (1999). Immunopathogenesis of multiple sclerosis: the role of T cells. *Curr Opin Neurol* **12**, 309–321.

Mason, J. L., Jones, J. J., Taniike, M., Morell, P., Suzuki, K., and Matsushima, G. K. (2000). Mature oligodendrocyte apoptosis precedes IGF-1 production and oligodendrocyte progenitor accumulation and differentiation during demyelination/remyelination. *J Neurosci Res* **61**, 251–262.

Mason, J. L., Suzuki, K., Chaplin, D. D., and Matsushima, G. K. (2001). Interleukin-1beta promotes repair of the CNS. *J Neurosci* **21**, 7046–7052.

Mason, J. L., Toews, A., Hostettler, J. D., *et al.* (2004). Oligodendrocytes and progenitors become progressively depleted within chronically demyelinated lesions. *Am J Pathol* **164**, 1673–1682.

Mata, M., Fink, D. J., Ernst, S. A., and Siegel, G. J. (1991). Immunocytochemical demonstration of Na$^+$, K(+)-ATPase in internodal axolemma of myelinated fibers of rat sciatic and optic nerves. *J Neurochem* **57**, 184–192.

Mathey, E. K., Derfuss, T., Storch, M. K., *et al.* (2007). Neurofascin as a novel target for autoantibody-mediated axonal injury. *J Exp Med* **204**, 2363–2372.

Matloubian, M., Lo, C. G., Cinamon, G., *et al.* (2004). Lymphocyte egress from thymus and peripheral lymphoid organs is dependent on S1P receptor 1. *Nature* **427**, 355–360.

Matsumoto, Y., Kohyama, K., Aikawa, Y., *et al.* (1998). Role of natural killer cells and TCR gamma delta T cells in acute autoimmune encephalomyelitis. *Eur J Immunol* **28**, 1681–1688.

Matute, C. (1998). Characteristics of acute and chronic kainate excitotoxic damage to the optic nerve. *Proc Natl Acad Sci USA* **95**, 10229–10234.

Matute, C., Alberdi, E., Domercq, M., *et al.* (2007). Excitotoxic damage to white matter. *J Anat* **210**, 693–702.

Matute, C., Sanchez-Gomez, M. V., Martinez-Millan, L., and Miledi, R. (1997). Glutamate receptor-mediated toxicity in optic nerve oligodendrocytes. *Proc Natl Acad Sci USA* **94**, 8830–8835.

Maurel, P., Einheber, S., Galinska, J., *et al.* (2007). Nectin-like proteins mediate axon Schwann cell interactions along the internode and are essential for myelination. *J Cell Biol* **178**, 861–874.

Maurer, M., Muller, M., Kobsar, I., Leonhard, C., Martini, R., and Kiefer, R. (2003). Origin of pathogenic macrophages and endoneurial fibroblast-like cells in an animal model of inherited neuropathy. *Mol Cell Neurosci* **23**, 351–359.

Mayer, M., Bhakoo, K., and Noble, M. (1994). Ciliary neurotrophic factor and leukemia inhibitory factor promote the generation, maturation and survival of oligodendrocytes in vitro. *Development* **120**, 143–153.

Maysami, S., Nguyen, D., Zobel, F., Heine, S., Hopfner, M., and Stangel, M. (2006a). Oligodendrocyte precursor cells express a functional chemokine receptor CCR3: implications for myelination. *J Neuroimmunol* **178**, 17–23.

Maysami, S., Nguyen, D., Zobel, F., *et al.* (2006b). Modulation of rat oligodendrocyte precursor cells by the chemokine CXCL12. *NeuroReport* **17**, 1187–1190.

McCarran, W. J. and Goldberg, M. P. (2007). White matter axon vulnerability to AMPA/kainate receptor-mediated ischemic injury is developmentally regulated. *J Neurosci* **27**, 4220–4229.

McDonald, J. W., Althomsons, S. P., Hyrc, K. L., Choi, D. W., and Goldberg, M. P. (1998a). Oligodendrocytes from forebrain are highly vulnerable to AMPA/kainate receptor-mediated excitotoxicity. *Nat Med* **4**, 291–297.

McDonald, J. W., Levine, J. M., and Qu, Y. (1998b). Multiple classes of the oligodendrocyte lineage are highly vulnerable to excitotoxicity. *NeuroReport* **9**, 2757–2762.

McDonald, W. I. and Ohlrich, G. D. (1971). Quantitative anatomical measurements on single isolated fibres from the cat spinal cord. *J Anat* **110**, 191–202.

McFarland, H. F. and Martin, R. (2007). Multiple sclerosis: a complicated picture of autoimmunity. *Nat Immunol* **8**, 913–919.

McGee, A. W., Yang, Y., Fischer, Q. S., Daw, N. W., and Strittmatter, S. M. (2005). Experience-driven plasticity of visual cortex limited by myelin and Nogo receptor. *Science* **309**, 2222–2226.

McKinnon, R. D., Piras, G., Ida, J. A., Jr., and Dubois-Dalcq, M. (1993). A role for TGF-beta in oligodendrocyte differentiation. *J Cell Biol* **121**, 1397–1407.

McMorris, F. A. and Dubois-Dalcq, M. (1988). Insulin-like growth factor I promotes cell proliferation and oligodendroglial commitment in rat glial progenitor cells developing in vitro. *J Neurosci Res* **21**, 199–209.

McQuaid, S. and Cosby, S. L. (2002). An immunohistochemical study of the distribution of the measles virus receptors, CD46 and SLAM, in normal human tissues and subacute sclerosing panencephalitis. *Lab Invest* **82**, 403–409.

McTigue, D. M., Wei, P., and Stokes, B. T. (2001). Proliferation of NG2-positive cells and altered oligodendrocyte numbers in the contused rat spinal cord. *J Neurosci* **21**, 3392–3400.

Mead, R. J., Singhrao, S. K., Neal, J. W., Lassmann, H., and Morgan, B. P. (2002). The membrane attack complex of complement causes severe demyelination associated with acute axonal injury. *J Immunol* **168**, 458–465.

Medzhitov, R. and Janeway, C. A., Jr. (1997). Innate immunity: impact on the adaptive immune response. *Curr Opin Immunol* **9**, 4–9.

Mei, L. and Xiong, W. C. (2008). Neuregulin 1 in neural development, synaptic plasticity and schizophrenia. *Nat Rev Neurosci* **9**, 437–452.

Meier, C., Parmantier, E., Brennan, A., Mirsky, R., and Jessen, K. R. (1999). Developing Schwann cells acquire the ability to survive without axons by establishing an autocrine circuit involving insulin-like growth factor, neurotrophin-3, and platelet-derived growth factor-BB. *J Neurosci* **19**, 3847–3859.

Mekki-Dauriac, S., Agius, E., Kan, P., and Cochard, P. (2002). Bone morphogenetic proteins negatively control oligodendrocyte precursor specification in the chick spinal cord. *Development* **129**, 5117–5130.

Melendez-Vasquez, C., Carey, D. J., Zanazzi, G., Reizes, O., Maurel, P., and Salzer, J. L. (2005). Differential expression of proteoglycans at central and peripheral nodes of Ranvier. *Glia* **52**, 301–308.

Melendez-Vasquez, C. V., Rios, J. C., Zanazzi, G., Lambert, S., Bretscher, A., and Salzer, J. L. (2001). Nodes of Ranvier form in association with ezrin-radixin-moesin (ERM)-positive Schwann cell processes. *Proc Natl Acad Sci USA* **98**, 1235–1240.

Meletis, K., Barnabe-Heider, F., Carlen, M., *et al.* (2008). Spinal cord injury reveals multilineage differentiation of ependymal cells. *PLoS Biol* **6**, e182.

Menegoz, M., Gaspar, P., Le Bert, M., *et al.* (1997). Paranodin, a glycoprotein of neuronal paranodal membranes. *Neuron* **19**, 319–331.

Menichella, D. M., Goodenough, D. A., Sirkowski, E., Scherer, S. S., and Paul, D. L. (2003). Connexins are critical for normal myelination in the CNS. *J Neurosci* **23**, 5963–5973.

Menon, K. K., Piddlesden, S. J., and Bernard, C. C. A. (1997). Demyelinating antibodies to myelin oligodendrocyte glycoprotein and galactocerebroside induce degradation of myelin basic protein in isolated human myelin. *J Neurochem* **69**, 214–222.

Merkler, D., Boretius, S., Stadelmann, C., *et al.* (2005). Multicontrast MRI of remyelination in the central nervous system. *NMR Biomed* 23, 7710–7718.

Merkler, D., Ernsting, T., Kerschensteiner, M., Bruck, W., and Stadelmann, C. (2006). A new focal EAE model of cortical demyelination: multiple sclerosis-like lesions with rapid resolution of inflammation and extensive remyelination. *Brain* **129**, 1972–1983.

Merkler, D., Metz, G. A., Raineteau, O., Dietz, V., Schwab, M. E., and Fouad, K. (2001). Locomotor recovery in spinal cord-injured rats treated with an antibody neutralizing the myelin-associated neurite growth inhibitor Nogo-A. *J Neurosci* **21**, 3665–3673.

Merrill, J. E. and Benveniste, E. N. (1996). Cytokines in inflammatory brain lesions: helpful and harmful. *Trends Neurosci* **19**, 331–338.

Merrill, J. E. and Zimmerman, R. P. (1991). Natural and induced cytotoxicity of oligodendrocytes by microglia is inhibitable by TGF beta. *Glia* **4**, 327–331.

Merrill, J. E., Ignarro, L. J., Sherman, M. P., Melinek, J., and Lane, T. E. (1993). Microglial cell cytotoxicity of oligodendrocytes is mediated through nitric oxide. *J Immunol* **151**, 2132–2141.

Meucci, O., Fatatis, A., Holzwarth, J. A., and Miller, R. J. (1996). Developmental regulation of the toxin sensitivity of Ca(2+)-permeable AMPA receptors in cortical glia. *J Neurosci* **16**, 519–530.

MeyerFranke, A., Kaplan, M. R., Pfrieger, F. W., and Barres, B. A. (1995). Characterization of the signaling interactions that promote the survival and growth of developing retinal ganglion cells in culture. *Neuron* **15**, 805–819.

Mi, S., Hu, B., Hahm, K., *et al.* (2007). LINGO-1 antagonist promotes spinal cord remyelination and axonal integrity in MOG-induced experimental autoimmune encephalomyelitis. *Nature Med* **10**, 1228–1233.

Mi, S., Lee, X., Shao, Z., *et al.* (2004). LINGO-1 is a component of the Nogo-66 receptor/p75 signaling complex. *Nat Neurosci* **7**, 221–228.

Mi, S., Miller, R. H., Lee, X., *et al.* (2005). LINGO-1 negatively regulates myelination by oligodendrocytes. *Nat Neurosci* **8**, 745–751.

Micevych, P. E. and Abelson, L. (1991). Distribution of mRNAs coding for liver and heart gap junction proteins in the rat central nervous system. *J Comp Neurol* **305**, 96–118.

Michailov, G. V., Sereda, M. W., Brinkmann, B. G., *et al.* (2004). Axonal neuregulin-1 regulates myelin sheath thickness. *Science* **304**, 700–703.

Micu, I., Jiang, Q., Coderre, E., *et al.* (2006). NMDA receptors mediate calcium accumulation in myelin during chemical ischaemia. *Nature* **439**, 988–992.

Miller, D. J. and Rodriguez, M. (1995). A monoclonal autoantibody that promotes central nervous system remyelination in a model of multiple sclerosis is a natural autoantibody encoded by germline immunoglobulin genes. *J Immunol* **154**, 2460–2469.

Miller, R. H. (2002). Regulation of oligodendrocyte development in the vertebrate CNS. *Prog Neurobiol* **67**, 451–467.

Miller, R. H. (2005). Dorsally derived oligodendrocytes come of age. *Neuron* **45**, 1–3.

Miller, R. H., Dinsio, K. J., Wang, R. Z., Geertman, R., Maier, C. E., and Hall, A. K. (2004). Patterning of spinal cord oligodendrocyte development by dorsally derived BMP4. *J Neurosci Res* **76**, 9–19.

Miller, S. P., Cozzio, C. C., Goldstein, R. B., *et al.* (2003). Comparing the diagnosis of white matter injury in premature newborns with serial MR imaging and transfontanel ultrasonography findings. *AJNR Am J Neuroradiol* **24**, 1661–1669.

Milner, R. (1997). Understanding the molecular basis of cell migration; implications for clinical therapy in multiple sclerosis. *Clin Sci (Lond)* **92**, 113–122.

Milner, R. and Ffrench-Constant, C. (1994). A developmental analysis of oligodendroglial integrins in primary cells: changes in alpha v-associated beta subunits during differentiation. *Development* **120**, 3497–3506.

Mimeault, M. and Batra, S. K. (2008). Recent progress on tissue-resident adult stem cell biology and their therapeutic implications. *Stem Cell Rev* **4**, 27–49.

Minuk, J. and Braun, P. E. (1996). Differential intracellular sorting of the myelin-associated glycoprotein isoforms. *J Neurosci Res* **44**, 411–420.

Mirsky, R., Winter, J., Abney, E. R., Pruss, R. M., Gavrilovic, J., and Raff, M. C. (1980). Myelin-specific proteins and glycolipids in rat Schwann cells and oligodendrocytes in culture. *J Cell Biol* **84**, 483–494.

Miska, E. A., Alvarez-Saavedra, E., Townsend, M., *et al.* (2004). Microarray analysis of microRNA expression in the developing mammalian brain. *Genome Biol* **5**, R68.

Mitani, A. and Tanaka, K. (2003). Functional changes of glial glutamate transporter GLT-1 during ischemia: an in vivo study in the hippocampal CA1 of normal mice and mutant mice lacking GLT-1. *J Neurosci* **23**, 7176–7182.

Mitrovic, B., Ignarro, L. J., Montestruque, S., Smoll, A., and Merrill, J. E. (1994). Nitric oxide as a potential pathological mechanism in demyelination: its differential effects on primary glial cells in vitro. *Neuroscience* **61**, 575–585.

Mitsunaga, Y., Ciric, B., Van Keulen, V., *et al.* (2002). Direct evidence that a human antibody derived from patient serum can promote myelin repair in a mouse model of chronic-progressive demyelinating disease. *FASEB J* **16**, 1325–1327.

Miura, M., Asou, H., Kobayashi, M., and Uyemura, K. (1992). Functional expression of a full-length cDNA coding for rat neural cell adhesion molecule L1 mediates homophilic intercellular adhesion and migration of cerebellar neurons. *J Biol Chem* **267**, 10752–10758.

Miyamoto, E., Kakiuchi, S., and Kakimoto, Y. (1974). In vitro and in vivo phosphorylation of myelin basic protein by cerebral protein kinase. *Nature* **249**, 150–151.

Miyamoto, Y., Yamauchi, J., and Tanoue, A. (2008). Cdk5 phosphorylation of WAVE2 regulates oligodendrocyte precursor cell migration through non-receptor tyrosine kinase Fyn. *J Neurosci* **28**, 8326–8337.

Mizuno, T., Sawada, M., Suzumura, A., and Marunouchi, T. (1994). Expression of cytokines during glial differentiation. *Brain Res* **656**, 141–146.

Moffett, J. R., Ross, B., Arun, P., Madhavarao, C. N., and Namboodiri, A. M. (2007). N-Acetylaspartate in the CNS: from neurodiagnostics to neurobiology. *Prog Neurobiol* **81**, 89–131.

Monje, M. L., Toda, H., and Palmer, T. D. (2003). Inflammatory blockade restores adult hippocampal neurogenesis. *Science* **302**, 1760–1765.

Montag, D., Giese, K. P., Bartsch, U., *et al.* (1994). Mice deficient for the myelin-associated glycoprotein show subtle abnormalities in myelin. *Neuron* **13**, 229–246.

Montague, P., McCallion, A. S., Davies, R. W., and Griffiths, I. R. (2006). Myelin-associated oligodendrocytic basic protein: a family of abundant CNS myelin proteins in search of a function. *Dev Neurosci* **28**, 479–487.

Moreau-Fauvarque, C., Kumanogoh, A., Camand, E., *et al.* (2003). The transmembrane semaphorin Sema4D/CD100, an inhibitor of axonal growth, is expressed on oligodendrocytes and upregulated after CNS lesion. *J Neurosci* **23**, 9229–9239.

Moretto, G., Xu, R. Y., and Kim, S. U. (1993). CD44 expression in human astrocytes and oligodendrocytes in culture. *J Neuropathol Exp Neurol* **52**, 419–423.

Morita, K., Sasaki, H., Fujimoto, K., Furuse, M., and Tsukita, S. (1999). Claudin-11/OSP-based tight junctions of myelin sheaths in brain and Sertoli cells in testis. *J Cell Biol* **145**, 579–588.

Moriya, T., Hassan, A. Z., Young, W., and Chesler, M. (1994). Dynamics of extracellular calcium activity following contusion of the rat spinal cord. *J Neurotrauma* **11**, 255–263.

Morris, J. K., Lin, W., Hauser, C., Marchuk, Y., Getman, D., and Lee, K. F. (1999). Rescue of the cardiac defect in ErbB2 mutant mice reveals essential roles of ErbB2 in peripheral nervous system development. *Neuron* **23**, 273–283.

Morrissey, T. K., Kleitman, N., and Bunge, R. P. (1995). Human Schwann cells in vitro. II. Myelination of sensory axons following extensive purification and heregulin-induced expansion. *J Neurobiol* **28**, 190–201.

Moscoso, L. M. and Sanes, J. R. (1995). Expression of four immunoglobulin superfamily adhesion molecules (L1, Nr-CAM/Bravo, neurofascin/ABGP, and N-CAM) in the developing mouse spinal cord. *J Comp Neurol* **352**, 321–334.

Moser, H. W., Mahmood, A., and Raymond, G. V. (2007). X-linked adrenoleuko-dystrophy. *Nat Clin Pract Neurol* **3**, 140–151.

Moser, H. W., Raymond, G. V., and Dubey, P. (2005). Adrenoleukodystrophy: new approaches to a neurodegenerative disease. *J Am Med Assoc* **294**, 3131–3134.

Mostov, K. E., Verges, M., and Altschuler, Y. (2000). Membrane traffic in polarized epithelial cells. *Curr Opin Cell Biol* **12**, 483–490.

Mronga, T., Stahnke, T., Goldbaum, O., and Richter-Landsberg, C. (2004). Mitochondrial pathway is involved in hydrogen-peroxide-induced apoptotic cell death of oligodendrocytes. *Glia* **46**, 446–455.

Mueller, M., Leonhard, C., Wacker, K., *et al.* (2003). Macrophage response to peripheral nerve injury: the quantitative contribution of resident and hematogenous macrophages. *Lab Invest* **83**, 175–185.

Mukhopadhyay, G., Doherty, P., Walsh, F. S., Crocker, P. R., and Filbin, M. T. (1994). A novel role for myelin-associated glycoprotein as an inhibitor of axonal regeneration. *Neuron* **13**, 757–767.

Munro, T. P., Magee, R. J., Kidd, G. J., *et al.* (1999). Mutational analysis of a heterogeneous nuclear ribonucleoprotein A2 response element for RNA trafficking. *J Biol Chem* **274**, 34389–34395.

Murru, M. R., Vannelli, A., Marrosu, G., *et al.* (2006). A novel Cx32 mutation causes X-linked Charcot-Marie-Tooth disease with brainstem involvement and brain magnetic resonance spectroscopy abnormalities. *Neurol Sci* **27**, 18–23.

Nagy, J. I., Ionescu, A. V., Lynn, B. D., and Rash, J. E. (2003). Connexin29 and connexin32 at oligodendrocyte and astrocyte gap junctions and in myelin of the mouse central nervous system. *J Comp Neurol* **464**, 356–370.

Nagy, Z., Westerberg, H., and Klingberg, T. (2004). Maturation of white matter is associated with the development of cognitive functions during childhood. *J Cogn Neurosci* **16**, 1227–1233.

Nait-Oumesmar, B., Picard-Riera, N., Kerninon, C., *et al.* (2007). Activation of the subventricular zone in multiple sclerosis: evidence for early glial progenitors. *Proc Natl Acad Sci USA* **104**, 4694–4699.

Nakagawa, M., Koyanagi, M., Tanabe, K., *et al.* (2008). Generation of induced pluripotent stem cells without Myc from mouse and human fibroblasts. *Nat Biotechnol* **26**, 101–106.

Nakahara, J., Seiwa, C., Tan-Takeuchi, K., *et al.* (2005). Involvement of CD45 in central nervous system myelination. *Neurosci Lett.* **379**, 116–121.

Nakajima, K. and Kohsaka, S. (2001). Microglia: activation and their significance in the central nervous system. *J Biochem* **130**, 169–175.

Namboodiri, A. M., Peethambaran, A., Mathew, R., *et al.* (2006). Canavan disease and the role of *N*-acetylaspartate in myelin synthesis. *Mol Cell Endocrinol* **252**, 216–223.

Narayanan, S. P., Flores, A. I., Wang, F., and Macklin, W. B. (2009). Akt signals through the mammalian target of rapamycin pathway to regulate CNS myelination. *J Neurosci* **29**, 6860–6870.

Naruse, M., Nakahira, E., Miyata, T., Hitoshi, S., Ikenaka, K., and Bansal, R. (2006). Induction of oligodendrocyte progenitors in dorsal forebrain by intraventricular microinjection of FGF-2. *Dev Biol* **297**, 262–273.

Nataf, S., Carroll, S. L., Wetsel, R. A., Szalai, A. J., and Barnum, S. R. (2000). Attenuation of experimental autoimmune demyelination in complement-deficient mice. *J Immunol* **165**, 5867–5873.

Nave, K. A. (2008). Neuroscience: an ageing view of myelin repair. *Nature* **455**, 478–479.

Nave, K. A. and Griffiths, I. (2004). Models of Pelizaeus-Merzbacher disease. In *Myelin Biology and Disorders*, R. A. Lazzarini, ed. (Amsterdam: Elsevier Academic Press), pp. 1125–1142.

Nave, K. A. and Salzer, J. L. (2006). Axonal regulation of myelination by neuregulin 1. *Curr Opin Neurobiol* **16**, 492–500.

Nave, K. A. and Trapp, B. D. (2008). Axon-glial signaling and the glial support of axon function. *Annu Rev Neurosci* **31**, 535–561.

Nave, K. A., Lai, C., Bloom, F. E., and Milner, R. J. (1987). Splice site selection in the proteolipid protein (PLP) gene transcript and primary structure of the DM-20 protein of central nervous system myelin. *Proc Natl Acad Sci USA* **84**, 5665–5669.

Nave, K. A., Sereda, M. W., and Ehrenreich, H. (2007). Mechanisms of disease: inherited demyelinating neuropathies – from basic to clinical research. *Nat Clin Pract Neurol* **3**, 453–464.

Nedergaard, M., Takano, T., and Hansen, A. J. (2002). Beyond the role of glutamate as a neurotransmitter. *Nat Rev Neurosci* **3**, 748–755.

Neuhaus, O., Kieseier, B. C., and Hartung, H. P. (2006). Mitoxantrone in multiple sclerosis. *Adv Neurol* **98**, 293–302.

Neumann, B., Machleidt, T., Lifka, A., *et al.* (1996). Crucial role of 55-kilodalton TNF receptor in TNF-induced adhesion molecule expression and leukocyte organ infiltration. *J Immunol* **156**, 1587–1593.

Nicolay, D. J., Doucette, J. R., and Nazarali, A. J. (2007). Transcriptional control of oligodendrogenesis. *Glia* **55**, 1287–1299.

Niederlander, C. and Lumsden, A. (1996). Late emigrating neural crest cells migrate specifically to the exit points of cranial branchiomotor nerves. *Development* **122**, 2367–2374.

Niederost, B., Oertle, T., Fritsche, J., McKinney, R. A., and Bandtlow, C. E. (2002). Nogo-A and myelin-associated glycoprotein mediate neurite growth inhibition by antagonistic regulation of RhoA and Rac1. *J Neurosci* **22**, 10368–10376.

Niehaus, A., Shi, J., Grzenkowski, M., *et al.* (2000). Patients with active relapsing-remitting multiple sclerosis synthesize antibodies recognizing oligodendrocyte progenitor cell surface protein: implications for remyelination. *Ann Neurol* **48**, 362–371.

Nielsen, J. A., Maric, D., Lau, P., Barker, J. L., and Hudson, L. D. (2006). Identification of a novel oligodendrocyte cell adhesion protein using gene expression profiling. *J Neurosci* **26**, 9881–9891.

Niemann, A., Berger, P., and Suter, U. (2006). Pathomechanisms of mutant proteins in Charcot-Marie-Tooth disease. *Neuromolecular Med* **8**, 217–242.

Nikizad, H., Yon, J. H., Carter, L. B., and Jevtovic-Todorovic, V. (2007). Early exposure to general anesthesia causes significant neuronal deletion in the developing rat brain. *Ann N Y Acad Sci* **1122**, 69–82.

Nimmerjahn, A., Kirchhoff, F., and Helmchen, F. (2005). Resting microglial cells are highly dynamic surveillants of brain parenchyma in vivo. *Science* **308**, 1314–1318.

Nishiyama, A. (2007). Polydendrocytes: NG2 cells with many roles in development and repair of the CNS. *Neuroscientist* **13**, 62–76.

Nishiyama, A., Komitova, M., Suzuki, R., and Zhu, X. (2009). Polydendrocytes (NG2 cells): multifunctional cells with lineage plasticity. *Nat Rev Neurosci* **10**, 9–22.

Nishiyama, A., Watanabe, M., Yang, Z., and Bu, J. (2002). Identity, distribution, and development of polydendrocytes: NG2-expressing glial cells. *J Neurocytol* **31**, 437–455.

Noakes, P. G. and Bennett, M. R. (1987). Growth of axons into developing muscles of the chick forelimb is preceded by cells that stain with Schwann cell antibodies. *J Comp Neurol* **259**, 330–347.

Noble, L. J. and Wrathall, J. R. (1989). Correlative analyses of lesion development and functional status after graded spinal cord contusive injuries in the rat. *Exp Neurol* **103**, 34–40.

Nodari, A., Previtali, S. C., Dati, G., *et al.* (2008). Alpha6beta4 integrin and dystroglycan cooperate to stabilize the myelin sheath. *J Neurosci* **28**, 6714–6719.

Nodari, A., Zambroni, D., Quattrini, A., *et al.* (2007). Beta1 integrin activates Rac1 in Schwann cells to generate radial lamellae during axonal sorting and myelination. *J Cell Biol* **177**, 1063–1075.

Norenberg, M. D., Smith, J., and Marcillo, A. (2004). The pathology of human spinal cord injury: defining the problems. *J Neurotrauma* **21**, 429–440.

Northington, F. J., Traystman, R. J., Koehler, R. C., and Martin, L. J. (1999). GLT1, glial glutamate transporter, is transiently expressed in neurons and develops astrocyte specificity only after midgestation in the ovine fetal brain. *J Neurobiol* **39**, 515–526.

Norton, W. T. (1984). *Oligodendroglia*. (New York: Plenum Press.)

Norton, W. T. (1996). Do oligodendrocytes divide? *Neurochem Res* **21**, 495–503.

Norton, W. T. and Cammer, W. (1984). Isolation and characterization of myelin. In *Myelin*, P. Morell, ed. (New York: Plenum Press), pp. 146–196.

Novgorodov, A. S., El-Alwani, M., Bielawski, J., Obeid, L. M., and Gudz, T. I. (2007). Activation of sphingosine-1-phosphate receptor S1P5 inhibits oligodendrocyte progenitor migration. *FASEB J* **21**, 1503–1514.

Nunes, M. C., Roy, N. S., Keyoung, H. M., *et al.* (2003). Identification and isolation of multipotential neural progenitor cells from the subcortical white matter of the adult human brain. *Nat Med* **9**, 439–447.

Nygren, J. M., Liuba, K., Breitbach, M., *et al.* (2008). Myeloid and lymphoid contribution to non-haematopoietic lineages through irradiation-induced heterotypic cell fusion. *Nat Cell Biol* **10**, 584–592.

Occhi, S., Zambroni, D., Del Carro, U., *et al.* (2005). Both laminin and Schwann cell dystroglycan are necessary for proper clustering of sodium channels at nodes of Ranvier. *J Neurosci* **25**, 9418–9427.

Odermatt, B., Wellershaus, K., Wallraff, A., *et al.* (2003). Connexin 47 (Cx47)-deficient mice with enhanced green fluorescent protein reporter gene reveal predominant oligodendrocytic expression of Cx47 and display vacuolized myelin in the CNS. *J Neurosci* **23**, 4549–4559.

Oertle, T., van der Haar, M. E., Bandtlow, C. E., *et al.* (2003). Nogo-A inhibits neurite outgrowth and cell spreading with three discrete regions. *J Neurosci* **23**, 5393–5406.

Ogata, J. and Feigin, I. (1975). Schwann cells and regenerated peripheral myelin in multiple sclerosis: an ultrastructural study. *Neurology* **25**, 713–716.

Oka, A., Belliveau, M. J., Rosenberg, P. A., and Volpe, J. J. (1993). Vulnerability of oligodendroglia to glutamate: pharmacology, mechanisms, and prevention. *J Neurosci* **13**, 1441–1453.

Oka, S., Honmou, O., Akiyama, Y., *et al.* (2004). Autologous transplantation of expanded neural precursor cells into the demyelinated monkey spinal cord. *Brain Res* **1030**, 94–102.

Oleszak, E. L., Zaczynska, E., Bhattacharjee, C., Butunoi, C., Ledigo, A., and Katsetos, C. (1998). Inducible nitric oxide synthase and nitrotyrosine are found in monocytes/macrophages and/or astrocytes in acute, but not in chronic multiple sclerosis. *Clin Diagn Lab Immunol* **5**, 438–445.

Olney, J. W., Labruyere, J., Wang, G., Wozniak, D. F., Price, M. T., and Sesma, M. A. (1991). NMDA antagonist neurotoxicity: mechanism and prevention. *Science* **254**, 1515–1518.

Olson, J. K. and Miller, S. D. (2004). Microglia initiate central nervous system innate and adaptive immune responses through multiple TLRs. *J Immunol* **173**, 3916–3924.

Omari, K. M., John, G., Lango, R., and Raine, C. S. (2006). Role for CXCR2 and CXCL1 on glia in multiple sclerosis. *Glia* **53**, 24–31.

Omari, K. M., John, G. R., Sealfon, S. C., and Raine, C. S. (2005). CXC chemokine receptors on human oligodendrocytes: implications for multiple sclerosis. *Brain* **128**, 1003–1015.

Omlin, F. X., Webster, H. D., Palkovits, C. G., and Cohen, S. R. (1982). Immunocytochemical localization of basic protein in major dense line regions of central and peripheral myelin. *J Cell Biol* **95**, 242–248.

Ono, K., Bansal, R., Payne, J., Rutishauser, U., and Miller, R. H. (1995). Early development and dispersal of oligodendrocyte precursors in the embyonic chick spinal cord. *Development* **121**, 1743–1754.

Ono, K., Fujisawa, H., Hirano, S., Norita, M., Tsumori, T., and Yasui, Y. (1997). Early development of the oligodendrocyte in the embryonic chick metencephalon. *J Neurosci Res* **48**, 1–14.

van Oosten, B. W., Barkhof, F., Truyen, L., Boringa, J. B., Bertelsmann, F. W., von Blomberg, B. M., Woody, J. N., Hartung, H. P., and Polman, C. H *et al.* (1996). Increased MRI activity and immune activation in two multiple sclerosis patients treated with the monoclonal anti-tumor necrosis factor antibody cA2. *Neurology* **47**, 1531–1534.

Openshaw, H., Lund, B. T., Kashyap, A., *et al.* (2000). Peripheral blood stem cell transplantation in multiple sclerosis with busulfan and cyclophosphamide conditioning: report of toxicity and immunological monitoring. *Biol Blood Marrow Transplant* **6**, 563–575.

Orentas, D. M. and Miller, R. H. (1996). The origin of spinal cord oligodendrocytes is dependent on local influences from the notochord. *Developmental Biology* **177**, 43–53.

Orentas, D. M., Hayes, J. E., Dyer, K. L., and Miller, R. H. (1999). Sonic hedgehog signaling is required during the appearance of spinal cord oligodendrocyte precursors. *Development* **126**, 2419–2429.

Orthmann-Murphy, J. L., Abrams, C. K., and Scherer, S. S. (2008). Gap junctions couple astrocytes and oligodendrocytes. *J Mol Neurosci* **35**, 101–116.

Ota, K., Matsui, M., Milford, E., Mackin, G., Weiner, H., and Hafler, D. (1990). T-cell recognition of an immunodominant myelin basic protein epitope in multiple sclerosis. *Nature* **346**, 183–187.

Ozawa, K., Suchanek, G., Breitschopf, H., *et al.* (1994). Patterns of oligodendroglia pathology in multiple sclerosis. *Brain* **117**, 1311–1322.

Padgett, B. L. and Walker, D. L. (1973). Prevalence of antibodies in human sera against JC virus, an isolate from a case of progressive multifocal leukoencephalopathy. *J Infect Dis* **127**, 467–470.

Padovani-Claudio, D., Lui, L., Ransohoff, R. M., and Miller, R. H. (2006). Alterations in the oligodendrocyte lineage, myelin and white matter in adult mice lacking the chemokine receptor CXCR2. *Glia* **54**, 471–483.

Pan, B., Fromholt, S. E., Hess, E. J., *et al.* (2005). Myelin-associated glycoprotein and complementary axonal ligands, gangliosides, mediate axon stability in the CNS and PNS: neuropathology and behavioral deficits in single- and double-null mice. *Exp Neurol* **195**, 208–217.

Pang, Y., Cai, Z., and Rhodes, P. G. (2005). Effect of tumor necrosis factor-alpha on developing optic nerve oligodendrocytes in culture. *J Neurosci Res* **80**, 226–234.

Panitch, H. S., Hirsch, R. L., Haley, A. S., and Johnson, K. P. (1987). Exacerbations of multiple sclerosis in patients treated with gamma interferon. *Lancet* **1** (8538), 893–895.

Papastefanaki, F., Chen, J., Lavdas, A. A., Thomaidou, D., Schachner, M., and Matsas, R. (2007). Grafts of Schwann cells engineered to express PSA-NCAM promote functional recovery after spinal cord injury. *Brain* **130**, 2159–2174.

Park, E., Liu, Y., and Fehlings, M. G. (2003). Changes in glial cell white matter AMPA receptor expression after spinal cord injury and relationship to apoptotic cell death. *Exp Neurol* **182**, 35–48.

Park, H. J., Lee, P. H., Bang, O. Y., Lee, G., and Ahn, Y. H. (2008). Mesenchymal stem cells therapy exerts neuroprotection in a progressive animal model of Parkinson's disease. *J Neurochem* **107**, 141–151.

Park, J. B., Yiu, G., Kaneko, S., *et al.* (2005). A TNF receptor family member, TROY, is a coreceptor with Nogo receptor in mediating the inhibitory activity of myelin inhibitors. *Neuron* **45**, 345–351.

Park, S. K., Miller, R., Krane, I., and Vartanian, T. (2001). The erbB2 gene is required for the development of terminally differentiated spinal cord oligodendrocytes. *J Cell Biol* **154**, 1245–1258.

Parker, R. and Sheth, U. (2007). P bodies and the control of mRNA translation and degradation. *Mol Cell* **25**, 635–646.

Parkinson, D. B., Bhaskaran, A., Arthur-Farraj, P., *et al.* (2008). c-Jun is a negative regulator of myelination. *J Cell Biol* **181**, 625–637.

Parmantier, E., Cabon, F., Braun, C., D'Urso, D., Muller, H. W., and Zalc, B. (1995). Peripheral myelin protein-22 is expressed in rat and mouse brain and spinal cord motoneurons. *Eur J Neurosci* **7**, 1080–1088.

Parpura, V., Basarsky, T. A., Liu, F., Jeftinija, K., Jeftinija, S., and Haydon, P. G. (1994). Glutamate-mediated astrocyte-neuron signalling. *Nature* **369**, 744–747.

Patani, R., Balaratnam, M., Vora, A., and Reynolds, R. (2007). Remyelination can be extensive in multiple sclerosis despite a long disease course. *Neuropathol Appl Neurobiol* **33**, 277–287.

Patneau, D. K., Wright, P. W., Winters, C., Mayer, M. L., and Gallo, V. (1994). Glial cells of the oligodendrocyte lineage express both kainate- and AMPA-preferring subtypes of glutamate receptor. *Neuron* **12**, 357–371.

Patrikios, P., Stadelmann, C., Kutzelnigg, A., *et al.* (2006). Remyelination is extensive in a subset of multiple sclerosis patients. *Brain* **129**, 3165–3172.

Paty, D. W. and Li, D. K. (1993). Interferon beta-1b is effective in relapsing-remitting multiple sclerosis. II. MRI analysis results of a multicenter, randomized, double-blind, placebo-controlled trial. UBC MS/MRI Study Group and the IFNB Multiple Sclerosis Study Group. *Neurology* **43**, 662–667.

Paul, F., Jarius, S., Aktas, O., *et al.* (2007). Antibody to aquaporin 4 in the diagnosis of neuromyelitis optica. *PLoS Med* **4**, e133.

Pearse, D. D., Pereira, F. C., Marcillo, A. E., *et al.* (2004). cAMP and Schwann cells promote axonal growth and functional recovery after spinal cord injury. *Nat Med* **10**, 610–616.

Peebles, D. M., Miller, S., Newman, J. P., Scott, R., and Hanson, M. A. (2003). The effect of systemic administration of lipopolysaccharide on cerebral haemodynamics and oxygenation in the 0.65 gestation ovine fetus in utero. *Br J Obstet Gynaecol* **110**, 735–743.

Peirce, T. R., Bray, N. J., Williams, N. M., *et al.* (2006). Convergent evidence for 2′,3′-cyclic nucleotide 3′-phosphodiesterase as a possible susceptibility gene for schizophrenia. *Arch Gen Psychiatry* **63**, 18–24.

Pellissier, F., Gerber, A., Bauer, C., Ballivet, M., and Ossipow, V. (2007). The adhesion molecule Necl-3/SynCAM-2 localizes to myelinated axons, binds to oligodendrocytes and promotes cell adhesion. *BMC Neurosci* **8**, 90.

Pellkofer, H., Schubart, A. S., Hoftberger, R., *et al.* (2004). Modelling paraneoplastic CNS disease: T-cells specific for the onconeuronal antigen PNMA1 mediate autoimmune encephalomyelitis in the rat. *Brain* **127**, 1822–1830.

Pende, M., Holtzclaw, L. A., Curtis, J. L., Russell, J. T., and Gallo, V. (1994). Glutamate regulates intracellular calcium and gene expression in oligodendrocyte progenitors through the activation of DL-α-amino-3-hydroxy-5-methyl-4-isoxazolepropionic acid receptors. *Proc Natl Acad Sci USA* **91**, 3215–3219.

Penderis, J., Shields, S. A., and Franklin, R. J. (2003). Impaired remyelination and depletion of oligodendrocyte progenitors does not occur following repeated episodes of focal demyelination in the rat central nervous system. *Brain* **126**, 1382–1391.

Penfield, W. (1924). Oligodendroglia and its relation to classical neuroglia. *Brain* **47**, 430–452.

Peress, N. S., Perillo, E., and Seidman, R. J. (1996). Glial transforming growth factor (TGF)-beta isotypes in multiple sclerosis: differential glial expression of TGF-beta 1, 2 and 3 isotypes in multiple sclerosis. *J Neuroimmunol* **71**, 115–123.

Perez Villages, E. M., Olivier, C., Spassky, N., *et al.* (1999). Early specification of oligodendrocytes in the chick embryonic brain. *Dev Biol* **216**, 98–113.

Perier, O. and Gregoire, A. (1965). Electron microscopic features of multiple sclerosis lesions. *Brain* **88**, 937–952.

Perkins, D. O., Jeffries, C. D., Jarskog, L. F., *et al.* (2007). microRNA expression in the prefrontal cortex of individuals with schizophrenia and schizoaffective disorder. *Genome Biol* **8**, R27.

Perron, H., Jouvin-Marche, E., Michel, M., *et al.* (2001). Multiple sclerosis retrovirus particles and recombinant envelope trigger an abnormal immune response in vitro, by inducing polyclonal Vbeta16 T-lymphocyte activation. *Virology* **287**, 321–332.

Perron, H., Lazarini, F., Ruprecht, K., *et al.* (2005). Human endogenous retrovirus (HERV)-W ENV and GAG proteins: physiological expression in human brain and pathophysiological modulation in multiple sclerosis lesions. *J Neurovirol* **11**, 23–33.

Perry, V. H., Brown, M. C., and Andersson, P. B. (1993). Macrophage responses to central and peripheral nerve injury. *Adv Neurol* **59**, 309–314.

Peters, A. and Sethares, C. (2002). Aging and the myelinated fibers in prefrontal cortex and corpus callosum of the monkey. *J Comp Neurol* **442**, 277–291.

Peters, A. and Sethares, C. (2003). Is there remyelination during aging of the primate central nervous system? *J Comp Neurol* **460**, 238–254.

Peters, A. and Sethares, C. (2004). Oligodendrocytes, their progenitors and other neuroglial cells in the aging primate cerebral cortex. *Cereb Cortex* **14**, 995–1007.

Peters, A., Moss, M. B., and Sethares, C. (2000). Effects of aging on myelinated nerve fibers in monkey primary visual cortex. *J Comp Neurol* **419**, 364–376.

Peters, A., Palay, S. L., and Webster, H. D. (1991). *The Fine Structure of the Nervous System: Neurons and their Supporting Cells.* (New York: Oxford University Press.)

Peters, A., Rosene, D. L., Moss, M. B., *et al.* (1996). Neurobiological bases of age-related cognitive decline in the rhesus monkey. *J Neuropathol Exp Neurol* **55**, 861–874.

Peters, A., Sethares, C., and Killiany, R. J. (2001). Effects of age on the thickness of myelin sheaths in monkey primary visual cortex. *J Comp Neurol* **435**, 241–248.

Pfeiffer, S. E., Warrington, A. E., and Bansal, R. (1993). The oligodendrocyte and its many cellular processes. *Trends Cell Biol* **3**, 191–197.

Picard-Riera, N., Decker, L., Delarasse, C., *et al.* (2002). Experimental autoimmune encephalomyelitis mobilizes neural progenitors from the subventricular zone to undergo oligodendrogenesis in adult mice. *Proc Natl Acad Sci USA* **99**, 13211–13216.

Piddlesden, S. J. and Morgan, B. P. (1993). Killing of rat glial cells by complement: deficiency of the rat analogue of CD59 is the cause of oligodendrocyte susceptibility to lysis. *J Neuroimmunol* **48**, 169–176.

Pierson, C. R., Folkerth, R. D., Billiards, S. S., *et al.* (2007). Gray matter injury associated with periventricular leukomalacia in the premature infant. *Acta Neuropathol* **114**, 619–631.

Pines, G., Danbolt, N. C., Bjørås, M., *et al.* (1992). Cloning and expression of a rat brain L-glutamate transporter. *Nature* **360**, 464–467.

Pitt, D., Nagelmeier, I. E., Wilson, H. C., and Raine, C. S. (2003). Glutamate uptake by oligodendrocytes: implications for excitotoxicity in multiple sclerosis. *Neurology* **61**, 1113–1120.

Pitt, D., Werner, P., and Raine, C. S. (2000). Glutamate excitotoxicity in a model of multiple sclerosis. *Nature Med* **6**, 67–70.

Pizzi, M., Sarnico, I., Boroni, F., *et al.* (2004). Prevention of neuron and oligodendrocyte degeneration by interleukin-6 (IL-6) and IL-6 receptor/IL-6 fusion protein in organotypic hippocampal slices. *Mol Cell Neurosci* **25**, 301–311.

Pluchino, S., Quattrini, A., Brambilla, E., *et al.* (2003). Injection of adult neurospheres induces recovery in a chronic model of multiple sclerosis. *Nature* **422**, 688–694.

Pluchino, S., Zanotti, L., Deleidi, M., and Martino, G. (2005a). Neural stem cells and their use as therapeutic tool in neurological disorders. *Brain Res Brain Res Rev* **48**, 211–219.

Pluchino, S., Zanotti, L., Rossi, B., *et al.* (2005b). Neurosphere-derived multipotent precursors promote neuroprotection by an immunomodulatory mechanism. *Nature* **436**, 266–271.

Poliak, S. and Peles, E. (2003). The local differentiation of myelinated axons at nodes of Ranvier. *Nat Rev Neurosci* **4**, 968–980.

Poliak, S., Gollan, L., Martinez, R., *et al.* (1999). Caspr2, a new member of the neurexin superfamily, is localized at the juxtaparanodes of myelinated axons and associates with K$^+$ channels. *Neuron* **24**, 1037–1047.

Polito, A. and Reynolds, R. (2005). NG2-expressing cells as oligodendrocyte progenitors in the normal and demyelinated adult central nervous system. *J Anat* **207**, 707–716.

Poltorak, M., Sadoul, R., Keilhauer, G., Landa, C., Fahrig, T., and Schachner, M. (1987). Myelin-associated glycoprotein, a member of the L2/HNK-1 family of neural cell adhesion molecules, is involved in neuron-oligodendrocyte and oligodendrocyte-oligodendrocyte interaction. *J Cell Biol* **105**, 1893–1899.

Popko, B. and Baerwald, K. D. (1999). Oligodendroglial response to the immune cytokine interferon gamma. *Neurochem Res* **24**, 331–338.

Pot, C., Simonen, M., Weinmann, O., *et al.* (2002). Nogo-A expressed in Schwann cells impairs axonal regeneration after peripheral nerve injury. *J Cell Biol* **159**, 29–35.

Pouly, S., Becher, B., Blain, M., and Antel, J. P. (2000). Interferon-γ modulates human oligodendrocyte susceptibility to Fas-mediated apoptosis. *J Neuropathol Exp Neurol* **59**, 280–286.

Prestoz, L., Chatzopoulou, E., Lemkine, G., *et al.* (2004). Control of axonophilic migration of oligodendrocyte precursor cells by Eph-ephrin interaction. *Neuron Glia Biol* **1**, 73–83.

Prineas, J. W. and Connell, F. (1979). Remyelination in multiple sclerosis. *Ann Neurol* **5**, 22–31.

Prineas, J. W. and Graham, J. S. (1981). Multiple sclerosis: capping of surface immunoglobulin G on macrophages engaged in myelin breakdown. *Ann Neurol* **10**, 149–158.

Prineas, J. W., Barnard, R. O., Kwon, E. E., Sharer, L. R., and Cho, E. S. (1993a). Multiple sclerosis: remyelination of nascent lesions. *Ann Neurol* **33**, 137–151.

Prineas, J. W., Barnard, R. O., Revesz, T., Kwon, E. E., Sharer, L., and Cho, E. S. (1993b). Multiple sclerosis. Pathology of recurrent lesions. *Brain* **116**, 681–693.

Pringle, N. P. and Richardson, W. D. (1993). A singularity of PDGF alpha-receptor expression in the dorsoventral axis of the neural tube may define the origin of the oligodendrocyte lineage. *Development* **117**, 525–533.

Pringle, N. P., Mudhar, H. S., Collarini, E. J., and Richardson, W. D. (1992). PDGF receptors in the rat CNS: during late neurogenesis, PDGF alpha-receptor expression appears to be restricted to glial cells of the oligodendrocyte lineage. *Development* **115**, 535–551.

Pringle, N. P., Yu, W. P., Guthrie, S., *et al.* (1996). Determination of neuroepithelial cell fate: induction of the oligodendrocyte lineage by ventral midline cells and sonic hedgehog. *Dev Biol* **177**, 30–42.

Prinjha, R., Moore, S. E., Vinson, M., *et al.* (2000). Inhibitor of neurite outgrowth in humans. *Nature* **403**, 383–384.

Privat, A., Jacque, C., Bourre, J. M., Dupouey, P., and Baumann, N. (1979). Absence of the major dense line in myelin of the mutant mouse "shiverer". *Neurosci Lett* **12**, 107–112.

Proudfoot, A. E. (2002). Chemokine receptors: multifaceted therapeutic targets. *Nat Rev Immunol* **2**, 106–115.

Puchalski, R. B., Louis, J. C., Brose, N., *et al.* (1994). Selective RNA editing and subunit assembly of native glutamate receptors. *Neuron* **13**, 131–147.

Puckett, C., Hudson, L., Ono, K., *et al.* (1987). Myelin-specific proteolipid protein is expressed in myelinating Schwann cells but is not incorporated into myelin sheaths. *J Neurosci Res* **18**, 511–518.

Pujol, J., Soriano-Mas, C., Ortiz, H., Sebastian-Galles, N., Losilla, J. M., and Deus, J. (2006). Myelination of language-related areas in the developing brain. *Neurology* **66**, 339–343.

Rabchevsky, A. G., Sullivan, P. G., and Scheff, S. W. (2007). Temporal-spatial dynamics in oligodendrocyte and glial progenitor cell numbers throughout ventrolateral white matter following contusion spinal cord injury. *Glia* **55**, 831–843.

Racke, M. K. (2008). The role of B cells in multiple sclerosis: rationale for B-cell-targeted therapies. *Curr Opin Neurol* **21** Suppl 1, S9–S18.

Radi, R., Beckman, J.S., Bush, K.M., and Freeman, B.A. (1991). Peroxynitrite-induced membrane lipid peroxidation: the cytotoxic potential of superoxide and nitric oxide. *Arch Biochem Biophys* **288**, 481–487.

Raff, M.C. (1989). Glial cell diversification in the rat optic nerve. *Science* **243**, 1450–1455.

Raff, M.C., Miller, R.H., and Noble, M. (1983). A glial progenitor cell that develops in vitro into an astrocyte or an oligodendrocyte depending on culture medium. *Nature* **303**, 390–396.

Raff, M.C., Mirsky, R., Fields, K.L., *et al.* (1978). Galactocerebroside is a specific cell-surface antigenic marker for oligodendrocytes in culture. *Nature* **274**, 813–816.

Raine, C.S. (1991). Multiple sclerosis: a pivotal role for the T cell in lesion development. *Neuropathol Appl Neurobiol* **17**, 265–274.

Raine, C.S. and Cross, A.H. (1989). Axonal dystrophy as a consequence of long-term demyelination. *Lab Invest* **60**, 714–725.

Raine, C.S. and Wu, E. (1993). Multiple sclerosis: remyelination in acute lesions. *J Neuropathol Exp Neurol* **52**, 199–204.

Raine, C.S., Scheinberg, L., and Waltz, J.M. (1981). Multiple sclerosis. Oligodendrocyte survival and proliferation in an active established lesion. *Lab Invest* **45**, 534–546.

Raisman, G. (2004). Olfactory ensheathing cells and repair of brain and spinal cord injuries. *Cloning Stem Cells* **6**, 364–368.

Ranscht, B. and Dours, M.T. (1988). Sequence of contactin, a 130-kD glycoprotein concentrated in areas of interneuronal contact, defines a new member of the immunoglobulin supergene family in the nervous system. *J Cell Biol* **107**, 1561–1573.

Ranvier, L.A. (1878). *Leçons sur l'Histologie du Système Nerveux.* (Paris: Librarie F. Savy.)

Rasband, M.N., Park, E.W., Zhen, D., *et al.* (2002). Clustering of neuronal potassium channels is independent of their interaction with PSD-95. *J Cell Biol* **159**, 663–672.

Rasband, M.N., Tayler, J., Kaga, Y., *et al.* (2005). CNP is required for maintenance of axon-glia interactions at nodes of Ranvier in the CNS. *Glia* **50**, 86–90.

Rasband, M.N., Trimmer, J.S., Schwarz, T.L., *et al.* (1998). Potassium channel distribution, clustering, and function in remyelinating rat axons. *J Neurosci* **18**, 36–47.

Rash, J.E., Yasumura, T., Davidson, K.G., Furman, C.S., Dudek, F.E., and Nagy, J.I. (2001). Identification of cells expressing Cx43, Cx30, Cx26, Cx32 and Cx36 in gap junctions of rat brain and spinal cord. *Cell Commun Adhes* **8**, 315–320.

Rauer, S., Euler, B., Reindl, M., and Berger, T. (2006). Antimyelin antibodies and the risk of relapse in patients with a primary demyelinating event. *J Neurol Neurosurg Psychiatry* **77**, 739–742.

Readhead, C., Popko, B., Takahashi, N., *et al.* (1987). Expression of a myelin basic protein gene in shiverer transgenic mice: correction of the dysmyelinating phenotype. *Cell* **48**, 703–712.

Readhead, C., Schneider, A., Griffiths, I., and Nave, K.-A. (1994). Premature arrest of myelin formation in transgenic mice with increased proteolipid protein gene dosage. *Neuron* **12**, 583–595.

Redwine, J.M., Buchmeier, M.J., and Evans, C.F. (2001). In vivo expression of major histocompatibility complex molecules on oligodendrocytes and neurons during viral infection. *Am J Pathol* **159**, 1219–1224.

Reier, J. P. (1988). The glial scar: its bearing on axonal elongation and transplantation approaches to CNS repair. In *Functional Recovery in Neurological Disease*, S. G. Waxman, ed. (New York: Raven), pp. 87–138.

Relvas, J. B., Setzu, A., Baron, W., *et al.* (2001). Expression of dominant-negative and chimeric subunits reveals an essential role for beta1 integrin during myelination. *Curr Biol* **11**, 1039–1043.

Remahl, S. and Hildebrand, C. (1990). Relation between axons and oligodendroglial cells during initial myelination. I. The glial unit. *J Neurocytol* **19**, 313–328.

Reynolds, B. A. and Weiss, S. (1992). Generation of neurons and astrocytes from isolated cells of the adult mammalian central nervous system. *Science* **255**, 1707–1710.

Reynolds, B. A., Tetzlaff, W., and Weiss, S. (1992). A multipotent EGF-responsive striatal embryonic progenitor cell produces neurons and astrocytes. *J Neurosci* **12**, 4565–4574.

Reynolds, R. and Hardy, R. (1997). Oligodendroglial progenitors labeled with the O4 antibody persist in the adult rat cerebral cortex in vivo. *J Neurosci Res* **47**, 455–470.

Reynolds, R., Dawson, M., Papadopoulos, D., *et al.* (2002). The response of NG2-expressing oligodendrocyte progenitors to demyelination in MOG-EAE and MS. *J Neurocytol* **31**, 523–536.

Ricci-Vitiani, L., Conticello, C., Zeuner, A., and De Maria, R. (2000). CD95/CD95L interactions and their role in autoimmunity. *Apoptosis* **5**, 419–424.

Rice, C. M. and Scolding, N. J. (2004). Adult stem cells – reprogramming neurological repair? *Lancet* **364**, 193–199.

Rice, C. M., and Scolding, N. J. (2008). Autologous bone marrow stem cells – properties and advantages. *J Neurol Sci* **15**, 59–62.

Rice, C. M., Whone, A. L., Marks, D. I., Butler, S. B., Brooks, D. J., and Scolding, N. J. (2007). A safety and feasibility study of intravenous autologous bone marrow stem cells in multiple sclerosis. *J Neurol Neurosurg Psychiatry* **78**, 1014–1038.

Rice, G. P., Hartung, H. P., and Calabresi, P. A. (2005). Anti-alpha4 integrin therapy for multiple sclerosis: mechanisms and rationale. *Neurology* **64**, 1336–1342.

Richardson, P. M., McGuinness, U. M., and Aguayo, A. J. (1980). Axons from CNS neurons regenerate into PNS grafts. *Nature* **284**, 264–265.

Richardson, W. D., Kessaris, N., and Pringle, N. (2006). Oligodendrocyte wars. *Nat Rev Neurosci* **7**, 11–18.

Richardson, W. D., Pringle, N., Mosley, M. J., Westermark, B., and Dubois-Dalcq, M. (1988). A role for platelet-derived growth factor in normal gliogenesis in the central nervous system. *Cell* **53**, 309–319.

Richter-Landsberg, C. and Gorath, M. (1999). Developmental regulation of alternatively spliced isoforms of mRNA encoding MAP2 and tau in rat brain oligodendrocytes during culture maturation. *J Neurosci Res* **56**, 259–270.

Riethmacher, D., Sonnenberg-Riethmacher, E., Brinkmann, V., Yamaai, T., Lewin, G. R., and Birchmeier, C. (1997). Severe neuropathies in mice with targeted mutations in the ErbB3 receptor. *Nature* **389**, 725–730.

Rincon-Orozco, B., Kunzmann, V., Wrobel, P., Kabelitz, D., Steinle, A., and Herrmann, T. (2005). Activation of V gamma 9V delta 2 T cells by NKG2D. *J Immunol* **175**, 2144–2151.

Rios, J. C., Melendez-Vasquez, C. V., Einheber, S., *et al.* (2000). Contactin-associated protein (Caspr) and contactin form a complex that is targeted to the paranodal junctions during myelination. *J Neurosci* **20**, 8354–8364.

Rivera, F. J., Couillard-Despres, S., Pedre, X., *et al.* (2006). Mesenchymal stem cells instruct oligodendrogenic fate decision on adult neural stem cells. *Stem Cells* **24**, 2209–2219.

Rivers, L. E., Young, K. M., Rizzi, M., *et al.* (2008). PDGFRA/NG2 glia generate myelinating oligodendrocytes and piriform projection neurons in adult mice. *Nat Neurosci* **11**, 1392–1401.

Robinson, S., Tani, M., Strieter, R. M., Ransohoff, R. M., and Miller, R. H. (1998). The chemokine growth-regulated oncogene-alpha promotes spinal cord oligodendrocyte precursor proliferation. *J Neurosci* **18**, 10457–10463.

Rodriguez, M. (2003). A function of myelin is to protect axons from subsequent injury: implications for deficits in multiple sclerosis. *Brain* **126**, 751–752.

Rodriguez, M., Scheithauer, B. W., Forbes, G., and Kelly, P. J. (1993). Oligodendrocyte injury is an early event in lesions of multiple sclerosis. *Mayo Clin Proc* **68**, 627–636.

Roettger, V. and Lipton, P. (1996). Mechanism of glutamate release from rat hippocampal slices during in vitro ischemia. *Neuroscience* **75**, 677–685.

Rosenberg, P. A. and Aizenman, E. (1989). Hundred-fold increase in neuronal vulnerability to glutamate toxicity in astrocyte-poor cultures of rat cerebral cortex. *Neurosci Lett* **103**, 162–168.

Rosenberg, P. A., Amin, S., and Leitner, M. (1992). Glutamate uptake disguises neurotoxic potency of glutamate agonists in cerebral cortex in dissociated cell culture. *J Neurosci* **12**, 56–61.

Rosenberg, P. A., Dai, W. M., Gan, X. D., *et al.* (2003). Mature myelin basic protein-expressing oligodendrocytes are insensitive to kainate toxicity. *J Neurosci Res* **71**, 237–245.

Rosenbluth, J. (1980a). Central myelin in the mouse mutant shiverer. *J Comp Neurol* **194**, 639–648.

Rosenbluth, J. (1980b). Peripheral myelin in the mouse mutant Shiverer. *J Comp Neurol* **193**, 729–739.

Rosenbluth, J., Schiff, R., and Lam, P. (2009). Effects of osmolality on PLP-null myelin structure: implications re axon damage. *Brain Res* **1253**, 191–197.

Rossi, D. and Zlotnik, A. (2000). The biology of chemokines and their receptors. *Annu Rev Immunol* **18**, 217–242.

Rossi, D. J., Oshima, T., and Attwell, D. (2000). Glutamate release in severe brain ischaemia is mainly by reversed uptake. *Nature* **403**, 316–321.

Roth, A. D., Ivanova, A., and Colman, D. R. (2006). New observations on the compact myelin proteome. *Neuron Glia Biol* **2**, 15–21.

Rothman, R. H., and Simeone, F. A. (1992). *The Spine.* (Philadelphia, PA: Saunders.)

Rousset, C. I., Kassem, J., Olivier, P., Chalon, S., Gressens, P., and Saliba, E. (2008). Antenatal bacterial endotoxin sensitizes the immature rat brain to postnatal excitotoxic injury. *J Neuropathol Exp Neurol* **67**, 994–1000.

Rowitch, D. H. (2004). Glial specification in the vertebrate neural tube. *Nat Rev Neurosci* **5**, 409–419.

Rowitch, D. H., Lu, Q. R., Kessaris, N., and Richardson, W. D. (2002). An "oligarchy" rules neural development. *Trends Neurosci* **25**, 417–422.

Roy, K., Murtie, J. C., El Khodor, B. F., *et al.* (2007). Loss of erbB signaling in oligodendrocytes alters myelin and dopaminergic function, a potential mechanism for neuropsychiatric disorders. *Proc Natl Acad Sci USA* **104**, 8131–8136.

Roy, N. S., Cleren, C., Singh, S. K., Yang, L., Beal, M. F., and Goldman, S. A. (2006). Functional engraftment of human ES cell-derived dopaminergic neurons enriched by coculture with telomerase-immortalized midbrain astrocytes. *Nat Med* **12**, 1259–1268.

Ruijs, T. C., Freedman, M. S., Grenier, Y. G., Olivier, A., and Antel, J. P. (1990). Human oligodendrocytes are susceptible to cytolysis by major histocompatibility complex class I-restricted lymphocytes. *J Neuroimmunol* **27**, 89–97.

Rutkowski, J. L., Kirk, C. J., Lerner, M. A., and Tennekoon, G. I. (1995). Purification and expansion of human schwann cells in vitro. *Nature Med* **1**, 80–83.

Saher, G., Brugger, B., Lappe-Siefke, C., *et al.* (2005). High cholesterol level is essential for myelin membrane growth. *Nat Neurosci* **8**, 468–475.

Saikali, P., Antel, J. P., Newcombe, J., *et al.* (2007). NKG2D-mediated cytotoxicity toward oligodendrocytes suggests a mechanism for tissue injury in multiple sclerosis. *J Neurosci* **27**, 1220–1228.

Salter, M. G. and Fern, R. (2005). NMDA receptors are expressed in developing oligodendrocyte processes and mediate injury. *Nature* **438**, 1167–1171.

Salviati, L., Trevisson, E., Baldoin, M. C., *et al.* (2007). A novel deletion in the GJA12 gene causes Pelizaeus-Merzbacher-like disease. *Neurogenetics* **8**, 57–60.

Salzer, J. L. (2003). Polarized domains of myelinated axons. *Neuron* **40**, 297–318.

Salzer, J. L., Brophy, P. J., and Peles, E. (2008). Molecular domains of myelinated axons in the peripheral nervous system. *Glia* **56**, 1532–1540.

Salzer, J. L., Holmes, W. P., and Colman, D. R. (1987). The amino acid sequences of the myelin-associated glycoproteins: homology to the immunoglobulin gene superfamily. *J Cell Biol* **104**, 957–965.

Sandler, A. N. and Tator, C. H. (1976). Effect of acute spinal cord compression injury on regional spinal cord blood flow in primates. *J Neurosurg* **45**, 660–676.

Sasaki, M., Honmou, O., Akiyama, Y., Uede, T., Hashi, K., and Kocsis, J. D. (2001). Transplantation of an acutely isolated bone marrow fraction repairs demyelinated adult rat spinal cord axons. *Glia* **35**, 26–34.

Sasaki, Y. F., Rothe, T., Premkumar, L. S., *et al.* (2002). Characterization and comparison of the NR3A subunit of the NMDA receptor in recombinant systems and primary cortical neurons. *J Neurophysiol* **87**, 2052–2063.

Satoh, J., Kastrukoff, L. F., and Kim, S. U. (1991). Cytokine-induced expression of intercellular adhesion molecule-1 (ICAM-1) in cultured human oligodendrocytes and astrocytes. *J Neuropathol Exp Neurol* **50**, 215–226.

Savio, T. and Schwab, M. E. (1990). Lesioned corticospinal tract axons regenerate in myelin-free rat spinal cord. *Proc Natl Acad Sci USA* **87**, 4130–4133.

Sawada, M., Itoh, Y., Suzumura, A., and Marunouchi, T. (1993). Expression of cytokine receptors in cultured neuronal and glial cells. *Neurosci Lett* **160**, 131–134.

Schabitz, W. R., Li, F., and Fisher, M. (2000). The N-methyl-D-aspartate antagonist CNS 1102 protects cerebral gray and white matter from ischemic injury following temporary focal ischemia in rats. *Stroke* **31**, 1709–1714.

Schachner, M. and Bartsch, U. (2000). Multiple functions of the myelin-associated glycoprotein MAG (siglec-4a) in formation and maintenance of myelin. *Glia* **29**, 154–165.

Schaefer, A., O'Carroll, D., Tan, C. L., *et al.* (2007). Cerebellar neurodegeneration in the absence of microRNAs. *J Exp Med* **204**, 1553–1558.

Schaeren-Wiemers, N., Schaefer, C., Valenzuela, D. M., Yancopoulos, G. D., and Schwab, M. E. (1995). Identification of new oligodendrocyte- and myelin-specific genes by a differential screening approach. *J Neurochem* **65**, 10–22.

Schafer, D. P. and Rasband, M. N. (2006). Glial regulation of the axonal membrane at nodes of Ranvier. *Curr Opin Neurobiol* **16**, 508–514.

Schafer, M., Fruttiger, M., Montag, D., Schachner, M., and Martini, R. (1996). Disruption of the gene for the myelin-associated glycoprotein improves axonal regrowth along myelin in C57BL/Wlds mice. *Neuron* **16**, 1107–1113.

Scheinman, R. I., Cogswell, P. C., Lofquist, A. K., and Baldwin, A. S., Jr. (1995). Role of transcriptional activation of I kappa B alpha in mediation of immuno-suppression by glucocorticoids. *Science* **270**, 283–286.

Scheld, W. M., Whitley, R. J., and Marra, C. M. eds. (2004). *Infections of the Central Nervous System*, 3rd edn. (Philadelphia, PA: Lippincott Williams & Wilkins.)

Scherer, S. S. and Arroyo, E. J. (2002). Recent progress on the molecular organization of myelinated axons. *J Peripher Nerv Syst* **7**, 1–12.

Scherer, S. S. and Easter, S. S., Jr. (1984). Degenerative and regenerative changes in the trochlear nerve of goldfish. *J Neurocytol* **13**, 519–565.

Scherer, S. S. and Wrabetz, L. (2008). Molecular mechanisms of inherited demyelinating neuropathies. *Glia* **56**, 1578–1589.

Scherer, S. S., Deschenes, S. M., Xu, Y. T., Grinspan, J. B., Fischbeck, K. H., and Paul, D. L. (1995). Connexin32 is a myelin-related protein in the PNS and CNS. *J Neurosci* **15**, 8281–8294.

Scherer, S. S., Vogelbacker, H. H., and Kamholz, J. (1992). Axons modulate the expression of proteolipid protein in the CNS. *J Neurosci Res* **32**, 138–148.

Scherer, S. S., Xu, Y. T., Nelles, E., Fischbeck, K., Willecke, K., and Bone, L. J. (1998). Connexin32-null mice develop demyelinating peripheral neuropathy. *Glia* **24**, 8–20.

Schlag, B. D., Vondrasek, J. R., Munir, M., *et al.* (1998). Regulation of the glial Na$^+$-dependent glutamate transporters by cyclic AMP analogs and neurons. *Mol Pharmacol* **53**, 355–369.

Schliwa, M. and Woehlke, G. (2003). Molecular motors. *Nature* **422**, 759–765.

Schlomann, U., Rathke-Hartlieb, S., Yamamoto, S., Jockusch, H., and Bartsch, J. W. (2000). Tumor necrosis factor alpha induces a metalloprotease-disintegrin, ADAM8 (CD 156): implications for neuron-glia interactions during neurodegeneration. *J Neurosci* **20**, 7964–7971.

Schmitz, T., Heep, A., Groenendaal, F., *et al.* (2007). Interleukin-1beta, interleukin-18, and interferon-gamma expression in the cerebrospinal fluid of premature infants with posthemorrhagic hydrocephalus – markers of white matter damage? *Pediatr Res* **61**, 722–726.

Schnapp, B. and Mugnaini, E. (1976). Freeze-fracture properties of central myelin in the bullfrog. *Neuroscience* **1**, 459–467.

Schneider, A. and Mandelkow, E. (2008). Tau-based treatment strategies in neurodegenerative diseases. *Neurotherapeutics* **5**, 443–457.

Schnell, L. and Schwab, M. E. (1990). Axonal regeneration in the rat spinal cord produced by an antibody against myelin-associated neurite growth inhibitors. *Nature* **343**, 269–272.

Scholz, J., Klein, M. C., Behrens, T. E., and Johansen-Berg, H. (2009). Training induces changes in white-matter architecture. *Nat Neurosci* **12**, 1370–1371.

Schonberg, D. L., Popovich, P. G., and McTigue, D. M. (2007). Oligodendrocyte generation is differentially influenced by toll-like receptor (TLR) 2 and TLR4-mediated intraspinal macrophage activation. *J Neuropathol Exp Neurol* **66**, 1124–1135.

Schroder, M. and Kaufman, R. J. (2005). The mammalian unfolded protein response. *Annu Rev Biochem* **74**, 739–789.

Schultz, R. L. and Pease, D. C. (1959). Cicatrix formation in rat cerebral cortex as revealed by electron microscopy. *Am J Pathol* **35**, 1017–1041.

Schwab, C. and McGeer, P. L. (2002). Complement activated C4d immunoreactive oligodendrocytes delineate small cortical plaques in multiple sclerosis. *Exp Neurol* **174**, 81–88.

Schwab, M. E. (2004). Nogo and axon regeneration. *Curr Opin Neurobiol* **14**, 118–124.

Schwab, M. E. and Bartholdi, D. (1996). Degeneration and regeneration of axons in the lesioned spinal cord. *Physiol Rev* **76**, 319–370.

Schwab, M. E. and Caroni, P. (1988). Oligodendrocytes and CNS myelin are non-permissive substrates for neurite growth and fibroblast spreading in vitro. *J Neurosci* **8**, 2381–2393.

Schwab, M. E. and Thoenen, H. (1985). Dissociated neurons regenerate into sciatic but not optic nerve explants in culture irrespective of neurotrophic factors. *J Neurosci* **5**, 2415–2423.

Schwarz, S., Knauth, M., Schwab, S., Walter-Sack, I., Bonmann, E., and Storch-Hagenlocher, B. (2000). Acute disseminated encephalomyelitis after parenteral therapy with herbal extracts: a report of two cases. *J Neurol Neurosurg Psychiatry* **69**, 516–518.

Schweigreiter, R., Roots, B. I., Bandtlow, C. E., and Gould, R. M. (2006). Understanding myelination through studying its evolution. *Int Rev Neurobiol* **73**, 219–273.

Schweitzer, J., Becker, T., Schachner, M., Nave, K. A., and Werner, H. (2006). Evolution of myelin proteolipid proteins: gene duplication in teleosts and expression pattern divergence. *Mol Cell Neurosci* **31**, 161–177.

Scolding, N. (2005). Stem-cell therapy: hope and hype. *Lancet* **365**, 2073–2075.

Scolding, N. J. and Compston, D. A. (1991). Oligodendrocyte-macrophage interactions in vitro triggered by specific antibodies. *Immunology* **72**, 127–132.

Scolding, N. J. and Dubois-Dalcq, M. (2008). Moving toward remyelinating and neuroprotective therapies in MS. In *Multiple Sclerosis: A Comprehensive Text*, C. S. Raine, H. McFarland, and R. Hohlfeld, eds. (Philadelphia, PA: Saunders Elsevier), pp. 366–382.

Scolding, N. J. and Rice, C. (2008). Autologous mesenchymal bone marrow stem cells: practical considerations. *J Neurol Sci* **15**, 111–115.

Scolding, N. J., Franklin, R. J. M., Stevens, S., Heldin, C. H., Compston, D. A. S., and Newcombe, J. (1998a). Oligodendrocyte progenitors are present in the normal adult human CNS and in the lesions of multiple sclerosis. *Brain* **121**, 2221–2228.

Scolding, N. J., Jones, J., Compston, D. A. S., and Morgan, B. P. (1990). Oligodendrocyte susceptibility to injury by T-cell perforin. *Immunology* **70**, 6–10.

Scolding, N. J., Morgan, B. P., and Compston, D. A. (1998b). The expression of complement regulatory proteins by adult human oligodendrocytes. *J Neuroimmunol* **84**, 69–75.

Scolding, N. J., Morgan, B. P., Houston, W. A. J., Linington, C., Campbell, A. K., and Compston, D. A. S. (1989). Vesicular removal by oligodendrocytes of membrane attack complexes formed by activated complement. *Nature* **339**, 620–622.

Scolding, N. J., Rayner, P. J., and Compston, D. A. (1999). Identification of A2B5-positive putative oligodendrocyte progenitor cells and A2B5-positive astrocytes in adult human white matter. *Neuroscience* **89**, 1–4.

Scolding, N. J., Rayner, P. J., Sussman, J., Shaw, C., and Compston, D. A. S. (1995). A proliferative adult human oligodendrocyte progenitor. *NeuroReport* **6**, 441–445.

Scott, G. S., Spitsin, S. V., Kean, R. B., Mikheeva, T., Koprowski, H., and Hooper, D. C. (2002). Therapeutic intervention in experimental allergic encephalomyelitis by administration of uric acid precursors. *Proc Natl Acad Sci USA* **99**, 16303–16308.

Scott, G. S., Virag, L., Szabo, C., and Hooper, D. C. (2003). Peroxynitrite-induced oligodendrocyte toxicity is not dependent on poly(ADP-ribose) polymerase activation. *Glia* **41**, 105–116.

Seeman, P., Mazanec, R., Ctvrteckova, M., and Smilkova, D. (2001). Charcot-Marie-Tooth type X: a novel mutation in the Cx32 gene with central conduction slowing. *Int J Mol Med* **8**, 461–468.

Segal, D., Koschnick, J. R., Slegers, L. H., and Hof, P. R. (2007). Oligodendrocyte pathophysiology: a new view of schizophrenia. *Int J Neuropsychopharmacol* **10**, 503–511.

Segovia, K. N., McClure, M., Moravec, M., *et al.* (2008). Arrested oligodendrocyte lineage maturation in chronic perinatal white matter injury. *Ann Neurol* **63**, 520–530.

Seilheimer, B. and Schachner, M. (1988). Studies of adhesion molecules mediating interactions between cells of peripheral nervous system indicate a major role for L1 in mediating sensory neuron growth on Schwann cells in culture. *J Cell Biol* **107**, 341–351.

Seilheimer, B., Persohn, E., and Schachner, M. (1989). Antibodies to the L1 adhesion molecule inhibit Schwann cell ensheathment of neurons in vitro. *J Cell Biol* **109**, 3095–3103.

Seki, Y., Feustel, P. J., Keller, R. W., Jr., Tranmer, B. I., and Kimelberg, H. K. (1999). Inhibition of ischemia-induced glutamate release in rat striatum by dihydrokinate and an anion channel blocker. *Stroke* **30**, 433–440.

Sellers, D. L., Maris, D. O., and Horner, P. J. (2009). Postinjury niches induce temporal shifts in progenitor fates to direct lesion repair after spinal cord injury. *J Neurosci* **29**, 6722–6733.

Selmaj, K. W. (2000). Tumour necrosis factor and anti-tumour necrosis factor approach to inflammatory demyelinating diseases of the central nervous system. *Ann Rheum Dis* **59** Suppl 1, i94–102.

Selmaj, K., Brosnan, C. F., and Raine, C. S. (1991a). Colocalization of lymphocytes bearing gamma/delta T-cell receptor and heat shock protein hsp 65+ oligodendrocytes in multiple sclerosis. *Proc Natl Acad Sci USA* **88**, 6452–6456.

Selmaj, K., Raine, C. S., and Cross, A. H. (1991b). Anti-tumor necrosis factor therapy abrogates autoimmune demyelination. *Ann Neurol* **30**, 694–700.

Shao, Z., Browning, J. L., Lee, X., *et al.* (2005). TAJ/TROY, an orphan TNF receptor family member, binds Nogo-66 receptor 1 and regulates axonal regeneration. *Neuron* **45**, 353–359.

Sharp, F. R. and Bernaudin, M. (2004). HIF1 and oxygen sensing in the brain. *Nat Rev Neurosci* **5**, 437–448.

Sheikh, K. A., Sun, J., Liu, Y., *et al.* (1999). Mice lacking complex gangliosides develop Wallerian degeneration and myelination defects. *Proc Natl Acad Sci USA* **96**, 7532–7537.

Sherman, D. L. and Brophy, P. J. (2005). Mechanisms of axon ensheathment and myelin growth. *Nat Rev Neurosci* **6**, 683–690.

Sherman, D. L., Tait, S., Melrose, S., *et al.* (2005). Neurofascins are required to establish axonal domains for saltatory conduction. *Neuron* **48**, 737–742.

Shi, Y., Do, J. T., Desponts, C., Hahm, H. S., Scholer, H. R., and Ding, S. (2008). A combined chemical and genetic approach for the generation of induced pluripotent stem cells. *Cell Stem Cell* **2**, 525–528.

Siegel, G. J., Agranoff, B. W., Fisher, S. K., Albers, R. W., and Uhler, M. D. (1999). *Basic Neurochemistry: Molecular, Cellular and Medical Aspects.* (Philadelphia, PA: Lippincott–Raven Publishers.)

Silver, J. and Miller, J. H. (2004). Regeneration beyond the glial scar. *Nat Rev Neurosci* **5**, 146–156.

Silverstein, F. S., Naik, B., and Simpson, J. (1991). Hypoxia-ischemia stimulates hippocampal glutamate efflux in perinatal rat brain: an in vivo microdialysis study. *Pediatr Res* **30**, 587–590.

Simard, A. R. and Rivest, S. (2006). Neuroprotective properties of the innate immune system and bone marrow stem cells in Alzheimer's disease. *Mol Psychiatry* **11**, 327–335.

Simonen, M., Pedersen, V., Weinmann, O., *et al.* (2003). Systemic deletion of the myelin-associated outgrowth inhibitor Nogo-A improves regenerative and plastic responses after spinal cord injury. *Neuron* **38**, 201–211.

Simons, M. and Trajkovic, K. (2006). Neuron-glia communication in the control of oligodendrocyte function and myelin biogenesis. *J Cell Sci* **119**, 4381–4389.

Simons, M. and Trotter, J. (2007). Wrapping it up: the cell biology of myelination. *Curr Opin Neurobiol* **17**, 533–540.

Simpson, P. B. and Armstrong, R. C. (1999). Intracellular signals and cytoskeletal elements involved in oligodendrocyte progenitor migration. *Glia* **26**, 22–35.

Singec, I. and Snyder, E. Y. (2008). Inflammation as a matchmaker: revisiting cell fusion. *Nat Cell Biol* **10**, 503–505.

Singh, A. K., Wilson, M. T., Hong, S., *et al.* (2001). Natural killer T cell activation protects mice against experimental autoimmune encephalomyelitis. *J Exp Med* **194**, 1801–1811.

Sinibaldi, L., De Luca, A., Bellacchio, E., *et al.* (2004). Mutations of the Nogo-66 receptor (RTN4R) gene in schizophrenia. *Hum Mutat* **24**, 534–535.

Sloane, J. A. and Vartanian, T. K. (2007a). Myosin Va controls oligodendrocyte morphogenesis and myelination. *J Neurosci* **27**, 11366–11375.

Sloane, J. A. and Vartanian, T. K. (2007b). WAVE1 and regulation of actin nucleation in myelination. *Neuroscientist* **13**, 486–491.

Sloane, J. A., Hinman, J. D., Lubonia, M., Hollander, W., and Abraham, C. R. (2003). Age-dependent myelin degeneration and proteolysis of oligodendrocyte proteins is associated with the activation of calpain-1 in the rhesus monkey. *J Neurochem* **84**, 157–168.

Smirnova, L., Grafe, A., Seiler, A., Schumacher, S., Nitsch, R., and Wulczyn, F. G. (2005). Regulation of miRNA expression during neural cell specification. *Eur J Neurosci* **21**, 1469–1477.

Smith, K. J., Blakemore, W. F., and McDonald, W. I. (1979). Central remyelination restores secure conduction. *Nature* **280**, 395–396.

Smith, K. J., Blakemore, W. F., and McDonald, W. I. (1981). The restoration of conduction by central remyelination. *Brain* **104**, 383–404.

Smith, K. J., Bostock, H., and Hall, S. M. (1982). Saltatory conduction precedes remyelination in axons demyelinated with lysophosphatidyl choline. *J Neurol Sci* **54**, 13–31.

Smith, T., Groom, A., Zhu, B., and Turski, L. (2000). Autoimmune encephalomyelitis ameliorated by AMPA antagonists. *Nat Med* **6**, 62–66.

Snethen, H., Love, S., and Scolding, N. (2008). Disease-responsive neural precursor cells are present in multiple sclerosis lesions. *Regenerative Med* **3**, 835–847.

Soane, L., Cho, H. J., Niculescu, F., Rus, H., and Shin, M. L. (2001). C5b-9 terminal complement complex protects oligodendrocytes from death by regulating Bad through phosphatidylinositol 3-kinase/Akt pathway. *J Immunol* **167**, 2305–2311.

Sohn, J., Natale, J., Chew, L. J., *et al.* (2006). Identification of Sox17 as a transcription factor that regulates oligodendrocyte development. *J Neurosci* **26**, 9722–9735.

Sokolov, B. P. (2007). Oligodendroglial abnormalities in schizophrenia, mood disorders and substance abuse. Comorbidity, shared traits, or molecular phenocopies? *Int J Neuropsychopharmacol* **10**, 547–555.

Soldan, M. M., Warrington, A. E., Bieber, A. J., *et al.* (2003). Remyelination-promoting antibodies activate distinct Ca^{2+} influx pathways in astrocytes and oligodendrocytes: relationship to the mechanism of myelin repair. *Mol Cell Neurosci* **22**, 14–24.

Somjen, G. G. (1988). Nervenkitt: notes on the history of the concept of neuroglia. *Glia* **1**, 2–9.

Song, J., Goetz, B. D., Baas, P. W., and Duncan, I. D. (2001). Cytoskeletal reorganization during the formation of oligodendrocyte processes and branches. *Mol Cell Neurosci* **17**, 624–636.

Song, J., O'Connor, L. T., Yu, W., Baas, P. W., and Duncan, I. D. (1999). Microtubule alterations in cultured taiep rat oligodendrocytes lead to deficits in myelin membrane formation. *J Neurocytol* **28**, 671–683.

Song, S. K., Sun, S. W., Ramsbottom, M. J., Chang, C., Russell, J., and Cross, A. H. (2002). Dysmyelination revealed through MRI as increased radial (but unchanged axial) diffusion of water. *Neuroimage* **17**, 1429–1436.

Song, S. K., Yoshino, J., Le, T. Q., *et al.* (2005). Demyelination increases radial diffusivity in corpus callosum of mouse brain. *Neuroimage* **26**, 132–140.

Sontheimer, H. (1991). Astrocytes, as well as neurons, express a diversity of ion channels. *Can J Physiol Pharmacol* **70**, s223–s238.

Southwood, C. M., Peppi, M., Dryden, S., Tainsky, M. A., and Gow, A. (2007). Microtubule deacetylases, SirT2 and HDAC6, in the nervous system. *Neurochem Res* **32**, 187–195.

Spassky, N., Goujet-Zalc, C., Parmantier, E., *et al.* (1998). Multiple restricted origin of oligodendrocytes. *J Neurosci* **18**, 8331–8343.

Spiegel, I. and Peles, E. (2002). Cellular junctions of myelinated nerves (Review). *Mol Membr Biol* **19**, 95–101.

Spiegel, I., Adamsky, K., Eshed, Y., *et al.* (2007). A central role for Necl4 (SynCAM4) in Schwann cell-axon interaction and myelination. *Nat Neurosci* **10**, 861–869.

Spillantini, M. G., Goedert, M., Crowther, R. A., Murrell, J. R., Farlow, M. R., and Ghetti, B. (1997). Familial multiple system tauopathy with presenile dementia: a disease with abundant neuronal and glial tau filaments. *Proc Natl Acad Sci USA* **94**, 4113–4118.

Spillmann, A. A., Bandtlow, C. E., Lottspeich, F., Keller, F., and Schwab, M. E. (1998). Identification and characterization of a bovine neurite growth inhibitor (bNI-220). *J Biol Chem* **273**, 19283–19293.

Squier, T. C. (2001). Oxidative stress and protein aggregation during biological aging. *Exp Gerontol* **36**, 1539–1550.

Srinivasan, R., Sailasuta, N., Hurd, R., Nelson, S., and Pelletier, D. (2005). Evidence of elevated glutamate in multiple sclerosis using magnetic resonance spectroscopy at 3 T. *Brain* **128**, 1016–1025.

Stadelmann, C., Ludwin, S., Tabira, T., *et al.* (2005). Tissue preconditioning may explain concentric lesions in Balo's type of multiple sclerosis. *Brain* **128**, 979–987.

Stefansson, H., Sigurdsson, E., Steinthorsdottir, V., *et al.* (2002). Neuregulin 1 and susceptibility to schizophrenia. *Am J Hum Genet* **71**, 877–892.

Steinman, L. (1996). A few autoreactive cells in an autoimmune infiltrate control a vast population of nonspecific cells: a tale of smart bombs and the infantry. *Proc Natl Acad Sci USA* **93**, 2253–2256.

Sternberger, N. H., Itoyama, Y., Koco, M. W., and Webster, H. D. (1978). Myelin basic protein demonstrated immunocytochemically in oligodendroglia prior to myelin sheath formation. *Proc Natl Acad Sci USA* **75**, 2521–2524.

Sternberger, N. H., Quarles, R. H., Itoyama, Y., and Webster, H. D. (1979). Myelin-associated glycoprotein demonstrated immunocytochemically in myelin and myelin-forming cells of developing rats. *Proc Natl Acad Sci USA* **76**, 1510–1514.

Stevens, B. and Fields, R. D. (2000). Response of Schwann cells to action potentials in development. *Science* **287**, 2267–2271.

Stevens, B., Porta, S., Haak, L. L., Gallo, V., and Fields, R. D. (2002). Adenosine: a neuron-glial transmitter promoting myelination in the CNS in response to action potentials. *Neuron* **36**, 855–868.

Stidworthy, M. F., Genoud, S., Suter, U., Mantei, N., and Franklin, R. J. (2003). Quantifying the early stages of remyelination following cuprizone-induced demyelination. *Brain Pathol* **13**, 329–339.

Stoffel, W., Boison, D., and Bussow, H. (1997). Functional analysis in vivo of the double mutant mouse deficient in both proteolipid protein (PLP) and myelin basic protein (MBP) in the central nervous system. *Cell Tissue Res* **289**, 195–206.

Stokes, B. T. and Jakeman, L. B. (2002). Experimental modelling of human spinal cord injury: a model that crosses the species barrier and mimics the spectrum of human cytopathology. *Spinal Cord* **40**, 101–109.

Stokes, B. T., Garwood, M., and Walters, P. (1981). Oxygen fields in specific spinal loci of the canine spinal cord. *Am J Physiol* **240**, H761–H766.

Stoll, G. and Muller, H. W. (1999). Nerve injury, axonal degeneration and neural regeneration: basic insights. *Brain Pathol* **9**, 313–325.

Stoll, G., Schroeter, M., Jander, S., *et al.* (2004). Lesion-associated expression of transforming growth factor-beta-2 in the rat nervous system: evidence for down-regulating the phagocytic activity of microglia and macrophages. *Brain Pathol* **14**, 51–58.

Stoll, G., Trapp, B. D., and Griffin, J. W. (1989). Macrophage function during Wallerian degeneration of rat optic nerve: clearance of degenerating myelin and Ia expression. *J Neurosci* **9**, 2327–2335.

Storck, T., Schulte, S., Hofmann, K., and Stoffel, W. (1992). Structure, expression, and functional analysis of a Na⁺-dependent glutamate/aspartate transporter from rat brain. *Proc Natl Acad Sci USA* **89**, 10955–10959.

Stys, P. K. (2004). White matter injury mechanisms. *Curr Mol Med* **4**, 113–130.

Sugai, T., Kawamura, M., Iritani, S., *et al.* (2004). Prefrontal abnormality of schizophrenia revealed by DNA microarray: impact on glial and neurotrophic gene expression. *Ann N Y Acad Sci* **1025**, 84–91.

Sulaiman, O. A. R., Boyd, J. G., and Gordon, T. (2005). Axonal regeneration in the peripheral nervous system of mammals. In *Neuroglia*, H. Kettenmann and B. R. Ransom, eds. (New York: Oxford University Press), pp. 454–466.

Sullivan, C. D. and Geisert, E. E., Jr. (1998). Expression of rat target of the anti-proliferative antibody (TAPA) in the developing brain. *J Comp Neurol* **396**, 366–380.

Suzuki, K. (2003). Globoid cell leukodystrophy (Krabbe's disease): update. *J Child Neurol* **18**, 595–603.

Svaren, J. and Meijer, D. (2008). The molecular machinery of myelin gene transcription in Schwann cells. *Glia* **56**, 1541–1551.

Swanson, R. A., Miller, J. W., Rothstein, J. D., Farrell, K., Stein, B. A., and Longuemare, M. C. (1997). Neuronal regulation of glutamate transporter subtype expression in astrocytes. *J Neurosci* **17**, 932–940.

Szatkowski, M., Barbour, B., and Attwell, D. (1990). Non-vesicular release of glutamate from glial cells by reversed electrogenic glutamate uptake. *Nature* **348**, 443–446.

Tabira, T., Cullen, M. J., Reier, P. J., and Webster, H. D. (1978). An experimental analysis of interlamellar tight junctions in amphibian and mammalian CNS myelin. *J Neurocytol* **7**, 489–503.

Tait, S., Gunn-Moore, F., Collinson, J. M., *et al.* (2000). An oligodendroctye cell adhesion molecule at the site of assembly of the paranodal axo-glial junction. *J Cell Biol* **150**, 657–666.

Takahashi, K., Tanabe, K., Ohnuki, M., *et al.* (2007). Induction of pluripotent stem cells from adult human fibroblasts by defined factors. *Cell* **131**, 861–872.

Takano, R., Misu, T., Takahashi, T., Izumiyama, M., Fujihara, K., and Itoyama, Y. (2008). A prominent elevation of glial fibrillary acidic protein in the cerebrospinal fluid during relapse in neuromyelitis optica. *Tohoku J Exp Med* **215**, 55–59.

Takebayashi, H., Nabeshima, Y., Yoshida, S., Chisaka, O., and Ikenaka, K. (2002). The basic helix-loop-helix factor olig2 is essential for the development of motoneuron and oligodendrocyte lineages. *Curr Biol* **12**, 1157–1163.

Takeda, Y., Asou, H., Murakami, Y., Miura, M., Kobayashi, M., and Uyemura, K. (1996). A nonneuronal isoform of cell adhesion molecule L1: tissue-specific expression and functional analysis. *J Neurochem* **66**, 2338–2349.

Talbott, J. F., Loy, D. N., Liu, Y., *et al.* (2005). Endogenous Nkx2.2+/Olig2+ oligodendrocyte precursor cells fail to remyelinate the demyelinated adult rat spinal cord in the absence of astrocytes. *Exp Neurol* **192**, 11–24.

Talos, D. M., Fishman, R. E., Park, H., *et al.* (2006). Developmental regulation of alpha-amino-3-hydroxy-5-methyl-4-isoxazole-propionic acid receptor subunit expression in forebrain and relationship to regional susceptibility to hypoxic/ischemic injury. I. Rodent cerebral white matter and cortex. *J Comp Neurol* **497**, 42–60.

Tambuyzer, B. R., Ponsaerts, P., and Nouwen, E. J. (2009). Microglia: gatekeepers of central nervous system immunology. *J Leukoc Biol* **85**, 352–370.

Tanaka, J. and Sobue, K. (1994). Localization and characterization of gelsolin in nervous tissues: gelsolin is specifically enriched in myelin-forming cells. *J Neurosci* **14**, 1038–1052.

Tanaka, K., Watase, K., Manabe, T., *et al.* (1997). Epilepsy and exacerbation of brain injury in mice lacking the glutamate transporter GLT-1. *Science* **276**, 1699–1702.

Targett, M., Sussman, J., Scolding, N., O'Leary, M. T., Compston, D. A., and Blakemore, W. F. (1996). Failure to achieve remyelination of demyelinated rat axons following transplantation of glial cells obtained from the adult human brain. *Neuropathol Appl Neurobiol* **22**, 199–206.

Tator, C. H. (1995). Update on the pathophysiology and pathology of acute spinal cord injury. *Brain Pathol* **5**, 407–413.

Taveggia, C., Thaker, P., Petrylak, A., *et al.* (2008). Type III neuregulin-1 promotes oligodendrocyte myelination. *Glia* **56**, 284–293.

Taveggia, C., Zanazzi, G., Petrylak, A., *et al.* (2005). Neuregulin-1 type III determines the ensheathment fate of axons. *Neuron* **47**, 681–694.

Tekkök, S. B. and Goldberg, M. P. (2001). AMPA/Kainate receptor activation mediates hypoxic oligodendrocyte death and axonal injury in cerebral white matter. *J Neurosci* **21**, 4237–4248.

Temple, S. and Raff, M. C. (1986). Clonal analysis of oligodendrocyte development in culture: evidence for a developmental clock that counts cell divisions. *Cell* **44**, 773–779.

Teng, F. Y. and Tang, B. L. (2005). Why do Nogo/Nogo-66 receptor gene knockouts result in inferior regeneration compared to treatment with neutralizing agents? *J Neurochem* **94**, 865–874.

Terada, N., Baracskay, K., Kinter, M., *et al.* (2002a). The tetraspanin protein, CD9, is expressed by progenitor cells committed to oligodendrogenesis and is linked to beta1 integrin, CD81, and Tspan-2. *Glia* **40**, 350–359.

Terada, N., Hamazaki, T., Oka, M., *et al.* (2002b). Bone marrow cells adopt the phenotype of other cells by spontaneous cell fusion. *Nature* **416**, 542–545.

Terada, N., Kidd, G. J., Kinter, M., Bjartmar, C., Moran-Jones, K., and Trapp, B. D. (2005). Beta(IV) tubulin is selectively expressed by oligodendrocytes in the central nervous system. *Glia* **50**, 212–222.

Thomson, J. M., Parker, J., Perou, C. M., and Hammond, S. M. (2004). A custom microarray platform for analysis of microRNA gene expression. *Nat Methods* **1**, 47–53.

Thorburne, S. K. and Juurlink, B. J. H. (1996). Low gluthathione and high iron govern the susceptibility of oligodendroglial precursosrs to oxidative stress. *J Neuroimmunol* **67**, 1014–1022.

Timsit, S., Martinez, S., Allinquant, B., Peyron, F., Puelles, L., and Zalc, B. (1995). Oligodendrocytes originate in a restricted zone of the embryonic ventral neural tube defined by DM-20 mRNA expression. *J Neurosci* **15**, 1012–1024.

Timsit, S., Sinoway, M. P., Levy, L., *et al.* (1992). The DM20 protein of myelin: intracellular and surface expression patterns in transfectants. *J Neurochem* **58**, 1936–1942.

Ting, A. E., Mays, R. W., Frey, M. R., Hof, W. V., Medicetty, S., and Deans, R. (2008). Therapeutic pathways of adult stem cell repair. *Crit Rev Oncol Hematol* **65**, 81–93.

Tkachev, D., Mimmack, M. L., Ryan, M. M., *et al.* (2003). Oligodendrocyte dysfunction in schizophrenia and bipolar disorder. *Lancet* **362**, 798–805.

Tofaris, G. K., Patterson, P. H., Jessen, K. R., and Mirsky, R. (2002). Denervated Schwann cells attract macrophages by secretion of leukemia inhibitory factor (LIF) and monocyte chemoattractant protein-1 in a process regulated by interleukin-6 and LIF. *J Neurosci* **22**, 6696–6703.

Tom, V. J., Steinmetz, M. P., Miller, J. H., Doller, C. M., and Silver, J. (2004). Studies on the development and behavior of the dystrophic growth cone, the hallmark of regeneration failure, in an in vitro model of the glial scar and after spinal cord injury. *J Neurosci* **24**, 6531–6539.

Tomonari, A., Tojo, A., Adachi, D., *et al.* (2003). Acute disseminated encephalo-myelitis (ADEM) after allogeneic bone marrow transplantation for acute myeloid leukemia. *Ann Hematol* **82**, 37–40.

Torcia, M., Bracci-Laudiero, L., Lucibello, M., *et al.* (1996). Nerve growth factor is an autocrine survival factor for memory B lymphocytes. *Cell* **85**, 345–356.

Tornatore, C., Berger, J. R., Houff, S. A., *et al.* (1992). Detection of JC virus DNA in peripheral lymphocytes from patients with and without progressive multi-focal leukoencephalopathy. *Ann Neurol* **31**, 454–462.

Totoiu, M. O. and Keirstead, H. S. (2005). Spinal cord injury is accompanied by chronic progressive demyelination. *J Comp Neurol* **486**, 373–383.

Traka, M., Dupree, J. L., Popko, B., and Karagogeos, D. (2002). The neuronal adhesion protein TAG-1 is expressed by Schwann cells and oligodendrocytes and is localized to the juxtaparanodal region of myelinated fibers. *J Neurosci* **22**, 3016–3024.

Traka, M., Goutebroze, L., Denisenko, N., *et al.* (2003). Association of TAG-1 with Caspr2 is essential for the molecular organization of juxtaparanodal regions of myelinated fibers. *J Cell Biol* **162**, 1161–1172.

Tran, P. B. and Miller, R. J. (2003). Chemokine receptors: signposts to brain development and disease. *Nat Rev Neurosci* **4**, 444–455.

Trapp, B. and Kidd, G. (2004). Structure of the myelinated axon. In *Myelin Biology and Disorders*, Volume 1, R. A. Lazzarini, J. W. Griffin, H. Lassmann, K. A. Nave, R. Miller, and B. Trapp, eds. (San Diego, CA: Academic Press), pp. 3–27.

Trapp, B. D. and Nave, K. A. (2008). Multiple sclerosis: an immune or neuro-degenerative disorder? *Annu Rev Neurosci* **31**, 247–269.

Trapp, B. D. and Stys, P. K. (2009). Virtual hypoxia and chronic necrosis of demyelinated axons in multiple sclerosis. *Lancet Neurol* **8**, 280–291.

Trapp, B. D., Andrews, S. B., Cootauco, C., and Quarles, R. H. (1989). The myelin-associated glycoprotein is enriched in multivesicular bodies and periaxonal membranes of actively myelinating oligodendrocytes. *J Cell Biol* **109**, 2417–2426.

Trapp, B. D., Bernier, L., Andrews, S. B., and Colman, D. R. (1988). Cellular and subcellular distribution of 2′,3′ cyclic nucleotide 3′ phosphodiesterase and its mRNA in the rat nervous system. *J Neurochem* **51**, 859–868.

Trapp, B. D., Itoyama, Y., MacIntosh, T. D., and Quarles, R. H. (1983). P2 protein in oligodendrocytes and myelin of the rabbit central nervous system. *J Neurochem* **40**, 47–54.

Trapp, B. D., Moench, T., Pulley, M., Barbosa, E., Tennekoon, G., and Griffin, J. W. (1987). Spatial segregation of mRNA encoding myelin-specific proteins. *Proc Natl Acad Sci USA* **84**, 7773–7777.

Trapp, B. D., Nishiyama, A., Cheng, D., and Macklin, W. (1997). Differentiation and death of premyelinating oligodendrocytes in developing rodent brain. *J Cell Biol* **137**, 459–468.

Trapp, B. D., Peterson, J., Ransohoff, R. M., Rudick, R. A., Mork, S., and Bo, L. (1998). Axon transection in the lesions of multiple sclerosis. *N Engl J Med* **338**, 278–285.

Trebst, C., Heine, S., Lienenklaus, S., *et al.* (2007). Lack of interferon-beta leads to accelerated remyelination in a toxic model of central nervous system demyelination. *Acta Neuropathol* **114**, 587–596.

Trotter, J. (2005). NG2-positive cells in CNS function and the pathological role of antibodies against NG2 in demyelinating diseases. *J Neurol Sci* **233**, 37–42.

Trotter, J., Bitter-Suermann, D., and Schachner, M. (1989). Differentiation-regulated loss of the polysialylated embryonic form and expression of the different polypeptides of the neural cell adhesion molecule by cultured oligodendrocytes and myelin. *J Neurosci Res* **22**, 369–383.

Trotter, J. L., Collins, K. G., and van der Veen, R. (1991). Serum cytokine levels in chronic progressive multiple sclerosis: interleukin-2 levels parallel tumor necrosis factor-α levels. *J Neuroimmunol* **33**, 29–36.

Tsai, H., Macklin, W. B., and Miller, R. H. (2006). Netrin 1 is required for the normal development of spinal cord oligodendrocytes. *J Neurosci* **26**, 1913–1922.

Tsai, H. H., Frost, E., To, V., *et al.* (2002). The chemokine receptor CXCR2 controls positioning of oligodendrocyte precursors in developing spinal cord by arresting their migration. *Cell* **110**, 373–383.

Tsai, H. H., Macklin, W. B., and Miller, R. H. (2009). Distinct modes of migration position oligodendrocyte precursors for localized cell division in the developing spinal cord. *J Neurosci Res.* **87**, 3320–3330.

Tsai, H. H., Tessier-Lavigne, M., and Miller, R. H. (2003). Netrin 1 mediates spinal cord oligodendrocyte precursor dispersal. *Development* **130**, 2095–2105.

Tsuru, T., Mizuguchi, M., Ohkubo, Y., Itonaga, N., and Momoi, M. Y. (2000). Acute disseminated encephalomyelitis after live rubella vaccination. *Brain Dev* **22**, 259–261.

Tzingounis, A. V. and Wadiche, J. I. (2007). Glutamate transporters: confining runaway excitation by shaping synaptic transmission. *Nat Rev Neurosci* **8**, 935–947.

Ueda, H., Levine, J. M., Miller, R. H., and Trapp, B. D. (1999). Rat optic nerve oligodendrocytes develop in the absence of viable retinal ganglion cell axons. *J Cell Biol* **146**, 1365–1374.

Uhlenberg, B., Schuelke, M., Ruschendorf, F., *et al.* (2004). Mutations in the gene encoding gap junction protein alpha 12 (connexin 46.6) cause Pelizaeus-Merzbacher-like disease. *Am J Hum Genet* **75**, 251–260.

Ulzheimer, J. C., Peles, E., Levinson, S. R., and Martini, R. (2004). Altered expression of ion channel isoforms at the node of Ranvier in P0-deficient myelin mutants. *Mol Cell Neurosci* **25**, 83–94.

Uschkureit, T., Sporkel, O., Stracke, J., Bussow, H., and Stoffel, W. (2000). Early onset of axonal degeneration in double (plp-/-mag-/-) and hypomyelinosis in triple (plp-/-mbp-/-mag-/-) mutant mice. *J Neurosci* **20**, 5225–5233.

Valerio, A., Ferrario, M., Dreano, M., Garotta, G., Spano, P., and Pizzi, M. (2002). Soluble interleukin-6 (IL-6) receptor/IL-6 fusion protein enhances in vitro differentiation of purified rat oligodendroglial lineage cells. *Mol Cell Neurosci* **21**, 602–615.

Vallstedt, A., Klos, J. M., and Ericson, J. (2005). Multiple dorsoventral origins of oligodendrocyte generation in the spinal cord and hindbrain. *Neuron* **45**, 55–67.

Van der Valk, P. and De Groot, C. J. (2000). Staging of multiple sclerosis (MS) lesions: pathology of the time frame of MS. *Neuropathol Appl Neurobiol* **26**, 2–10.

Vanderlugt, C. L. and Miller, S. D. (2002). Epitope spreading in immune-mediated diseases: implications for immunotherapy. *Nat Rev Immunol* **2**, 85–95.

Vanguri, P., Koski, C. L., Silverman, B., and Shin, M. L. (1982). Complement activation by isolated myelin: activation of the classical pathway in the absence of myelin-specific antibodies. *Proc Natl Acad Sci USA* **79**, 3290–3294.

Vargas, M. E. and Barres, B. A. (2007). Why is Wallerian degeneration in the CNS so slow? *Annu Rev Neurosci* **30**, 153–179.

Vartanian, T., Fischbach, G., and Miller, R. (1999). Failure of spinal cord oligodendrocyte development in mice lacking neuregulin. *Proc Natl Acad Sci USA* **96**, 731–735.

Vartanian, T., Goodearl, A., Viehover, A., and Fischbach, G. (1997). Axonal neuregulin signal cells of the oligodendrocyte lineage through activation of HER4 and Schwann cells through HER2 and HER3. *J Cell Biol* **137**, 211–220.

Vassilopoulos, G., Wang, P. R., and Russell, D. W. (2003). Transplanted bone marrow regenerates liver by cell fusion. *Nature* **422**, 901–904.

Vaughn, J. E. and Pease, D. C. (1970). Electron microscopic studies of wallerian degeneration in rat optic nerves. II. Astrocytes, oligodendrocytes and adventitial cells. *J Comp Neurol* **140**, 207–226.

Vela, J. M., Molina-Holgado, E., Arevalo-Martin, A., Almazan, G., and Guaza, C. (2002). Interleukin-1 regulates proliferation and differentiation of oligodendrocyte progenitor cells. *Mol Cell Neurosci* **20**, 489–502.

Venkatesh, K., Chivatakarn, O., Lee, H., *et al.* (2005). The Nogo-66 receptor homolog NgR2 is a sialic acid-dependent receptor selective for myelin-associated glycoprotein. *J Neurosci* **25**, 808–822.

Vergelli, M., Le, H., van Noort, J. M., Dhib-Jalbut, S., McFarland, H., and Martin, R. (1996). A novel population of CD4+CD56+ myelin-reactive T cells lyses target cells expressing CD56/neural cell adhesion molecule. *J Immunol* **157**, 679–688.

Villoslada, P., Hauser, S. L., Bartke, I., *et al.* (2000). Human nerve growth factor protects common marmosets against autoimmune encephalomyelitis by switching the balance of T helper cell type 1 and 2 cytokines within the central nervous system. *J Exp Med* **191**, 1799–1806.

Vincent, T., Saikali, P., Cayrol, R., *et al.* (2008). Functional consequences of neuromyelitis optica-IgG astrocyte interactions on blood-brain barrier permeability and granulocyte recruitment. *J Immunol* **181**, 5730–5737.

Vitkovic, L., Konsman, J. P., Bockaert, J., Dantzer, R., Homburger, V., and Jacque, C. (2000). Cytokine signals propagate through the brain. *Mol Psychiatry* **5**, 604–615.

Vogler, S., Pahnke, J., Rousset, S., *et al.* (2006). Uncoupling protein 2 has protective function during experimental autoimmune encephalomyelitis. *Am J Pathol* **168**, 1570–1575.

Volpe, J. J. (2003). Cerebral white matter injury of the premature infant – more common than you think. *Pediatrics* **112**, 176–180.

Volpe, J. J. (2008). Hypoxic-ischemic encephalopathy: neuropathology and pathogenesis. *In Neurology of the Newborn* (Philadelphia, PA: W.B. Saunders Co.)

Volpe, J. J. (2009). Brain injury in premature infants: a complex amalgam of destructive and developmental disturbances. *Lancet Neurol* **8**, 110–124.

Vourc'h, P. and Andres, C. (2004). Oligodendrocyte myelin glycoprotein (OMgp): evolution, structure and function. *Brain Res Brain Res Rev* **45**, 115–124.

Vouyiouklis, D. A. and Brophy, P. J. (1993). Microtubule-associated protein MAP1B expression precedes the morphological differentiation of oligodendrocytes. *J Neurosci Res* **35**, 257–267.

Vouyiouklis, D. A. and Brophy, P. J. (1995). Microtubule-associated proteins in developing oligodendrocytes: transient expression of a MAP2c isoform in oligodendrocyte precursors. *J Neurosci Res* **42**, 803–817.

Voyvodic, J. T. (1989). Target size regulates calibre and myelination of sympathetic axons. *Nature* **342**, 430–433.

Wakefield, C. L. and Eidelberg, E. (1975). Electron microscopic observations of the delayed effects of spinal cord compression. *Exp Neurol* **48**, 637–646.

Wallström, E., Diener, P., Ljungdahl, Ã., Khademi, M., Nilsson, C. G., and Olsson, T. (1996). Memantine abrogates neurological deficits, but not CNS inflammation, in Lewis rat experimental autoimmune encephalomyelitis. *J Neurol Sci* **137**, 89–96.

Wang Ip, C., Kroner, A., Fischer, S., Berghoff, M., Kobsar, I., Maurer, M., and Martini, R. (2006). Role of immune cells in animal models for inherited peripheral neuropathies. *Neuromolecular Med* **8**, 175–190.

Wang, H., Tewari, A., Einheber, S., Salzer, J. L., and Melendez-Vasquez, C. V. (2008). Myosin II has distinct functions in PNS and CNS myelin sheath formation. *J Cell Biol* **182**, 1171–1184.

Wang, K. C., Kim, J. A., Sivasankaran, R., Segal, R., and He, Z. (2002a). P75 interacts with the Nogo receptor as a co-receptor for Nogo, MAG and OMgp. *Nature* **420**, 74–78.

Wang, K. C., Koprivica, V., Kim, J. A., *et al.* (2002b). Oligodendrocyte-myelin glycoprotein is a Nogo receptor ligand that inhibits neurite outgrowth. *Nature* **417**, 941–944.

Wang, S., Sdrulla, A. D., diSibio, G., *et al.* (1998). Notch receptor activation inhibits oligodendrocyte differentiation. *Neuron* **21**, 63–75.

Wang, W., van Niekerk, E., Willis, D. E., and Twiss, J. L. (2007). RNA transport and localized protein synthesis in neurological disorders and neural repair. *Dev Neurobiol* **67**, 1166–1182.

Wang, W. X., Rajeev, B. W., Stromberg, A. J., *et al.* (2008). The expression of microRNA miR-107 decreases early in Alzheimer's disease, and may accelerate disease progression through regulation of beta-site amyloid precursor protein-cleaving enzyme 1. *J Neurosci* **28**, 1213–1223.

Wanner, I. B., Guerra, N. K., Mahoney, J., *et al.* (2006a). Role of N-cadherin in Schwann cell precursors of growing nerves. *Glia* **54**, 439–459.

Wanner, I. B., Mahoney, J., Jessen, K. R., Wood, P. M., Bates, M., and Bunge, M. B. (2006b). Invariant mantling of growth cones by Schwann cell precursors characterize growing peripheral nerve fronts. *Glia* **54**, 424–438.

Warrington, A. E., Asakura, K., Bieber, A. J., *et al.* (2000). Human monoclonal antibodies reactive to oligodendrocytes promote remyelination in a model of multiple sclerosis. *Proc Natl Acad Sci USA* **97**, 6820–6825.

Warrington, A. E., Barbarese, E., and Pfeiffer, S. E. (1993). Differential myelinogenic capacity of specific developmental stages of the oligodendrocyte lineage upon transplantation into hypomyelinating hosts. *J Neurosci Res* **34**, 1–13.

Warshawsky, I., Rudick, R. A., Staugaitis, S. M., and Natowicz, M. R. (2005). Primary progressive multiple sclerosis as a phenotype of a PLP1 gene mutation. *Ann Neurol* **58**, 470–473.

Watanabe, M., Hadzic, T., and Nishiyama, A. (2004). Transient upregulation of Nkx2.2 expression in oligodendrocyte lineage cells during remyelination. *Glia* **46**, 311–322.

Watkins, L. R., Hutchinson, M. R., Johnston, I. N., and Maier, S. F. (2005). Glia: novel counter-regulators of opioid analgesia. *Trends Neurosci* **28**, 661–669.

Waxman, S. G. (1989). Demyelination in spinal cord injury. *J Neurol Sci* **91**, 1–14.

Waxman, S. G. (2006). Axonal conduction and injury in multiple sclerosis: the role of sodium channels. *Nat Rev Neurosci* **7**, 932–941.

Waxman, S. G. and Ritchie, J. M. (1993). Molecular dissection of the myelinated axon. *Ann Neurol* **33**, 121–136.

Weber, P., Bartsch, U., Rasband, M. N., *et al.* (1999). Mice deficient for tenascin-R display alterations of the extracellular matrix and decreased axonal conduction velocities in the CNS. *J Neurosci* **19**, 4245–4262.

Wegner, M. (2000). Transcriptional control in myelinating glia: the basic recipe. *Glia* **29**, 118–123.

Wegner, M., Drolet, D. W., and Rosenfeld, M. G. (1993). Regulation of JC virus by the POU-domain transcription factor Tst-1: implications for progressive multifocal leukoencephalopathy. *Proc Natl Acad Sci USA* **90**, 4743–4747.

Wehrle-Haller, B., Koch, M., Baumgartner, S., Spring, J., and Chiquet, M. (1991). Nerve-dependent and -independent tenascin expression in the developing chick limb bud. *Development* **112**, 627–637.

Weimann, J. M., Charlton, C. A., Brazelton, T. R., Hackman, R. C., and Blau, H. M. (2003). Contribution of transplanted bone marrow cells to Purkinje neurons in human adult brains. *Proc Natl Acad Sci USA* **100**, 2088–2093.

Weimbs, T. and Stoffel, W. (1992). Proteolipid protein (PLP) of CNS myelin: positions of free, disulfide-bonded, and fatty acid thioester-linked cysteine residues and implications for the membrane topology of PLP. *Biochemistry* **31**, 12289–12296.

Weimbs, T., Low, S. H., Chapin, S. J., and Mostov, K. E. (1997). Apical targeting in polarized epithelial cells: there's more afloat than rafts. *Trends Cell Biol* **7**, 393–399.

Weinberg, H. J. and Spencer, P. S. (1975). Studies on the control of myelinogenesis. I. Myelination of regenerating axons after entry into a foreign unmyelinated nerve. *J Neurocytol* **4**, 395–418.

Werner, P., Pitt, D., and Raine, C. S. (2000). Glutamate excitotoxicity – a mechanism for axonal damage and oligodendrocyte death in multiple sclerosis? *J Neural Transm Suppl* (60), 375–385.

Werner, P., Pitt, D., and Raine, C. S. (2001). Multiple sclerosis: altered glutamate homeostasis in lesions correlates with oligodendrocyte and axonal damage. *Ann Neurol* **50**, 169–180.

Wiessner, C., Bareyre, F. M., Allegrini, P. R., *et al.* (2003). Anti-Nogo-A antibody infusion 24 hours after experimental stroke improved behavioral outcome and corticospinal plasticity in normotensive and spontaneously hypertensive rats. *J Cereb Blood Flow Metab* **23**, 154–165.

Wight, P. A., Duchala, C. S., Readhead, C., and Macklin, W. B. (1993). A myelin proteolipid protein-LacZ fusion protein is developmentally regulated and targeted to the myelin membrane in transgenic mice. *J Cell Biol* **123**, 443–454.

Wigley, R., Hamilton, N., Nishiyama, A., Kirchhoff, F., and Butt, A. M. (2007). Morphological and physiological interactions of NG2-glia with astrocytes and neurons. *J Anat* **210**, 661–670.

Wilkins, A. and Compston, A. (2005). Trophic factors attenuate nitric oxide mediated neuronal and axonal injury in vitro: roles and interactions of mitogen-activated protein kinase signalling pathways. *J Neurochem.* **92**, 1487–1496.

Wilkins, A. and Scolding, N. (2008). Protecting axons in multiple sclerosis. *Mult Scler* **14**, 1013–1025.

Wilkins, A., Chandran, S., and Compston, A. (2001). A role for oligodendrocyte-derived IGF-1 in trophic support of cortical neurons. *Glia* **36**, 48–57.

Wilkins, A., Majed, H., Layfield, R., Compston, A., and Chandran, S. (2003). Oligodendrocytes promote neuronal survival and axonal length by distinct intracellular mechanisms: a novel role for oligodendrocyte-derived glial cell line-derived neurotrophic factor. *J Neurosci* **23**, 4967–4974.

Wilkinson, D. G., Bhatt, S., Chavrier, P., Bravo, R., and Charnay, P. (1989). Segment-specific expression of a zinc-finger gene in the developing nervous system of the mouse. *Nature* **337**, 461–464.

Williams, A., Piaton, G., Aigrot, M. S., *et al.* (2007a). Semaphorin 3A and 3F: key players in myelin repair in multiple sclerosis? *Brain* **130**, 2554–2465.

Williams, A., Piaton, G., and Lubetzki, C. (2007b). Astrocytes – Friends or foes in multiple sclerosis? *Glia* **55**, 1300–1312.

Wilson, H., Scolding, N., and Raine, C. (2006). Co-expression of PDGF α receptor and NG2 by oligodendrocyte precursor cells in human CNS and multiple sclerosis lesions. *J Neuroimmunol* **176**, 162–173.

Wilson, R. and Brophy, P. J. (1989). Role of the oligodendrocyte cytoskeleton in myelination. *J Neurosci Res* **22**, 439–448.

Wilson, S. S., Baetge, E. E., and Stallcup, W. B. (1981). Antisera specific for cell lines with mixed neuronal and glial properties. *Dev Biol* **83**, 146–153.

Windrem, M. S., Nunes, M. C., Rashbaum, W. K., *et al.* (2004). Fetal and adult human oligodendrocyte progenitor cell isolates myelinate the congenitally dysmyelinated brain. *Nat Med* **10**, 93–97.

Wingerchuk, D. M. (2004). Neuromyelitis optica: current concepts. *Front Biosci* **9**, 834–840.

Wolman, L. (1965). The disturbance of circulation in traumatic paraplegia in acute and late stages: a pathological study. *Paraplegia* **2**, 213–226.

Wolswijk, G. (1998). Chronic stage multiple sclerosis lesions contain a relatively quiescent population of oligodendrocyte precursor cells. *J Neurosci* **18**, 601–609.

Wolswijk, G. (2002). Oligodendrocyte precursor cells in the demyelinated multiple sclerosis spinal cord. *Brain* **125**, 338–349.

Wolswijk, G. and Noble, M. (1989). Identification of an adult-specific glial progenitor cell. *Development* **105**, 387–400.

Wolswijk, G., Munro, P. M. G., Riddle, P. N., and Noble, M. (1991). Origin, growth factor responses, and ultrastructural characteristics of an adult-specific glial progenitor cell. *Ann New York Acad Sci* **633**, 502–504.

Wong, S. T., Henley, J. R., Kanning, K. C., Huang, K. H., Bothwell, M., and Poo, M. M. (2002). A p75(NTR) and Nogo receptor complex mediates repulsive signaling by myelin-associated glycoprotein. *Nat Neurosci* **5**, 1302–1308.

Wood, P. M., Schachner, M., and Bunge, R. P. (1990). Inhibition of Schwann cell myelination in vitro by antibody to the L1 adhesion molecule. *J Neurosci* **10**, 3635–3645.

Woodhoo, A. and Sommer, L. (2008). Development of the Schwann cell lineage: from the neural crest to the myelinated nerve. *Glia* **56**, 1481–1490.

Woodhoo, A., Sahni, V., Gilson, J., *et al.* (2007). Schwann cell precursors: a favourable cell for myelin repair in the central nervous system. *Brain* **130**, 2175–2185.

Woodruff, R. H., Fruttiger, M., Richardson, W. D., and Franklin, R. J. (2004). Platelet-derived growth factor regulates oligodendrocyte progenitor numbers in adult CNS and their response following CNS demyelination. *Mol Cell Neurosci* **25**, 252–262.

Woodward, L. J., Edgin, J. O., Thompson, D., and Inder, T. E. (2005). Object working memory deficits predicted by early brain injury and development in the preterm infant. *Brain* **128**, 2578–2587.

Wosik, K., Antel, J., Kuhlmann, T., Brück, W., Massie, B., and Nalbantoglu, J. (2003). Oligodendrocyte injury in multiple sclerosis: a role for p53. *J Neurochem* **85**, 635–644.

Wrathall, J. R., Li, W., and Hudson, L. D. (1998). Myelin gene expression after experimental contusive spinal cord injury. *J Neurosci* **18**, 8780–8793.

Wren, D., Wolswijk, G., and Noble, M. (1992). In vitro analysis of the origin and maintenance of O-2A(adult) progenitor cells. *J Cell Biol* **116**, 167–176.

Wu, Q., Miller, R. H., Ransohoff, R. M., Robinson, S., Bu, J., and Nishiyama, A. (2000). Elevated levels of the chemokine GRO-1 correlate with elevated oligodendrocyte progenitor proliferation in the jimpy mutant. *J Neurosci* **20**, 2609–2617.

Wucherpfennig, K. W., Newcombe, J., Li, H., Keddy, C., Cuzner, M. L., and Hafler, D. A. (1992). δ T-cell receptor repertoire in acute multiple sclerosis lesions. *Proc Natl Acad Sci USA* **89**, 4588–4592.

Xu, W., Fazekas, G., Hara, H., and Tabira, T. (2005). Mechanism of natural killer (NK) cell regulatory role in experimental autoimmune encephalomyelitis. *J Neuroimmunol* **163**, 24–30.

Xu, W., Shy, M., Kamholz, J., *et al.* (2001). Mutations in the cytoplasmic domain of P0 reveal a role for PKC-mediated phosphorylation in adhesion and myelination. *J Cell Biol* **155**, 439–446.

Yamada, K., Watanabe, M., Shibata, T., Nagashima, M., Tanaka, K., and Inoue, Y. (1998). Glutamate transporter GLT-1 is transiently localized on growing axons of the mouse spinal cord before establishing astrocytic expression. *J Neurosci* **18**, 5706–5713.

Yamada, M., Mizuguchi, M., Otsuka, N., Ikeda, K., and Takahashi, H. (1997). Ultrastructural localization of CD38 immunoreactivity in rat brain. *Brain Res* **756**, 52–60.

Yamamoto, S., Yamamoto, N., Kitamura, T., Nakamura, K., and Nakafuku, M. (2001). Proliferation of parenchymal neural progenitors in response to injury in the adult rat spinal cord. *Exp Neurol* **172**, 115–127.

Yamamoto, Y., Mizuno, R., Nishimura, T., *et al.* (1994). Cloning and expression of myelin-associated oligodendrocytic basic protein. A novel basic protein constituting the central nervous system myelin. *J Biol Chem* **269**, 31725–31730.

Yan, P., Liu, N., Kim, G. M., *et al.* (2003). Expression of the type 1 and type 2 receptors for tumor necrosis factor after traumatic spinal cord injury in adult rats. *Exp Neurol* **183**, 286–297.

Yang, D. P., Zhang, D. P., Mak, K. S., Bonder, D. E., Pomeroy, S. L., and Kim, H. A. (2008). Schwann cell proliferation during Wallerian degeneration is not necessary for regeneration and remyelination of the peripheral nerves: axon-dependent removal of newly generated Schwann cells by apoptosis. *Mol Cell Neurosci* **38**, 80–88.

Yang, Y., Ogawa, Y., Hedstrom, K. L., and Rasband, M. N. (2007). betaIV spectrin is recruited to axon initial segments and nodes of Ranvier by ankyrinG. *J Cell Biol* **176**, 509–519.

Ye, M., Chen, S., Wang, X., *et al.* (2005). Glial cell line-derived neurotrophic factor in bone marrow stromal cells of rat. *NeuroReport* **16**, 581–584.

Ye, P., Carson, J., and D'Ercole, A. J. (1995). In vivo actions of insulin-like growth factor-I (IGF-I) on brain myelination: studies of IGF-I and IGF binding protein-1 (IGFBP-1) transgenic mice. *J Neurosci* **15**, 7344–7356.

Yednock, T. A., Cannon, C., Fritz, L. C., Sanchez-Madrid, F., Steinman, L., and Karin, N. (1992). Prevention of experimental autoimmune encephalomyelitis by antibodies against alpha 4 beta 1 integrin. *Nature* **356**, 63–66.

Yin, X., Baek, R. C., Kirschner, D. A., *et al.* (2006). Evolution of a neuroprotective function of central nervous system myelin. *J Cell Biol* **172**, 469–478.

Yin, X., Crawford, T. O., Griffin, J. W., *et al.* (1998). Myelin-associated glycoprotein is a myelin signal that modulates the caliber of myelinated axons. *J Neurosci* **18**, 1953–1962.

Yin, X., Peterson, J., Gravel, M., Braun, P. E., and Trapp, B. D. (1997). CNP over-expression induces aberrant oligodendrocyte membranes and inhibits MBP accumulation and myelin compaction. *J Neurosci Res* **50**, 238–247.

Yiu, G. and He, Z. (2006). Glial inhibition of CNS axon regeneration. *Nat Rev Neurosci* **7**, 617–627.

Yool, D. A., Edgar, J. M., Montague, P., and Malcolm, S. (2000). The proteolipid protein gene and myelin disorders in man and animal models. *Hum Mol Genet* **9**, 987–992.

Yoon, B. H., Kim, C. J., Romero, R., *et al.* (1997). Experimentally induced intra-uterine infection causes fetal brain white matter lesions in rabbits. *Am J Obstet Gynecol* **177**, 797–802.

Yoshida, M. and Colman, D. R. (1996). Parallel evolution and coexpression of the proteolipid proteins and protein zero in vertebrate myelin. *Neuron* **16**, 1115–1126.

Yoshino, J. E., Mason, P. W., and DeVries, G. H. (1987). Developmental changes in myelin-induced proliferation of cultured Schwann cells. *J Cell Biol* **104**, 655–660.

Yoshioka, A., Hardy, M., Younkin, D. P., Grinspan, J. B., Stern, J. L., and Pleasure, D. (1995). α-Amino-3-hydroxy-5-methyl-4-isoxazolepropionate (AMPA) receptors mediate excitotoxicity in the oligodendroglial lineage. *J Neurochem* **64**, 2442–2448.

Yoshioka, A., Ikegaki, N., Williams, M., and Pleasure, D. (1996). Expression of *N*-methyl-D-aspartate (NMDA) and non-NMDA glutamate receptor genes in neuroblastoma, medulloblastoma, and other cell lines. *J Neurosci Res* **46**, 164–172.

Young, E. A., Fowler, C. D., Kidd, G. J., *et al.* (2008). Imaging correlates of decreased axonal Na^+/K^+ ATPase in chronic MS lesions. *Ann Neurol* **63**, 428–435.

Yousry, T. A., Major, E. O., Ryschkewitsch, C., *et al.* (2006). Evaluation of patients treated with natalizumab for progressive multifocal leukoencephalopathy. *N Engl J Med* **354**, 924–933.

Yu, J., Vodyanik, M. A., Smuga-Otto, K., *et al.* (2007). Induced pluripotent stem cell lines derived from human somatic cells. *Science* **318**, 1917–1920.

Yu, W. M., Feltri, M. L., Wrabetz, L., Strickland, S., and Chen, Z. L. (2005). Schwann cell-specific ablation of laminin gamma1 causes apoptosis and prevents proliferation. *J Neurosci* **25**, 4463–4472.

Yuan, X., Eisen, A. M., McBain, C. J., and Gallo, V. (1998). A role for glutamate and its receptors in the regulation of oligodendrocyte development in cerebellar tissue slices. *Development* **125**, 2901–2914.

Zai, L. J. and Wrathall, J. R. (2005). Cell proliferation and replacement following contusive spinal cord injury. *Glia* **50**, 247–257.

Zajicek, J., Wing, M., Skepper, J., and Compston, A. (1995). Human oligodendro-cytes are not sensitive to complement. A study of CD59 expression in the human central nervous system. *Lab Invest* **73**, 128–138.

Zajicek, J. P., Wing, M., Scolding, N. J., and Compston, D. A. (1992). Interactions between oligodendrocytes and microglia. A major role for complement and tumour necrosis factor in oligodendrocyte adherence and killing. *Brain* **115**, 1611–1631.

Zalc, B. (2006). The acquisition of myelin: a success story. *Novartis Found Symp* **276**, 15–21.

Zalc, B., Goujet, D., and Colman, D. (2008). The origin of the myelination pro-gram in vertebrates. *Curr Biol* **18**, R511–R512.

Zang, Y. C., Li, S., Rivera, V. M., *et al.* (2004). Increased CD8(+) cytotoxic T cell responses to myelin basic protein in multiple sclerosis. *J Immunol* **172**, 5120–5127.

Zappia, E., Casazza, S., Pedemonte, E., *et al.* (2005). Mesenchymal stem cells ameliorate experimental autoimmune encephalomyelitis inducing T-cell anergy. *Blood* **106**, 1755–1761.

Zeck-Kapp, G., Kroegel, C., Riede, U. N., and Kapp, A. (1995). Mechanisms of human eosinophil activation by complement protein C5a and platelet-activating factor: similar functional responses are accompanied by different morphologic alterations. *Allergy* **50**, 34–47.

Zeger, M., Popken, G., Zhang, J., *et al.* (2007). Insulin-like growth factor type 1 receptor signaling in the cells of oligodendrocyte lineage is required for normal in vivo oligodendrocyte development and myelination. *Glia* **55**, 400–411.

Zeis, T., Graumann, U., Reynolds, R., and Schaeren-Wiemers, N. (2008a). Normal-appearing white matter in multiple sclerosis is in a subtle balance between inflammation and neuroprotection. *Brain* **131**, 288–303.

Zeis, T., Kinter, J., Herrero-Herranz, E., Weissert, R., and Schaeren-Wiemers, N. (2008b). Gene expression analysis of normal appearing brain tissue in an animal model for multiple sclerosis revealed grey matter alterations, but only minor white matter changes. *J Neuroimmunol* **205**, 10–19.

Zeller, N. K., Hunkeler, M. J., Campagnoni, A. T., Sprague, J., and Lazzarini, R. A. (1984). Characterization of mouse myelin basic protein messenger RNAs with a myelin basic protein cDNA clone. *Proc Natl Acad Sci USA* **81**, 18–22.

Zerangue, N. and Kavanaugh, M. P. (1996). Flux coupling in a neuronal glutamate transporter. *Nature* **383**, 634–637.

Zhang, J., Li, Y., Chen, J., *et al.* (2005). Human bone marrow stromal cell treatment improves neurological functional recovery in EAE mice. *Exp Neurol* **195**, 16–26.

Zhang, J., Li, Y., Lu, M., *et al.* (2006). Bone marrow stromal cells reduce axonal loss in experimental autoimmune encephalomyelitis mice. *J Neurosci Res* **84**, 587–595.

Zhang, S. C., Ge, B., and Duncan, I. D. (1999). Adult brain retains the potential to generate oligodendroglial progenitors with extensive myelination capacity. *Proc Natl Acad Sci USA* **96**, 4089–4094.

Zhang, Y., Wang, H., Li, J., *et al.* (2006). Intracellular zinc release and ERK phosphorylation are required upstream of 12-lipoxygenase activation in peroxynitrite toxicity to mature rat oligodendrocytes. *J Biol Chem* **281**, 9460–9470.

Zheng, B., Atwal, J., Ho, C., *et al.* (2005). Genetic deletion of the Nogo receptor does not reduce neurite inhibition in vitro or promote corticospinal tract regeneration in vivo. *Proc Natl Acad Sci USA* **102**, 1205–1210.

Zheng, B., Ho, C., Li, S., Keirstead, H., Steward, O., and Tessier-Lavigne, M. (2003). Lack of enhanced spinal regeneration in Nogo-deficient mice. *Neuron* **38**, 213–224.

Zhou, D., Srivastava, R., Nessler, S., *et al.* (2006). Identification of a pathogenic antibody response to native myelin oligodendrocyte glycoprotein in multiple sclerosis. *Proc Natl Acad Sci USA* **103**, 19057–19062.

Zhou, Q. and Anderson, D. J. (2002). The bHLH transcription factors OLIG2 and OLIG1 couple neuronal and glial subtype specification. *Cell* **109**, 61–73.

Zhou, Q., Choi, G., and Anderson, D. J. (2001). The bHLH transcription factor Olig2 promotes oligodendrocyte differentiation in collaboration with Nkx2.2. *Neuron* **31**, 791–807.

Zhou, Q., Wang, S., and Anderson, D. J. (2000). Identification of a novel family of oligodendrocyte lineage-specific basic helix-loop-helix transcription factors. *Neuron* **25**, 331–343.

Zhu, X., Bergles, D. E., and Nishiyama, A. (2008). NG2 cells generate both oligo-dendrocytes and gray matter astrocytes. *Development* **135**, 145–157.

Ziak, D., Chvatal, A., and Sykova, E. (1998). Glutamate-, kainate- and NMDA-evoked membrane currents in identified glial cells in rat spinal cord slice. *Physiol Res* **47**, 365–375.

Ziskin, J. L., Nishiyama, A., Rubio, M., Fukaya, M., and Bergles, D. E. (2007). Vesicular release of glutamate from unmyelinated axons in white matter. *Nat Neurosci* **10**, 321–330.

Zuo, J., Ferguson, T. A., Hernandez, Y. J., Stetler-Stevenson, W. G., and Muir, D. (1998). Neuronal matrix metalloproteinase-2 degrades and inactivates a neurite-inhibiting chondroitin sulfate proteoglycan. *J Neurosci* **18**, 5203–5211.

Index